Manufactured in U.S.A.

8 7 6 5 4 3 2 1

ISBN: 0-7853-0951-9

Medical consultant: Ira J. Chasnoff, M.D.
Contributing consultation and editorial assistance: Richard J. Sagall, M.D.
Interior illustrations: Nan Brooks; Laura D'Argo; Dori Gordon; Ilene Robinette
Interior medical illustrations: Teri J. McDermott, M.A.; Mike Muir
Cover photography: Superstock

Notice
In this book, the authors, editors, and consultants have done their best to outline the indicated general treatment for various childhood conditions, diseases, and ailments and their symptoms. Different people react to the same treatment, medication, or preparation in different ways. This book does not attempt to answer all questions about all situations that you or your child may encounter. Always consult a physician if you suspect that your child may be allergic to a specific drug.

Neither the Editors of CONSUMER GUIDE® and Publications International, Ltd., nor the authors, consultants, or publisher take responsibility for any possible consequences from any treatment, action, or application of medication or preparation by any person reading or following the information in this book. The publication of this book does not constitute the practice of medicine, and this book does not attempt to replace your physician or other health-care provider. The authors, consultants, and publisher advise the reader to check with a physician before administering any medication or undertaking any course of prevention or treatment.

BY THE EDITORS OF CONSUMER GUIDE®
WITH IRA J. CHASNOFF, M.D.

YOUR CHILD:
A MEDICAL
G U I D E

THE ILLUSTRATED MEDICAL
AND HEALTH ADVISER

PUBLICATIONS INTERNATIONAL, LTD.

Contents

Introduction

Raising a healthy, happy child is always a challenge, and every parent knows that panicky feeling that comes with the knowledge—or even the suspicion—that a child is sick. Part of the problem is that it can be very difficult to assess the seriousness of a childhood illness. Does a stomachache indicate only that the child overate at a birthday party, or does it mean something more serious? How bad does a cold have to be before you need to keep the child home from school? Should you treat a cut knee yourself or let a doctor look at it? The questions are endless, and no parent avoids them all.

It's even harder for the first-time parent with a brand-new baby who suddenly breaks out in an unexplained rash or feels feverish. But even parents who have survived those first confusing months find that the childhood years hold all sorts of unexpected challenges. When a child gets hit on the head with a ball, could he or she have a concussion? How do you treat a minor burn? What does a fever really mean? What constitutes an emergency?

This book works on the principle that informed parents who have done their homework ahead of time are in the best possible position to deal with both the major and the minor crises of childhood. This book is a comprehensive guide to the problems that parents are most likely to encounter, and it provides practical advice on recognizing, assessing, and dealing with each one. You will learn how to spot the signs that may mean your child is sick and how to determine whether the child is tired as a result of playing hard or because the child is coming down with a virus. You will learn how to judge when the child needs a doctor's care and what information to give the doctor's office when you call. You will also learn how best to take care of your child when home treatment is appropriate and how to follow your doctor's instructions.

The opening section, Taking Care of Basics, provides information that every parent needs to know. There is sensible advice on how to choose a doctor for your child, what to expect from the doctor, and how to make sure that you and the doctor work well together to take good care of your child's health. You'll learn:

■ Why vaccinations are vital;
■ Why routine checkups are so important, and what the doctor looks for;
■ What you need in your medicine chest;
■ What kinds of medications the doctor may order, and why it's important to understand dosage directions;
■ What medical tests involve and why the doctor needs them.

There's also a reassuring discussion of what to expect of a newborn and how to tell if the baby is developing normally.

Following the opening section, you'll find the Quick-Reference Action Guide and Understanding Your Child's Condition. These two sections cover specific problems and diseases that parents may have to cope with before a child grows up and becomes responsible for his or her own health care. The Quick-Reference Action Guide includes instructions on giving mouth-to-mouth resuscitation; a chart of symptoms and possible causes; and quick-read pages that give you the essentials on more than 150 conditions, arranged alphabetically, so that you can assess your child's condition and, if necessary, act quickly. In Understanding Your Child's Condition, you will find those same conditions, again arranged alphabetically, but discussed in more detail, so that you can get a better grasp of the condition once any initial crisis is over. The information is provided in clear, nontechnical language. The subjects covered range from the sort of everyday problems that are an inevitable part of childhood—colds, sore throats, stomachaches, cuts—to potentially life-threatening diseases that, fortunately, affect far fewer children. Whether the condition is major or minor, you'll be better able to help your child if you understand what is involved and what you should do.

Your Child: A Medical Guide can be a parent's best friend in many of the medical situations that occur as any child is growing up. Use it to help you play an informed, competent role in caring for your child's good health.

Taking Care of Basics

Taking care of your child's health means more than acting quickly in an emergency or making sure your child gets the medical treatment he or she needs when ill. It means laying the groundwork for health by choosing and working with a competent, compassionate physician; having your child's health and development checked at regular intervals; making sure your child gets the immunizations that help ward off certain devastating diseases; understanding some of the common tests and procedures your child's doctor may need to perform; knowing what 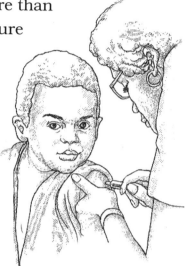 medical supplies to have on hand; knowing how to follow medication instructions given by your child's doctor; recognizing what's typical of a normal newborn; knowing how to monitor your child's temperature; and preparing for emergencies. That's what this section is all about—taking care of essentials that can help keep your child healthy and make you better prepared to help your child when disease or other problems strike.

The parent-physician partnership

Raising a child is a big responsibility, and it's always comforting to know that there's someone you can turn to when you have a problem. For advice on many of your concerns about your child, you can call on your own parents, your family and friends, other parents, or your child's teachers. But when it comes to your child's health, the person you need is a physician.

CHOOSING A DOCTOR

To get the best from your child's doctor, you must first select the best doctor for your child. Family practitioners and pediatricians care for children. Family practitioners are trained in all aspects of medicine, including pediatrics, adolescent care, and adult medicine. Since they often care for the entire family, they may be more aware of family dynamics and how one family member's health may affect the rest of the family. Pediatricians see only children. Like family practitioners, pediatricians spend three or more years after medical school in a residency program. Pediatricians are trained to handle all aspects of children's health but have an emphasis on special and complicated problems of children.

Many physicians work with a physician extender, either a nurse practitioner or a physician's assistant. Commonly called mid-level practitioners, these health-care providers have more training and experience than a registered nurse but not as much as a medical doctor. They frequently see children for routine health problems and usually work closely with a doctor.

The most important thing, however, is that you get along with the health-care provider who is caring for your child. If you feel more comfortable with your family physician than with any pediatrician in your area, you may decide to have the family physician take care of your child, too. You may, on the other hand, decide upon a pediatrician. You know what's best for your child, so trust your own decision.

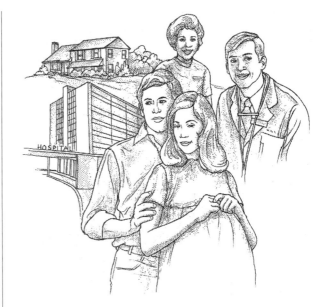

The physician and the nurse practitioner are your partners in caring for your child's health.

Your child's doctor, who is a trained and experienced professional, should be a reliable and sympathetic source of information and advice throughout your child's growing years. Remember, though, that the doctor is a medical adviser, not another parent. There are decisions about your child's well-being only you can make, and a good doctor does not try either to make child-rearing decisions for you or to make you feel that you're not a competent parent. A good parent-doctor relationship is one in which each partner respects the other.

How do you find a good doctor? That's a difficult question to answer because there are no hard-and-fast rules to follow. If you are a first-time parent, the doctor who delivered your baby may be able to give you names of local physicians and perhaps recommend someone who is well thought of by other new parents. You may have a friend or neighbor who has children and can recommend someone. If you've moved to a new area, consult a neighbor who has children, or call a local hospital or the state medical society. Professional organizations will not give you recommendations as such; they will give you names and expect you to make your own inquiries. However, a phone call and a visit to a doctor's office should be enough to tell you whether that doctor is right for you and your child. It is also a good idea to visit the doctor even before your baby is born to become acquainted and to arrange for your baby's medical care. If you live in a larger city with many hospitals, make sure the doctor you select cares for patients in your hospital of preference.

WORKING TOGETHER

Once you have found a doctor whose medical ability you trust, there are practical steps you can take to maintain a good working relationship between the two of you.

For example, don't feel slighted if you don't always speak directly with the doctor when you call the office because your child is sick. In many pediatricians' offices, a professional nurse acts as the go-between in communications with the doctor. You can have the same confidence in the nurse that you have in the doctor. The nurse is a qualified medical professional in his or her own right and is well able to handle many of your questions. This means you don't have to wait for the doctor to get through with a patient before he or she can talk to you. Of course, if your child's condition does require the doctor's attention, the nurse will arrange to have the doctor talk to you on the phone or will help you set up an appointment to see the doctor.

Whether you talk directly to the doctor or to the nurse when you call the office, be prepared to give the following information:

■ Your name and the child's name.

■ Your child's approximate weight. This is important because medications are prescribed by body weight, and the dosage that is appropriate for a 125-pound teenager is very different from that given to a 25-pound toddler.

■ Your child's temperature. Whether the child is running a fever—and if so, how high a fever—is a clue to the child's condition. Use a thermometer to take the child's temperature. A guess based on flushed cheeks or a hot forehead isn't good enough.

■ Information on any illnesses the child has been exposed to recently.

■ Details of medications to which your child is allergic.

■ The name, phone number, and business hours of your pharmacist, so that the doctor can phone in a prescription if necessary. (Although the nurse can handle many of your questions and perform some examinations and medical procedures, only a doctor can prescribe medication.)

Be sure to have a pencil and paper at hand so that you can write down any information or instructions the doctor or nurse gives you.

When you call the doctor's office, you probably know whether you just want some advice on the telephone or whether you want to bring the child in to see the doctor. Tell the doctor or nurse what you have in mind—don't expect him or her to guess. If the doctor or nurse thinks that it's not necessary for you to bring the child in, you'll be told the reason for that advice. However, the decision is yours, and if you still want a personal consultation, you're entitled to insist.

It's better to call early in the day rather than waiting until late in the afternoon. The longer you wait, the less likely the doctor will be able to see your child that day. And if you know you want your child seen, call and ask for an appointment rather than asking to speak with the doctor or nurse.

Another way to stay on good terms with your child's doctor is to plan ahead so that both you and the doctor know what an office visit is intended to achieve. A common cause of communication breakdown between parent and physician is the parent's complaint that the doctor was too busy, didn't answer questions, or cut the visit short. To avoid this, always tell the receptionist what the visit is for at the time you make the appointment. If you feel you're going to need extra time with the doctor, let the receptionist know so that enough time can be scheduled—in this way, neither you nor the doctor will feel rushed.

When you see the doctor, do not confuse the issue by trying to get a complete update on other family members' problems in the course of one appointment. Let the doctor examine your child and deal with the reason you brought the child into the office. If you have other concerns not directly related to the present one, make an appointment to come back another time.

ASKING QUESTIONS

One of the things you probably checked out when you chose your doctor was his or her ability to use language you understand. Doctors, like specialists in any field, are so familiar with their professional language that they sometimes forget how confusing it is to other people. So if your child's doctor slips into medical jargon that you don't understand, ask for a translation. Don't feel uncomfortable about asking, either. You must know what the doctor's instructions are before you can carry them out, and it's part of the doctor's responsibility to make sure that you are fully informed about all matters that concern your child's health.

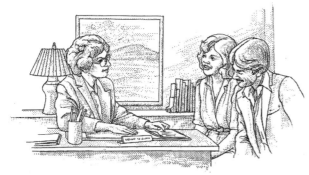

You should feel comfortable communicating with the doctor who is caring for your child.

Sometimes you may find that you understand what the doctor is saying—but you don't agree with it. In this case, don't hesitate to ask why the doctor has reached a certain decision, or what the alternatives are. If you still don't feel comfortable with the doctor's advice, don't argue. You may get the doctor to agree with your point of view, but this may not be in the child's best interests. If you and the doctor disagree on a diagnosis or a course of treatment, ask for a second opinion. This means going to another doctor and asking his or her professional advice on the issue. Your doctor may welcome this suggestion—or even make the suggestion before you do. A doctor may be hesitant to assume full responsibility for diagnosing and treating a difficult or unusual case. In such a situation, it is common to have two or more consultants working together to diagnose the condition and determine the best course of treatment.

When you ask for a second opinion, your doctor should be able to suggest names of possible consultants. If you trust the doctor, you'll trust his or her choice of other professionals. If you don't, you'll be looking for another doctor anyway.

It sometimes happens that when communication between parent and physician does break down, the only responsible course the parent can take is to find another doctor.

HOUSE CALLS

Many people who are now parents remember the days when doctors made house calls, and they wonder why doctors today don't make house calls. Your physician will probably tell you that many wrong diagnoses resulted from the old practice of examining sick children in their homes without adequate equipment. In the office, the doctor has a professionally set-up medical facility with the equipment necessary for an accurate diagnosis. So whether or not a doctor makes house calls—and most don't—should not affect your opinion of his or her competence. If you trust your doctor, and if you're confident that he or she will always be available in an emergency, you've made a good choice.

COMMUNICATION

A final word on the parent-physician partnership—and, again, it's partly a matter of courtesy. If your physician is taking good care of your child, express your appreciation—doctors like to be thanked, just like anyone else. However, if you're not satisfied with the health care your child is receiving, the doctor should know that, too. A physician's failure to please you may be due to many factors other than professional inadequacy. If you let the doctor know that there is a problem, he or she may be able to correct it. If not, your best plan may be to find another doctor.

Remember that although the doctor is your partner in caring for your child's health, you're still responsible for deciding just who this partner will be.

The physical examination

The medical care of a child is usually aimed at preventing serious illness. This is why children should be examined regularly by a doctor or other health professional. The child need not be ill at the time of these visits. In fact, if the child is sick, the routine examination may be delayed until the child has recovered. These routine visits to the doctor are sometimes called "well-child" or "well-baby" checkups. They are often scheduled to coincide with required immunizations.

Although they are extremely important, immunizations are only a small part of keeping your child healthy. At the time of the checkup, the child should be examined thoroughly, have routine tests, and have his or her physical and mental development evaluated.

The child will also be measured to find out if he or she is growing normally. Measurements include weight, length (or height), and head circumference (the distance around the head). The changes in these measurements as the child grows can then be charted on a graph and compared with the normal range of child development. If the child is not growing normally over a period of time, the doctor will check to see if the problem is caused by a growth disorder or by some other disease or abnormality. If such problems are found early, they can sometimes be corrected before any lasting damage is done.

THE FIRST VISIT

A baby's first visit to the doctor's office usually takes place two to four weeks after birth. This visit serves several purposes. For one thing, it gives the parent, the doctor, and the child an opportunity to meet and begin a relationship. The parent can get to know the doctor and the customs of the practice; the doctor can get basic information about the family, and the child's general health can be evaluated.

At this first visit, the doctor will take the baby's physical measurements and examine the baby for abnormalities. Some babies are born with physical problems and abnormalities that are obvious right away. Other inborn prob-

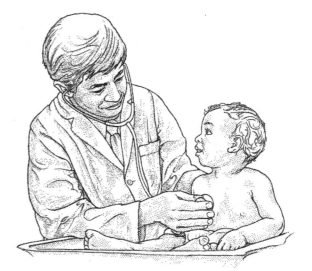

During regular checkups, a child should be examined thoroughly, have routine tests, and have his or her physical and mental development evaluated by a physician or other health professional.

lems do not show up until a few weeks after birth.

The doctor will also ask questions about the parents' health and medical histories. Some medical problems can be inherited, and some can run in families. It is important for the new baby's medical record to show such background information. If the child later shows signs of problems that have appeared before in the family, the doctor will be able to make a diagnosis more quickly.

The first visit will also include checking to see that the umbilical cord is healing as it should, that the circumcision (if one was done) is healing, and that the child has had no ill effects from labor and delivery. Feeding schedules, vitamins, and immunizations will be discussed as well.

Usually, regular return visits are scheduled at the first visit. The number and spacing of the visits will depend on the baby's health, the parents' needs and wishes, and the baby's scheduled immunizations.

If the baby's health and development seem normal, some or all of the later visits may be handled by a pediatric nurse practitioner or a physician's assistant. These health professionals are specially trained to be extensions of the doctor. They can work with you to clear up any questions you have about taking care of your baby. Of course, any question or problem that the nurse or assistant cannot handle is referred to the doctor.

LATER VISITS

As the child grows past babyhood, questions will come up about how to handle toilet training, rivalries with brothers and sisters, obedience, temper tantrums, and the like. These are areas where your doctor and his or her staff can help. Go ahead and ask about them. A child's doctor is concerned not only with the child's physical health and development, but also with his or her social and psychological development, which are a part of every child's growth and affect health in many ways.

THE DOCTOR'S PROCEDURES

In a complete physical examination, the doctor uses a combination of his or her senses and knowledge of the body to check over your child, system by system. The doctor uses instruments to extend the senses. For example, the stethoscope magnifies sounds, and the otoscope (for examining the ears) and ophthalmoscope (for examining the eyes) have lights and magnifying lenses in them to extend the doctor's vision.

In the process of an examination, the doctor will look at the child's skin, ears, eyes, nose, bone structure, and body openings. He or she will feel the lymph nodes and the organs that can be felt through the skin. The doctor will tap over body cavities and listen to the sounds that result. He or she will also listen to the sounds made by the heart, the lungs, and the digestive system. A blood pressure reading is an important part of the child's examination from an early age.

The doctor's senses are further extended by laboratory tests. Some of these tests such as vision and hearing tests, hemoglobin and hematocrit blood tests, and urinalysis, are routine. These tests are discussed elsewhere in this book. Other tests may be done if the doctor suspects that there may be a problem.

Each physical examination your child has will vary, depending on the child's age, stage of development, and state of health. During the first six months, the doctor will be paying particular attention to the baby's growth and development, including how well the baby is learning to move and control his or her muscles. The doctor will also check to be sure that the hips are properly developed and will listen for heart murmurs, which may be normal or may indicate heart problems. The doctor will take the pulse at the baby's groin (the femoral pulse) to be sure that there is no obstruction to blood flow in the aorta (the main artery of the body).

The baby's developing language skills are also an important part of growth, and the doctor will ask about progress in that area.

After the age of about six months, the child may begin to be afraid of the doctor. The child may cry and be actively uncooperative. This will, of course, make the physical examination and conversation more difficult for the doctor, but a doctor who deals with children every day knows what to expect. You can help make the examination go more smoothly by trying to reassure or distract your child. If the combined efforts of you and the doctor fail, the doctor will get as much information as possible under the circumstances.

THE PARENT'S ROLE

Especially with younger children and babies, you will play an important role in the examination. Most of the time, the doctor will want you to be present. Your presence has two main purposes: You can learn about your child's health, and you can comfort and reassure your child during the examination. An infant is often examined on the parent's lap, and the parent may also be asked to help with measuring the child and taking his or her temperature.

If you have questions during the examination, be sure to ask them, even if you think they may sound silly or feel that you ought to know the answers already. Part of the doctor's job is answering your questions. The more you know about how to care for your child, the better off both you and your child will be. After all, you will be responsible for carrying out the doctor's instructions. The doctor needs you to be well informed.

Immunizations

Despite the availability of vaccines that effectively protect children against diseases that used to be killers, surveys repeatedly indicate that almost 50 percent of American children are inadequately protected against these diseases.

The potentially devastating diseases against which all children can and should be properly immunized are diphtheria, tetanus, pertussis (whooping cough), polio, measles, mumps, and rubella (German measles). All children should also be immunized against Haemophilus influenzae b, which is a bacteria that causes a type of meningitis. Many doctors also believe that children should be immunized against hepatitis B.

There are two reasons why so many children go unprotected against these diseases. First, many parents believe that polio, diphtheria, and whooping cough no longer exist. Second, people don't realize how dangerous these diseases are. Children die or are permanently disabled each year as a result of these preventable diseases. The statistics prove that children *are* in danger from these diseases, and without immunization your child is also at risk.

Doctors use two types of immunization:

Active immunization is achieved by injecting a weakened or killed virus or bacterium into the body. This stimulates the body's natural defense system. The body produces substances known as antibodies, which are tailor-made to fight invading organisms. The antibodies, which are carried in the bloodstream, remain in the body for years, sometimes a lifetime, to protect it against that particular disease.

Passive immunization involves injecting ready-made antibodies—usually extracted from the blood of animals in which immunity has been induced for the sole purpose of producing a vaccine. Passive immunization is only temporary but serves to protect a person who may already be infected until the body has time to create its own antibodies.

The following sections explain how you can protect your child against these diseases. (Refer to the articles on each of these diseases for full

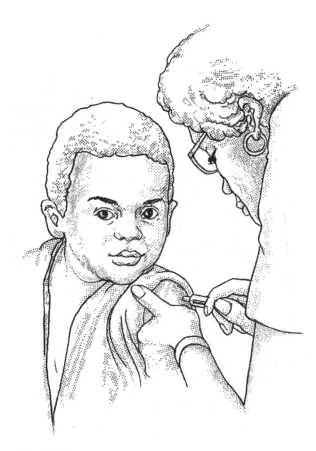

All children should be properly immunized. Consult your child's doctor for a schedule of immunizations.

information on symptoms, diagnosis, and treatment.) Keep in mind, however, that immunization schedules are always being reevaluated. So check with your child's doctor to be sure that the schedule shown on page 18 is appropriate for your child. You can also use the handy chart on page 19 to record the immunizations and boosters your child has received.

DIPHTHERIA, TETANUS, AND WHOOPING COUGH (PERTUSSIS)

To be protected against these three diseases, infants must receive three injections of the combined diphtheria-tetanus-pertussis (DTP) vaccine by the age of six months. The first injection is given at two months, followed by two more administered every other month. The child must receive a booster shot of DTP vaccine between ages 15 and 18 months and another booster shot at age four to six years. Thereafter, a booster of diphtheria-tetanus vaccine is necessary every ten years for life.

Diphtheria. Diphtheria is a bacterial disease that is frequently fatal. It causes infection of the nose, throat, tonsils, and lymph nodes of the neck. The bacterium responsible can produce a toxin (poison) that causes heart damage and paralysis. Cases of diphtheria are reported in every state each year. For every case reported, there are many carriers of the disease. (Carriers are people who harbor the organisms that cause a disease and can transmit the organisms to other people but who do not get sick themselves.)

Before the diphtheria vaccine came into general use 40 years ago, 80 percent of adult Americans were immune to diphtheria because they had had some form of the illness in childhood. This situation no longer exists, so adults should receive booster shots of diphtheria vaccine every ten years. Serious reactions to the diphtheria vaccine are rare.

Tetanus. Tetanus, or lockjaw, is a serious disease of the nervous system that is caused by a bacterium that can enter the body through a wound—even a minor wound like a scratch or an insect bite. Cases of tetanus are reported every year.

The vaccine is thoroughly safe and effective. However, its protection weakens over the years, and booster shots are necessary. Medical opinion differs as to how often boosters should be given. The American Academy of Pediatrics states that after receiving a booster at the age of four to six years, a person should receive a booster every ten years for life. The American College of Surgeons believes that boosters are necessary every five years to ensure protection from tetanus that results from the type of minor wound that is unlikely to be treated by a doctor.

As a general rule, if your child receives a relatively clean wound, such as one from a kitchen utensil, you should be sure that he or she has had a booster within the past ten years; but if the wound is a "dirty" one (for example, a wound from a nail or any wound that happens outdoors), you should check to see that your child has received a booster within the past five years. Adults should receive boosters at least every ten years.

Whooping cough. Whooping cough is more common than many parents (and doctors) realize. It is a highly contagious infection of the respiratory tract, which gets its name from the severe, strangling cough that develops as the disease progresses.

Whooping cough vaccine is the most uncertain of the three components of the DTP vaccine, because it does not give complete immunity. There have been extremely rare instances of brain damage following its use, but in some of these cases the damage was caused by faulty administration of the vaccine rather than by the vaccine itself. The vaccine may also cause a brief fever. For these reasons, routine boosters are not recommended after the child receives a booster at the age of four to six years. However, the mortality rate among infants under the age of one year who contract whooping cough and the possibility of complications in older children are high enough to exceed by far the minimal risk of the vaccine.

POLIO

Polio, also known as poliomyelitis and infantile paralysis, is an infection of the spinal cord that can, in one to two percent of cases, lead to paralysis or death.

Outbreaks of polio still occur in this country, and infants should receive two or three doses of the Sabin vaccine, which provides protection against all types of polio. The first dose should be given at two months, the second should be given two months later, and the third dose two months after that. This vaccine is given by mouth, not as an injection. A booster series should be given at the age of four to six years. Children who were not immunized in infancy should receive a total of three or four doses, depending on their ages. The Sabin vaccine is undoubtedly safe for children.

Adults who are not immune and who plan to travel to a country where polio is uncontrolled should also be immunized. In fact, all adults should be immunized against this disease if they were not immunized in childhood. Some medical authorities believe that the risk of an adult being exposed to polio within the United States is minimal, and therefore adult immunization is unnecessary. However, too many

(Continued on page 20)

IMMUNIZATION SCHEDULE

The following schedule summarizes the Advisory Committee on Immunization Practices (ACIP) recommendations for DTP, DTaP, Polio, MMR, Hib, and Hepatitis B vaccines. Ask your child's doctor if this schedule is appropriate for your child.

VACCINE	2 Months*	4 Months	6 Months	12–15 Months	15 Months	4–6 Years (before school entry)	14–16 Years and every 10 years thereafter
DTP	DTP	DTP	DTP		DTaP/DTP†	DTaP/DTP	Td
Polio	Polio	Polio	Polio			Polio	
MMR				MMR		MMR	
Hib Option 1‡ Option 2‡	Hib Hib	Hib Hib	Hib	Hib Hib			

VACCINE	At Birth (before hospital discharge)	1–2 Months	4 Months	6–18 Months
HBV Option 1 Option 2	HBV	HBV§ HBV§	HBV§	HBV§ HBV§

DTP: Diphtheria and Tetanus Toxoids, and Pertussis Vaccine
DTaP: Diphtheria and Tetanus Toxoids, and Acellular Pertussis Vaccine
Td: Tetanus and Diphtheria Toxoids—Adult
Polio: Live Oral Polio Vaccine drops (OPV) or Killed (inactivated) Polio Vaccine shots (IPV)
MMR: Measles, Mumps, and Rubella Vaccine
Hib: Haemophilus b Conjugate Vaccine
HBV: Hepatitis B Vaccine

*   Can be administered as early as six weeks of age.

†   This dose of DTP can be administered as early as 12 months of age provided that the interval since the previous dose of DTP is at least six months. *Diphtheria and tetanus toxoids and acellular pertussis vaccine (DTaP) is currently recommended only for use as the fourth and/or fifth doses of the DTP series among children aged 15 months through six years (before the seventh birthday).*

‡   Hib vaccine is given in either a four-dose schedule (option 1) or a three-dose schedule (option 2), depending on the types of vaccine used.

§   Hepatitis B vaccine can be given simultaneously with DTP, DTaP, Polio, MMR, and Hib vaccine at the same visit.

revised 3/94

IMMUNIZATION RECORD			
Type	Initial	Booster	Remarks
DTP/DTaP/Td			
Polio			
MMR			
Hib			
HBV			
Other			
Tuberculin Test*			

* Not an immunization but a test for the presence of tuberculosis.

(Continued from page 17)

cases of polio have occurred in adults over the age of 30 to make this argument acceptable.

Because the Sabin vaccine is a "live" vaccine (meaning that it contains live organisms), it does carry a slight risk of polio for adults. However, the Salk vaccine (a dead vaccine, prepared from inactivated organisms) does not. Adults who are not immune should receive an initial series of Salk vaccine to acquire temporary immunity, followed by a full series of Sabin vaccine for permanent protection.

MEASLES, MUMPS, AND RUBELLA

The live measles-mumps-rubella (MMR) combination vaccine should be given to children at age 12 to 15 months. A second dose is recommended at either four to six years of age or in early adolescence.

Measles. Measles is a contagious viral disease that affects mainly the respiratory system, the eyes, and the skin. It is considered dangerous mainly because its complications can include pneumonia (inflammation of the lungs), encephalitis (inflammation of the brain), and ear infections. Because most children are now vaccinated against it, measles is seldom seen today. The risk of a child contracting encephalitis from the vaccine is less than one in a million, and pneumonia and ear infections are never seen as a consequence of immunization.

Mumps. Mumps is a contagious viral disease that causes swelling of the parotid glands, which are the salivary glands beneath the ear. Mumps can be painful and uncomfortable but seldom has long-term complications. The most serious complication of mumps is encephalitis (inflammation of the brain), which can be followed by hearing loss or deafness. The mumps vaccine, which is included in the MMR vaccine, is harmless to the child and is 95 percent effective in preventing the disease.

Rubella. Rubella, or German measles, is a contagious viral disease that produces mild, cold-like symptoms and a short-lived rash. The disease is not usually dangerous except when it is contracted by a pregnant woman. In the first three to four months of a pregnancy, rubella can affect the fetus and cause serious, lifelong problems. Now that the vaccine is available and routinely given to young children, rubella is fairly uncommon. The last major outbreak was in 1964 to 1965. Still, a pregnant woman should take care to avoid exposure to the disease, and a child who contracts rubella should be kept away from any woman who is or might be pregnant. Very rarely, the vaccine causes temporary arthritis in older children.

SMALLPOX

Vaccination against smallpox, a highly contagious disease that used to appear in epidemics, is no longer practiced in the United States. According to the World Health Organization, smallpox has been eradicated throughout the world.

HAEMOPHILUS INFLUENZA TYPE B

Children are now routinely protected against this potentially life-threatening type of meningitis. The vaccine is given with the DTP at two, four, and six months of age; a booster is given at 12 to 15 months of age. Don't confuse this type of infection with other infections caused by different strains of the same bacteria. A different strain of Haemophilus influenza bacteria causes ear infections, but the vaccine offers no protection against it.

HEPATITIS B

This is the latest vaccine that many doctors consider part of the routine immunization schedule. Hepatitis (inflammation of the liver) is not common in childhood, but it can be deadly. If the doctor believes vaccination is warranted, the first dose will be given before the newborn is discharged from the hospital. The second dose is given one to two months later, followed by a dose at four months of age and another at 6 to 18 months of age.

OTHER VACCINES

A vaccine against pneumococcal infection is available for use in children in certain high-risk groups. A vaccine against meningococcal infection is still in the experimental stage and is used only in specific cases. A vaccine to prevent chicken pox has recently been developed but is not yet available for general use.

Vaccines against typhoid, typhus, yellow fever, and influenza are presently available. None of these is yet recommended for children unless a child will be at special risk. Consult your doctor if you are in doubt.

RELATED TOPICS:

Diphtheria; Hepatitis; Influenza; Measles; Meningitis; Mumps; Pneumonia; Polio; Rubella; Tetanus; Whooping cough

Medical tests

Laboratory tests are used by doctors to help identify illnesses, to determine what particular type of infectious organism is causing a problem, and to learn how serious a disease may be. Some procedures can be performed right in the doctor's office; others must be done in a laboratory, where more complex equipment is available. Some common tests and procedures are described here.

URINALYSIS

Urinalysis means analysis of a specimen of urine (the liquid form of body waste). Urine tests can reveal infections in the kidneys, the bladder, and the rest of the urinary tract. The chemical and cell content of urine can also show how well the digestive system is working.

Urine can be tested in four different ways. First, it can be examined visually for color and texture. Normal urine is a clear yellow; if it is cloudy, reddish, or some other color, an infection or an injury may be present in the body. Second, the water content of the urine can be measured. This shows how well the kidneys are doing their job of filtering the body's wastes. Third, the chemical content of the urine can be analyzed to find out if the body is discarding necessary chemicals that should be retained. Finally, the urine can be examined under a microscope to find out what cells, bacteria, and other material are present.

Chemical analysis of urine is often used as a screening test for diabetes, a disease in which the body does not properly use the carbohydrates (sugars and starches) that are its chief sources of energy. To test for diabetes, the amount of glucose (a form of sugar) in the urine is measured by dipping a chemically treated stick in the urine and comparing the color of the stick with a color chart. If the glucose concentration is above a certain level, diabetes may be the cause. Blood tests are then done to verify the diagnosis.

BLOOD TESTS

Blood circulates throughout the body, so the contents of the blood can provide information both about general health and about specific diseases. The blood to be tested is drawn out of

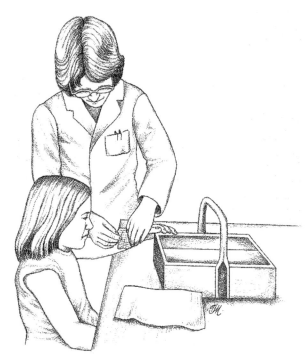

Doctors use laboratory tests to identify illnesses, to determine what organisms are causing a problem, and to learn how serious a disease may be.

a vein with a syringe or taken by pricking a finger. The method used to take a sample depends on how much blood is needed for the tests that are to be done and how "clean" the specimen needs to be. A finger-stick sample is more likely to be contaminated by contact with the surface of the finger than is a sample taken by putting a sterile needle into a vein.

Many different tests can be done on the blood, and a few of the most common ones are described here. More complex tests can be done to find out what chemicals are present in the blood.

Hematocrit. This test is done to find out how much of the blood is made up of red blood cells, which carry oxygen to the body tissues. This is one of two tests done to check for anemia (red blood cell deficiency). A blood sample is spun in a machine called a centrifuge, which makes it separate into red blood cells, white blood cells, and plasma. The red cells are the heaviest, so they sink to the bottom. The percentage of red cells is then determined and compared with the normal range.

Hemoglobin. Hemoglobin is a protein that gives red blood cells their red color; it combines with oxygen so that it can be carried in the blood. The amount of hemoglobin in the blood is tested by adding certain chemicals to the blood and then measuring the intensity of the red color that signifies the presence of hemoglobin. A hemoglobin test is often done at the same time as a hematocrit. (This is the other test always done to check for anemia.)

White blood cell count. White blood cells play a role in the body's defense against infection. Too many or too few of these cells in the blood may indicate an infection or a disorder. To count the white blood cells, a blood specimen is diluted and put in a counting chamber, which is a slide with a grid on it. The slide is examined under a microscope, and the cells are counted. This test can be done in most doctors' offices.

Differential blood cell count. There are five different types of normal white blood cells; each type has a distinctive shape and appearance, and each one has a different function. To get more precise information about a disease, the doctor may need to know how many of each type of white blood cell are present in the blood. To do this, a stain is added to a blood specimen. Because the stain affects each type of white blood cell differently, it is then easier to tell them apart. The stained specimen is examined under a microscope, and at least 100 white blood cells are identified and classified. The cells are also examined to see if they have a normal shape. In the course of this test, the red blood cells can also be counted and checked for abnormalities.

Sedimentation rate. The sedimentation rate reflects the speed at which red blood cells move through the blood and settle in the bottom of a container. To test the rate of settling, a chemical is added to a blood sample to keep it from clotting. Then the red cells are timed as they move to the bottom of a specially marked test tube.

This test is used to screen for diseases. A rapid sedimentation rate is a sign of disease, but the test does not identify what is causing the cells to fall more quickly than normal. Keeping track of the sedimentation rate in suc-

cessive tests can help a physician follow the progress of diseases that cause inflammation, including rheumatic fever and rheumatoid arthritis.

Monospot test. Infectious mononucleosis ("mono") is a viral disease that causes, among other symptoms, mild to severe fatigue. The monospot test is a blood test that determines if a child has mono (although sometimes a child with early mono will have a negative test). If the monospot is positive, it may remain positive for up to a few years after the disease has gone away.

THROAT CULTURES

A throat culture is done to find out if a throat infection is being caused by bacteria and, if so, to identify the specific type of bacterium. This can provide the doctor with important information. If the infection is due to a virus rather than to a bacterium, the doctor will know not to prescribe antibiotics (viruses don't respond to antibiotics); if a bacterium is the cause, knowing which one it is will enable the doctor to prescribe the correct antibiotic to combat it.

To collect material for the culture, the doctor uses a cotton-tipped swab to remove cells and discharge from the throat. This material is put into a growth medium (a special substance that encourages bacteria to grow). The specimen is watched carefully, and the bacteria are identified. Because throat cultures are often sent to a laboratory for analysis, it may take 48 hours to get the results.

Many doctors now use a rapid strep screening test to detect infection by streptococcus bacteria ("strep throat"). Most of these tests take only 10 to 20 minutes and, if positive, are a good indication that the child has strep throat. Some doctors don't trust a negative result from the test and order a throat culture to verify negative results.

OTHER CULTURES

Although throat cultures are the most commonly performed, cultures can also be made from blood, bowel movements, and urine, as well as from discharge coughed up from the lungs or obtained from an infected eye or ear or an infected cut or wound. As with a throat culture, material from the site is sent to a laboratory, where it is placed in a growth medium to see what types of bacteria grow.

ELECTROCARDIOGRAM

An electrocardiogram, or ECG, is a recording of the electrical impulses of the heart. These impulses are what make the heart beat in a regular rhythm. To make such a record, the patient is attached to an ECG machine with electrodes (metal plates that are placed on the arms, legs, and chest). These electrodes pick up the electrical impulses that move through the body. The impulses cause a needle in the machine to move on a piece of paper as the paper moves through the machine. Where the needle touches the paper, it makes a line. The physician studies the pattern on the paper to see if the heart rhythm is normal.

The ECG does not hurt the patient, but it is important for the patient to stay very still while the recording is being done. All muscle movements, not just movements of the heart muscle, are caused by electrical impulses. Therefore, any movement can affect the ECG recording and give an inaccurate picture of the heartbeat.

An ECG is done to check for arrhythmias (irregular heart rhythms), an enlarged heart, heart valve disorders, heart malformations, and many other heart disorders. The test can be done in a doctor's office or an outpatient laboratory.

ELECTROENCEPHALOGRAM

An electroencephalogram, or EEG, is a recording of electrical activity in the brain. It is a painless procedure similar to an ECG. The metal plates known as electrodes are attached to the patient's head and to an EEG machine. The electrodes pick up the brain's electrical impulses. These impulses activate a needle, which traces the pattern of the impulses on a piece of paper moving through the machine. The physician compares the pattern on the recording with patterns of normal brain activity and determines if there is an abnormality. Recordings from opposite sides of the brain can also be compared to see if the patterns match.

An EEG is done to test for epilepsy, brain tumors, encephalitis (inflammation of the brain), and other brain disorders.

LUMBAR PUNCTURE

A lumbar puncture, or spinal tap, is the method used to obtain a sample of cerebrospinal fluid for testing. Cerebrospinal fluid is a clear liquid that surrounds the brain and the spinal cord. In a lumbar puncture, a needle is used to penetrate into the area of the lumbar spine (the lower portion of the spine) between two vertebrae (the bones that make up the spine) and to draw out some fluid. The pressure in the spinal column can be measured at the same time. The fluid is examined to see if it is clear or cloudy and to see if it contains any blood. It is then tested for viruses, bacteria, and other signs of infection.

A lumbar puncture may be done to test for meningitis, encephalitis, brain hemorrhage (bleeding in the brain), polio, and other nervous system disorders. Under usual circumstances, there is no risk from a lumbar puncture. If the spinal fluid is under extreme pressure, however, the procedure carries some risk of complications; a different technique is then used to minimize risk.

COMPUTED TOMOGRAPHY

Computed tomography (also called computerized axial tomography, CT scan, or CAT scan) is a sophisticated X-ray study. A series of X-ray films is made of a part of the body, such as the head or the torso. The patient is placed in a tunnel-like opening in the scanning machine. The patient does not have to be repositioned for each picture, as would be necessary for ordinary X-ray films, because the scanning machine is capable of taking X-ray images from many different angles. A computer then assembles those X-ray images into cross-sectional pictures of that part of the body.

CT scans are used to find abnormal growths or other problems in areas that are inside the body and therefore impossible to see without potentially dangerous exploratory surgery. For example, the brain can be examined for an abnormal growth without opening up the skull.

MAGNETIC RESONANCE IMAGING

Magnetic resonance imaging (MRI) is a way to visualize parts of the body without using X rays. It provides doctors with an exceedingly clear picture of certain parts of the body. The actual machine is somewhat like a CT scanner. Many people believe an MRI is just a better CT scan, but that's not true. There are some situations in which a CT scan is better than an MRI, and a CT scan is much less expensive.

The medicine chest

Although most of the medications your child will take will be by a doctor's prescription, there are certain items every parent ought to have on hand at home. Some of these are medications that you can buy without a prescription at your drugstore. Other items, like a thermometer, are basics of a home health care kit. You'll also need antiseptics, ointments, gauze pads, and bandages in preparation for the inevitable bangs, scrapes, cuts, and other minor crises of childhood.

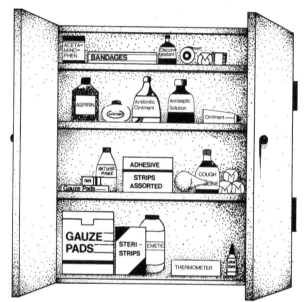

When you assemble a home medicine chest, buy only the most basic items without the advice of a doctor.

When you're assembling this kit, however, remember a few safety rules:
■ Do not buy or administer any but the most basic drugs without the advice of a doctor.
■ Only buy medications in containers that have childproof caps. Keep all medications in their original, clearly labeled containers. Periodically check expiration dates on over-the-counter medications, and throw out any that have expired.
■ Unless your child must take a prescription medication on a regular basis, do not keep left-over medicines. Flush liquids, pills, and cap-

sules down the toilet, and throw out the containers.
■ Keep all medications locked away from children. If you and your young child are visiting friends who do not have children, make sure that no dangerous substances are within reach of the child.
■ Don't keep medicines in your bathroom. The heat and steam from the shower affect many drugs, sometimes lessening their potency.

The following basic medical supplies should see you through most nonemergency situations:

    Acetaminophen (choose a form—liquid or pill—suited for your child's age)
    Adhesive bandages (assorted sizes, including "butterfly" bandages)
    Adhesive tape
    Antibiotic ointment
    Antiseptic solution and/or soap
    Aspirin
    Decongestant
    Emetic (syrup of ipecac)
    Rolls of knitted bandage
    Lubricant (petroleum jelly and/or a water-soluble gel)
    Nasal aspirator
    Nose drops
    Sterile gauze pads (various sizes)
    Thermometer

ASPIRIN AND ACETAMINOPHEN

Aspirin is probably the most commonly used home remedy of all and the one parents think of at once in the face of any crisis. Acetaminophen is a nonaspirin alternative with similar properties. Both are available as flavored, chewable tablets and as liquids. (Aspirin rectal suppositories are also available but are not recommended for children. Their rate of absorption is uneven, and they present a greater risk of aspirin poisoning than other forms of this drug.) Liquid ibuprofen has also been approved for use in children, but it is available only by prescription.

Because both acetaminophen and aspirin come in different strengths, you should check the label to make sure that the strength is appropriate to the age of your child. Acetaminophen and aspirin tablets can be crushed and mixed with a little applesauce, jelly, or ice cream to make them more acceptable to the child. Whenever you disguise a medicine in this way, however, you must make sure that the child takes the whole dose.

Until recently, acetaminophen was used primarily when a child couldn't take aspirin for one reason or another. There is now evidence, however, that the use of aspirin, especially when given to a child with chicken pox or the flu, may be associated with a condition known as Reye's syndrome. This is a relatively rare condition that combines encephalitis (inflammation of the brain) with liver disease.

Although it has not been proved that aspirin causes or promotes Reye's syndrome, it is recommended that aspirin not be given to children with a viral infection, particularly chicken pox or influenza. Acetaminophen, however, has not been linked to Reye's syndrome and is an acceptable substitute. If you are in any doubt about the use of aspirin or acetaminophen for your child, consult your doctor.

EMETIC

An emetic is a substance that is used to induce vomiting, which is desirable in certain cases of poisoning. Every medicine chest should contain an emetic—syrup of ipecac is recommended. It is a good idea to have two small bottles, each containing a single dose of two to three teaspoonfuls for immediate use. Note, however, that vomiting should not be induced automatically in a case of poisoning. If the poison is something that is not normally edible (for example, gasoline, turpentine, or cleaning fluid), you should *not* make the child vomit because the poison may do additional harm on the way back up. (See *Poisoning* for more information.)

NOSE DROPS, NASAL ASPIRATOR, AND DECONGESTANTS

Nose drops and oral decongestants and a nasal aspirator may be used to relieve nasal stuffiness and discharge. Ask your doctor to recommend types and uses.

THERMOMETER AND LUBRICANT

A stubby-bulb thermometer is the most practical because it can be used to take an oral, rec-

tal, or armpit temperature. Any lubricating ointment will serve to prepare a thermometer for rectal use, but a water-soluble gel is superior because it readily washes off in cold water.

ADDITIONS

The following are useful for treating minor injuries: antiseptic solution, antibiotic ointment, sterile gauze pads (two-by-two inches and three-by-three inches), rolls of knitted bandage (two inches wide and three inches wide), adhesive tape (one-quarter inch wide), "butterfly" bandages, and other adhesive bandages of assorted sizes.

Medications

Treating a sick child with medication is a two-way responsibility, and it's a perfect example of how parent and doctor work together in the interests of the child's health. The doctor is responsible for making an accurate diagnosis of the child's condition and prescribing the appropriate drug. But it is the parent's responsibility to make sure that the drug is administered correctly.

It has been estimated that in 10 to 30 percent of cases in which medication apparently failed to work, that failure occurred because the medication wasn't given properly. Whenever a doctor prescribes medication for your child, the doctor will also instruct you in how the medicine should be given. If you don't understand, ask. And don't rely on the scribble on the prescription. Prescriptions are written in a form of medical shorthand that is quite clear to a pharmacist but may not mean a thing to you. So make sure you know, before you leave the doctor's office or get off the phone, just how to give the child the medication.

HOW MUCH MEDICATION TO GIVE

The quantity of medication the doctor prescribes for your child depends on the child's weight and age. The dosage prescribed for a baby will be much different from that prescribed for an adolescent, even if the drug is the same and given for the same reason. It's important to give the child the exact amount prescribed, which means that you can't rely on hit-or-miss measurements. It's easy enough to give one or two pills, but liquid measures are trickier. You can't use a kitchen teaspoon to administer a teaspoonful of medication—you could be way off. One teaspoonful means 5.0 milliliters (ml) of liquid. Half a teaspoonful means 2.5 ml—not what looks like half of the teaspoon you use to stir your coffee.

You can buy a specially marked measuring spoon for medication from any pharmacy. Keep it in the medicine chest and be sure to use it any time you are giving your child liquid medication. If you have a child who insists on taking medication from his or her own special

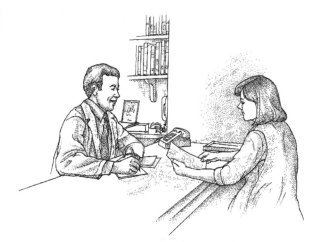

Before you leave the doctor's office or get off the phone, make sure you know how to give your child the prescribed medication.

spoon, transfer the medication from the measuring spoon to the child's spoon *after* measuring.

Make sure the child takes all the medication. If the child vomits within 20 minutes of receiving medication, you can assume that the medication was lost and should give another dose.

WHEN TO GIVE MEDICATION

It is also important to follow the doctor's instructions about *when* medicine should be given. Medications vary in the amount of time it takes for them to be absorbed by the body and start doing their work of helping the child. Some medications need to be given at very precisely regulated intervals. Therefore, make sure you fully understand the prescription. For example, "four times a day" and "every six hours" do *not* mean the same thing. If the label on the medication tells you to give the medicine four times a day, it means that the child should have four doses within the waking hours at fairly equally spaced intervals. On the other hand, "every six hours" means exactly what it says. Each dose must be given six hours after the last one, and the child must be awakened at the appropriate time if necessary. This instruction may also appear on the prescription as "every six hours around the clock."

HOW LONG TO GIVE MEDICATION

A mistake that is all too easy to make is to assume that because a child acts well, he or she *is* well. Stopping a child's medication too soon can cause a relapse and complications. The symptoms of an illness can subside long before the illness itself is over. The child's earache goes away, the fever drops, the appetite returns to normal, and the parent thinks the child is well again. In fact, the healing process may barely have begun. Strep infections, for example, require ten straight days of antibiotic treatment. Some infections—urinary tract and ear infections, for instance—often take even longer, even though the symptoms may disappear in a day. Therefore, such instructions as "Give for ten full days," "Continue for two weeks," and "Give until finished" are not just so many words. They are precise and necessary directions to you from the doctor. Consider such an instruction not as a request, but as an order.

HOW TO GIVE MEDICATION

It is best to let your child find out early that taking medication is just one of those things that children have to do now and then—a situation in which you are the boss and the child doesn't have a choice in the matter.

Every parent needs to know how to give a child medicine, and the parent who reports to the doctor that "my child just won't take the medication" is forcing the doctor to resort to another method of treatment that may be less effective. In extreme cases, a child who cannot be medicated at home must be hospitalized so that the appropriate medications can be given by professionals.

A young child, approached in a reassuring and matter-of-fact manner, will usually accept medication without any trouble. There are also some special techniques that may make it easier for both you and the child.

Liquid medicine can be given directly from the spoon (after careful measurement), and many medications designed for children are specially flavored so that they are not unpleasant to taste. An alternative method is to use a nonglass medicine dropper to squirt the liquid slowly into the child's mouth. If you use this method, you must be very careful not to direct the stream of liquid forcefully against the back of the throat and down the windpipe, but rather against the inside of the cheek.

If the medicine doesn't taste good, give the child a sweet treat afterward to take away the bad taste, or disguise the medicine in a little applesauce, ice cream, or juice. If you do this, however, make sure the child takes the entire portion.

Some young children will accept medicine in the form of chewable tablets or even regular tablets or capsules that can be swallowed whole. However, do not give pills and capsules to even a cooperative child under the age of five years. Small children can easily choke to death on a bulky pill. If the medication is not available in liquid form, a tablet may usually be mashed (or the contents of a capsule emptied) and mixed with a small quantity of juice or food. (Always check with your pharmacist or physician first, though, to be certain that the medication will be effective if given in this way.) Again, you must make sure that the child gets the whole dose.

After the age of five or six years, your child can probably swallow tablets or capsules whole. You can help the child learn how to do this by taking advantage of occasions when he or she needs a nonprescription remedy— aspirin for a slight headache, perhaps. If the child is willing, show him or her how to put the pill on the back of the tongue and swallow it with a drink or with a half-teaspoonful of ice cream, applesauce, or jelly. It's also possible to buy a special glass that delivers the pill into the mouth automatically with the first gulp of liquid. Whenever a child is taking a pill, watch to be sure that the medication goes down smoothly and that the child is in no danger of choking.

A final caution: Don't ever try to fool a child into taking medication by saying that it's candy or just like candy. Many cases of drug poisoning have occurred in children who helped themselves to medications that looked or tasted like candy. Many doctors even discourage the use of children's vitamin pills that are sweet, brightly colored, or shaped like cartoon characters. Such products blur the distinction in the child's mind between candy and drugs, and the child may make a tragic mistake.

Fever

Because fever is such a common sign of a variety of illnesses, parents need to learn ahead of time when to take their child's temperature, what method is most effective for children of various ages, how to read and handle a thermometer, when to be concerned about an abnormal reading, and whether or not they should make an effort to bring the fever down. By becoming familiar with these basics, you'll be better able to assess your child's condition quickly and effectively.

Everybody knows what a fever is, but many people don't know what it means. One common error is to assume that the higher the fever, the sicker the child. It is also commonly believed that fever is a child's enemy—that it should be fought and the temperature brought to normal as soon as possible.

The fact is that children past early infancy tend to develop high fevers with little provocation. Relatively harmless illnesses like roseola often cause temperatures as high as 106°F, whereas many serious diseases, such as leukemia and polio, may cause only a slight rise in temperature or none at all. And it is not true that high fever causes brain damage.

Remember that the degree of fever does not necessarily indicate the severity of the illness. A child with pneumonia or meningitis who has had a fever of 104°F is still quite ill even when the temperature has been artificially reduced to normal. A child with a strep throat and a fever of 101°F is no less sick than the same child with a strep throat and a temperature of 104°F. Other symptoms (such as exhaustion, confusion, and difficulty in breathing) indicate the severity of the illness.

It makes more sense, in fact, to regard a fever as a child's friend rather than as an enemy. A fever is an early warning signal that a child is ill. Fever also speeds up the body's metabolic processes (possibly including its resistance mechanisms) and, in some instances, may help the body's defenses overcome an illness.

Fever, together with other symptoms, also acts as a barometer to help you judge when an illness is ending. For example, the course of a fever may indicate whether an antibiotic is working effectively. Finally, the pattern of daily fluctuations in fever is characteristic of certain illnesses and may aid the physician in making a correct diagnosis.

A high fever does have disadvantages, however. It makes a child feel uncomfortable and, as it develops, may cause chills. If a fever continues for days, it may weaken a child so that it takes longer for the child to recuperate. In susceptible younger children, a fever may lead to convulsions (see *Convulsions with fever*). For all these reasons, it is sensible to reduce a fever. Nevertheless, it is important not to confuse treating the fever with treating the illness, not to panic as a fever rises, and not to harm the child in your anxiousness to fight the fever.

A MATTER OF DEGREE

No one can accurately estimate the degree of a fever by touch. If your child feels warm or appears ill, you must use a thermometer to accurately register the temperature, which your doctor needs to know in order to plan treatment.

At any given moment, different parts of the body are at different temperatures. Furthermore, normal body temperatures vary as much as 3°F over the course of a day even when a child is healthy. A rectal temperature of 99.8°F or lower, an oral temperature of 98.6°F or lower, and an armpit temperature (which is the least accurate) of 98°F or lower are all considered normal. Despite these variations, all thermometers are marked to indicate 98.6°F as the normal temperature.

For the most reliable readings at any age, the rectal thermometer is recommended, although it takes a little longer for the temperature to register. (A rectal thermometer differs from an oral one only in having a more rugged bulb.) The most practical instrument for home use is a stubby-bulb thermometer, which can be used to take a child's temperature either rectally or orally.

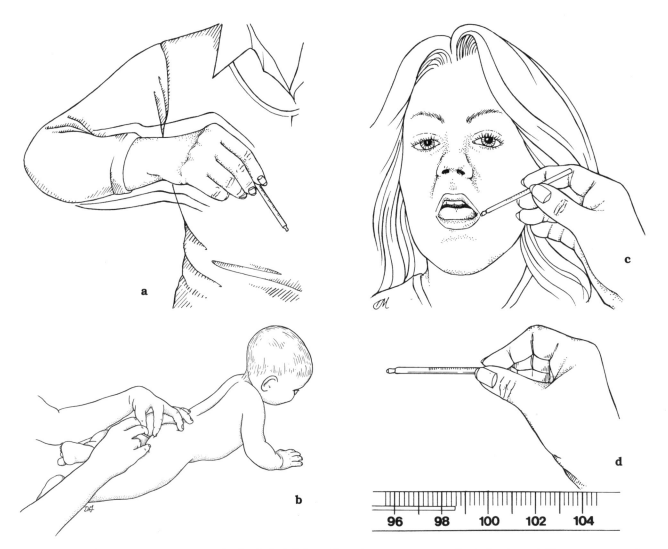

(a) Before using a thermometer, shake it briskly a few times to ensure that the top of the mercury column is below 96°F. (b) To take a rectal temperature, lubricate the bulb of the thermometer, spread the child's buttocks with the thumb and forefinger of one hand, and gently insert the bulb of the thermometer into the center of the anus; hold it there for at least two minutes. (c) To take an older child's oral temperature, place the thermometer under the child's tongue and have her hold it there (with her mouth closed) for three minutes. (d) A rectal temperature of 99.8°F or less and an oral temperature of 98.6°F or below are both considered normal.

USING THE THERMOMETER

Before using the thermometer, shake it briskly a few times to make certain that the top of the mercury column is below 98.6°F and that the bulb is intact.

To take a rectal temperature, first lubricate the bulb of the thermometer with petroleum jelly, and then spread the child's buttocks with the thumb and forefinger of one hand so that the anal opening is clearly visible. Insert the bulb of the thermometer gently into the center of the anus and hold it there for two to three minutes. (Only the bulb portion of the ther-

mometer needs to be inserted to get an accurate reading.)

The child should feel no pain or discomfort from having a rectal temperature taken, but he or she probably will not like being restrained. Nevertheless, it is important to keep the child from moving so that the thermometer will not break. To take a baby's rectal temperature, place the child facedown on a solid surface and put the heel of your hand firmly on the lower back. An unwilling toddler can be firmly clasped between your thighs and bent forward over one of your legs.

Although less reliable, an oral temperature reading is sufficient and can be taken in a child who is old enough to hold the bulb of the thermometer under the tongue with the mouth closed for three minutes. (If the thermometer breaks and the child accidentally swallows the mercury in the thermometer, don't worry. Thermometers contain elemental mercury, which is a nonpoisonous and harmless form of the metal.) Axillary temperatures (taken by putting a thermometer in the child's armpit) are very unreliable and shouldn't be used.

Two newer ways to measure a child's temperature are forehead strips and tympanic-membrane (eardrum) thermometers. Forehead strips are pieces of plastic containing chemicals that change color depending on their temperature. Unfortunately, they are not very accurate. The newest way to take a temperature is with a tympanic-membrane thermometer. This device makes temperature taking quick and painless. But if not used correctly (proper use usually requires some experience), it can easily give a false reading.

CARE OF YOUR THERMOMETER

After each use, the thermometer should be shaken so that the mercury level is below the "normal" level of 98.6°F and then washed with soap and cold water. You may want to wipe the thermometer with a tissue that has been moistened with rubbing alcohol before storing it. Place the thermometer back in the medicine cabinet where it will be handy the next time you need it. Do not let children treat the thermometer as a toy.

TREATMENT OF FEVER

The most reliable medications for lowering fever are acetaminophen (a nonaspirin pain reliever), aspirin, and ibuprofen. All of these medicines are labeled with the appropriate dose for children; the dose can generally be repeated every four hours. Read the directions carefully, since some medicines may look the same but may be dosed differently. For example, although acetaminophen liquid and acetaminophen syrup may look similar, the recommended amount to give to a child is different for each. Other basic guidelines for administering acetaminophen or aspirin include the following:

1. Do not awaken the child to give acetaminophen, aspirin, or ibuprofen.
2. Do not mix acetaminophen, aspirin, and ibuprofen or alternate them.
3. Call the doctor if fever persists longer than 48 hours or if other signs of illness are present.

Keep a feverish child only lightly clothed or covered to allow the body heat to escape, which will help lower a fever. Other traditional methods of reducing a fever, such as placing the child in a lukewarm bath or encasing the naked child in a wet sheet, only temporarily lower a child's temperature and are of little use. A child with a consistently high temperature should be under the care of a doctor.

Acetaminophen is the drug of choice for children with a fever. Although giving aspirin has long been the accepted home treatment for lowering a fever, aspirin should not be used if the child has a viral infection, particularly chicken pox or influenza. A condition called Reye's syndrome has been associated with the use of aspirin in the treatment of chicken pox or influenza (see *Reye's syndrome*). Reye's syndrome is a relatively rare type of encephalitis (inflammation of the brain) accompanied by changes in the liver. The condition usually starts after the child has begun to recover from chicken pox or influenza.

It has not been proved that aspirin causes or promotes Reye's syndrome, but it is recommended that aspirin not be given to children with chicken pox or influenza. Instead, acetaminophen (which has not been linked to Reye's syndrome) should be used to manage the fever and other symptoms.

RELATED TOPICS: Chicken pox; Convulsions with fever; Influenza; Reye's syndrome

Preparing for emergencies

In most situations involving your child's health, becoming knowledgeable about health and nutrition and obtaining the best professional advice you can on health matters will stand you in good stead. But there is always the chance of an emergency when no trained medical personnel are available and when a book—no matter how good—cannot answer your every question.

LEARNING WHAT TO DO IN AN EMERGENCY

Studies have shown that every person will be involved in an emergency situation at least twice in life. In such a situation, knowing what to do—and what not to do—can mean the difference between life and death. That is why it is recommended that everyone (and especially every parent) take a course in first aid, including training in cardiopulmonary resuscitation (CPR). While the quick-reference section of this book includes basic information about mouth-to-mouth resuscitation (which is only one aspect of CPR) and how to aid a child who is choking, it is no replacement for the skills and knowledge learned in a first-aid course. CPR, specifically, must be learned in a course. Such a course is available in virtually every town in the United States. Call your local chapter of the American Heart Association or the American Red Cross for further information.

GETTING HELP IN AN EMERGENCY

Knowing *when* to call for help is an important consideration in an emergency. In some situations, if you are the first person on the scene, your efforts must be devoted to the victim, and calling for medical assistance must wait until certain steps have been carried out or until a second person arrives. In less urgent situations, a call for help may be the appropriate first step. An approved first-aid class will teach you to differentiate between these situations. (The "Emergency Quick Reference" pages in this book will indicate when it is appropriate to summon help.)

Knowing *whom* to call for help is the next consideration in an emergency. In general,

don't waste time by calling your doctor—in a true emergency, his or her first instruction may well be to call an ambulance or paramedic squad. Post a list of emergency phone numbers near all phones in the house. That list should include the phone number for:
■ the paramedic squad
■ the local poison control center
■ the nearest major hospital with a fully equipped emergency department (ask your physician for a recommendation if you are uncertain)
■ the police department
■ the fire department
■ your child's doctor, including any emergency numbers provided by the doctor

Be certain that these phone numbers are current and accurate *before* you ever have to use them.

If you do have to call one of those emergency numbers, remember to give all necessary information—location, nature of the emergency, telephone number—and wait for the operator to tell you that it's OK to break the connection.

The normal newborn baby

Part of being able to recognize when a child is ill is knowing what to expect from a normal, healthy child. While every baby is different, there are some traits, behaviors, and developments that nearly all babies have in common. Although this section is especially intended for first-time parents, anyone who has a new baby may find a "refresher course" useful. If you expect your second baby to be just like your first, you may be in for a surprise.

One thing that is easy to forget is how tiny even the healthiest, heftiest baby really is. A newborn usually is only 18 to 21 inches long, stretched out. And very young babies often keep their legs in the fetal, or folded-up, position for several months, which makes them seem even smaller. The baby was in that position for many months before birth, and it takes a while to get used to an uncramped environment.

Remember that at birth the baby has left a warm, dark, still, safe environment; been pushed through a narrow birth canal; and been suddenly thrust into light, noise, and a new degree of independence. It's a difficult adjustment to make, even more difficult than the adjustment you must make as new parents.

There are some things about a new baby's appearance that may worry you if you're not prepared. For instance, it is perfectly normal for a newborn to have bluish-tinged skin (which soon turns to pinkish-red), a slightly lopsided head, and soft spots, called fontanelles, above the forehead and at the top of the head. It is also quite common for a newborn to have jaundice, which gives a yellowish color to the skin and the whites of the eyes.

Although the baby went through a period of incredible growth and development before birth, the newborn still has a lot of growing and developing to do. Many bones are still unformed; they are made of tough, elastic tissue called cartilage that will gradually harden into bone. The legs are often bowed and shorter than you might expect when you compare them with the arms. The head may seem too big for the body. The baby's face may seem abnormally plump in the cheeks and flat in the nose. The eyes will not move together well and may seem to be crossed. The genitals, especially on a boy, may seem abnormally large.

Be reassured that in a few months your baby will begin to look more "normal." Movements of the limbs, eyes, and neck will become more controlled as muscles develop, and the face will become more alert and expressive.

ROUTINE TESTS FOR A NEWBORN BABY

Certain tests are done on each new baby to check for abnormalities. Many minor problems can be taken care of before the baby leaves the hospital. Others can be treated by the parents at home. Some problems that appear at birth must be detected early so that they can be corrected before they become serious.

One test that is required in all states is a screening test on samples of the baby's blood and urine to check for phenylketonuria (PKU). This rare disorder can cause brain damage and mental retardation. If it is detected right away, however, changes can be made in the baby's diet to prevent such damage.

Also done routinely is a blood test for congenital hypothyroidism (a disorder of the thyroid gland that causes abnormalities of mental and physical development.) Other tests may be done as well, depending on the hospital routine and your doctor's recommendations.

SPECIAL SUPPLIES AND EQUIPMENT

Before you bring your baby home, you will want to have everything you need on hand.

Clothes. A newborn baby usually needs only diapers and soft nightgowns for sleeping and extra sheets or blankets. Overdressing a baby can cause heat rash. Babies spit up on and otherwise dirty their clothes, sometimes many times a day, so be sure you have plenty. You don't want to spend all your time washing.

Diapers. Diapers can be made of reusable cloth or disposable paper. The initial cost of new cloth diapers may be high, but they can be used for many years. Disposables cost more in the long run. Many parents use disposables for the first few weeks, for convenience in the initial adjustment period, and then switch to cloth when a routine has been established.

Skin cleanser. Many doctors recommend using just a mild soap and water to keep a baby clean. Do not use oils, lotions, or powders; clear water is best. A baby's skin can be very sensitive, and scented products can be irritating. Some babies are allergic to certain lotions and creams.

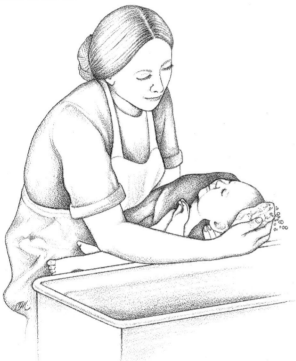

Many doctors recommend using only a mild soap and water to clean a baby's sensitive skin.

Bed. You can use a cradle or bassinet for a new baby, but your baby will soon outgrow it. A crib will work just as well and be useful for a longer time, making it a better investment. Choose a crib with one side that drops, so that you can easily reach the baby. Make sure the catch is out of the baby's reach; it won't be long before the child is standing up in bed. Also, be sure that the rails are close enough together that the baby's head won't fit through them; they should be no more than 2⅜ inches apart.

Mattress. The mattress should be firm and covered with a plastic or vinyl mattress protector and a regular fitted crib sheet. Make sure that the mattress is not too small for the crib; the edge of the mattress should be no more ·

than half an inch from the side of the crib all around (otherwise, the baby might get wedged between the mattress and the side of the crib).

Toys. Babies like toys that are brightly colored. Soft toys are safest in the early months. Avoid sharp edges. Remember that soon everything will go into the baby's mouth, so be sure that toys are safe and washable. Mobiles and music boxes are interesting and stimulating, but be sure they are either out of reach or safe for the baby to touch.

Car restraints. No baby should ever ride in a car unless protected by a car seat with a sturdy harness system and a shell made of molded plastic and steel tubing. A car seat that adapts to fit both infants and toddlers may be your best investment, and one that allows the child to recline is more comfortable for a napping child than is an upright model.

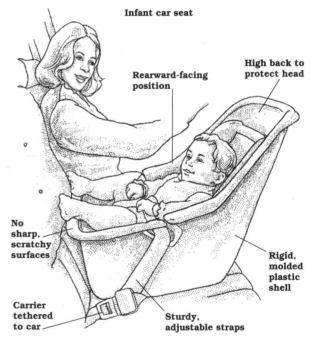

Infant car seat

Rearward-facing position

High back to protect head

No sharp, scratchy surfaces

Carrier tethered to car

Sturdy, adjustable straps

Rigid, molded plastic shell

No baby should ride in a car without the protection of a car seat.

COMING HOME

When you come home from the hospital with a new baby, a period of adjustment begins for all concerned. It may take several weeks, or even several months, for the mother to recover from the physical stress of labor and delivery. At the same time, the new baby is completely dependent on the parents for food, shelter, and comfort. To accommodate the mother's physical tiredness and the baby's constant needs, you may have to review what is most important to you as a family. For example, keeping the house spotless may have to take second place to caring for the baby and allowing the mother to get the extra rest she needs. Household jobs may have to be reassigned so that the mother can devote more time to the baby.

Your social schedule may have to change as well. You may find that your preferences have changed, and you would rather stay home with the baby than go to a party or a movie. This certainly does not mean you must—or should—give up going out or never do the things you enjoy. It only means that your priorities will probably change when you have an infant in your household.

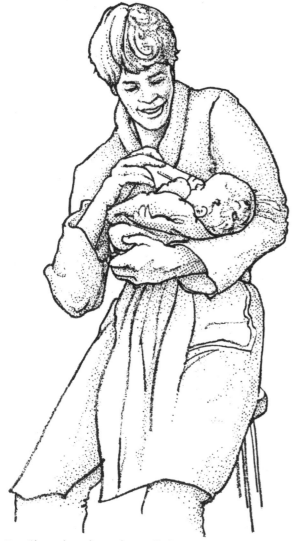

Feeding time is a time of closeness.

FEEDING

In the first months of life, eating is a major concern of your baby. This activity will take up a lot of your time and energy. But whether you breast-feed or bottle-feed your baby, feeding time is a time of closeness. You are giving the baby nourishment and thus meeting your child's most basic need. At the same time, you are holding and cuddling the baby, and he or she is getting to know your touch and your voice.

Whether you are breast-feeding or bottle-feeding, remember that your baby's appetite is generally a reliable measure of how much he or she needs to eat. A characteristic, demanding cry will let you know when the baby is hungry. After a few weeks or months, you'll probably be able to identify that hunger cry.

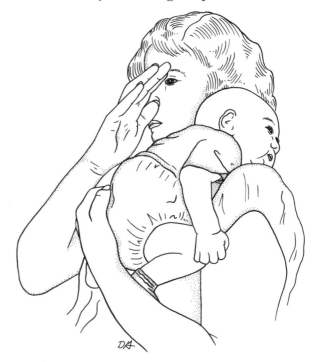

Burping the baby helps to expel excess air that the baby has swallowed while feeding.

BURPING THE BABY

As the baby nurses, from the bottle or the breast, air is swallowed along with the milk. Burping the baby helps to expel excess air and prevent discomfort. Interrupt the feeding once in the middle for a burp, and also burp the baby after a feeding. Expelling extra air in the middle of the meal ensures that the baby's stomach will not fill up with air rather than milk or formula.

To burp an infant, put the baby over your shoulder, sit the baby up on your lap, or place the baby facedown across your lap. Pat or rub the baby's back gently until you hear a good, solid burp. Some babies prefer one position, while others need to be moved around until they burp. If burping is difficult, experiment with different positions and combinations of patting and rubbing. Some babies will protest the interruption of the meal, but burp them anyway at mid-meal. They will get more nourishment, and your life will be easier.

SPITTING UP

Many babies spit up either as they are being burped or a little while after a feeding. This is normal. Check with your doctor if the baby is spitting up large amounts, is having projectile vomiting (forceful, explosive vomiting), or does not appear to be gaining weight. Also consult your doctor if the baby is spitting up and seems hungry all the time or becomes limp and not alert.

To reduce spitting up, try burping the baby more often during a feeding or changing the feeding position slightly so that the baby is more upright. It may help to have the baby rest quietly in an infant seat for a few minutes after feeding, rather than laying the baby down or encouraging active playing.

THE PACIFIER

Babies need to suck for a certain amount of time each day. If your baby acts hungry but takes only a small amount of food, he or she probably just needed to suck. If this happens consistently, a pacifier may be a great help. It meets the baby's need to suck. Most babies stop using pacifiers when they are ready to stop. This varies from six months to two years of age.

BREAST-FEEDING

Many doctors today recommend breast-feeding, if it is possible, for a number of reasons. First, breast milk is thought to pass on to the baby some of the mother's own resistance to infections. Second, many babies develop allergies to infant formulas, but it is rare for a baby to be allergic to breast milk. Third, breast-feeding is generally more convenient than bottle-feeding because it requires no sterilizing, mixing, or refrigeration. Fourth, the experience of breast-feeding is emotionally satisfying for both

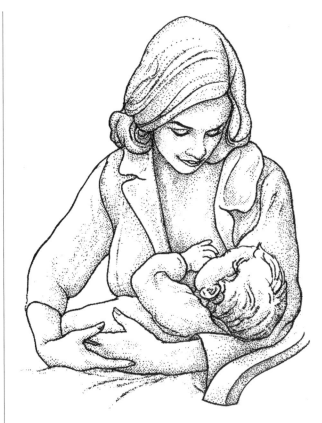

Many doctors recommend breast-feeding if it is possible.

mother and baby. Fifth, breast-feeding is less expensive than bottle-feeding.

In general, breast-fed babies are healthier than those who are bottle-fed. Breast-fed babies tend to have fewer illnesses such as ear infections and colds, they tend to have fewer hospitalizations, and they are less likely to become overweight.

Breast milk can be pumped and stored just like cow's milk. You can freeze it for later use or put it in bottles stored in the refrigerator.

You can give the baby an occasional bottle, if you choose. This can give the mother a chance to be away from the baby sometimes or to sleep through the night while the father gives a feeding. The breasts can be emptied with a breast pump if they become uncomfortably full.

BOTTLE-FEEDING

If you are bottle-feeding, you must have clean water and refrigeration available. Be sure to clean the top of the can before you open it, and follow the directions carefully when you're preparing the formula. Some formulas are concentrated, so you must add water. Others are "ready to feed," and if you dilute this type the baby will not get enough nourishment.

Bottles and nipples must be cleaned well with soap and water. Force water through the nipple to be sure the hole in the nipple is not clogged. There is no need to sterilize the bottles or the nipples.

Hold and rock the baby when you're bottle-feeding. Do not prop the bottle up and leave the baby alone to eat. Human contact is important to the baby's development, so don't rush the feeding time. However, try not to spend more than 30 to 45 minutes on each feeding.

WHY BABIES CRY

It's normal for babies to cry. It is, after all, their only way of letting you know that they need something. At first it may be difficult to figure out what the baby needs. In a newborn, though, there are only a few things a cry can signify—hunger, needing a diaper change, and needing to be held and comforted. As the baby grows up, he or she will find more reasons to complain—for example, boredom, frustration, loneliness, fear, overstimulation, and tiredness.

Sometimes you and your baby can get into a crying cycle. When the baby cries, you get anxious and nervous. The more the baby cries, the worse you feel, and nothing you do seems to help quiet the baby. It sometimes seems that the baby senses your feelings and responds by crying even more. If you find yourself getting into these cycles, talk about it with an experienced parent or your doctor, who may be able to suggest a solution.

Occasionally, a baby will cry because he or she is in pain. Check to see if you can figure out what is causing the pain. A sick baby may cry but will usually also have some other symptom of illness, such as a fever, diarrhea, or a runny nose. Generally, a healthy baby will have a strong, loud cry. If your baby's cry becomes weak, contact your doctor right away.

WHAT TO EXPECT OF YOUR BABY

For about the first month of life (longer if the baby was born prematurely and is catching up), the baby will do little besides eat, sleep, and dirty diapers. An infant has a small stomach and can't eat very much at a time, so feeding the baby the usual six to ten times a day is likely to be the biggest demand the baby makes on you. The rest of the time, the baby will probably sleep, and you may be able to catch up on your sleep, too.

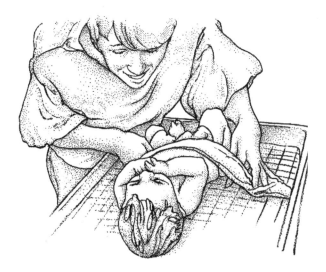

Getting to know your newborn baby is one of the joys of parenthood.

Babies develop at different rates, so the following description of a baby's development is only a guide. It will give you a general idea of what changes to expect in your baby over the first year or so of life. Many parents keep a baby book in which they note these events. But whether you record the baby's progress or not, it's fun to see a tiny infant that does nothing but eat and sleep develop into a person. Beware, though, of making comparisons between your child and your relatives' or neighbors' babies. Remember that each baby is unique. If a child is slow to talk or stand up, it doesn't mean that he or she is less intelligent than a cousin or a neighbor's child. However, if your child lags far behind other children of the same age, check with your doctor. Basically, here is what you can expect from your baby:
■ At six weeks, the baby may be awake and playful, without crying, for half an hour after each feeding. This is about the time when you can expect those first spontaneous smiles.
■ At three months, the baby will follow the movement of a favorite toy dangled in front of his or her eyes.
■ At four months, the baby will learn to roll over from front to back. At five months, the baby will be able to roll from back to front.
■ Between the ages of four and six months, the baby will learn to lift his or her head and shoulders, and by about six months will have enough muscle control to balance in a sitting position without support.

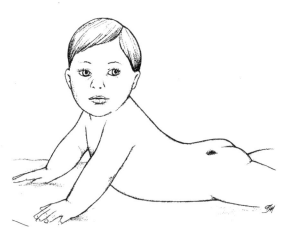

By six months, the baby will learn to lift the head and shoulders.

■ Most babies begin to make simple, recognizable sounds (such as "Da-da" and "Mama") at about eight months of age. This is also the stage at which they may try to use a spoon for the first time.

■ At nine months, most babies can get to a sitting position from lying down and can pull up to a stand and walk holding onto furniture and walls. The baby may begin to crawl, but some babies skip crawling altogether. This is the time to "childproof" your home and put harmful items out of reach.

■ At about a year old, the baby may be able to stand up for a few seconds and may be taking a few steps alone. Fortunately, this is also the time when a baby begins to understand a few simple commands, like "Stop!" and "Don't touch!" In most cases, it will be a few more

months before the baby is walking. By this time, your child will be eating only three to four times a day.

As your baby develops, her attention span and interests will also broaden. A very small baby may watch a mobile for a few minutes, but then fall asleep or cry. As the child learns how to use her arms and legs, she discovers the ability to make things move. The baby learns to grab for things, too. Her eyes begin to focus better, so she can see more things. Still, a toy may hold a baby's interest for only five minutes before she needs to look at something different. As you play with your baby, you can see how long a game remains satisfying. The complexities of the game and the time it holds the child's attention will gradually increase.

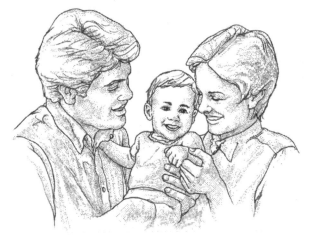

As a baby grows and develops, his or her attention span and interests will also broaden.

Quick-Reference Action Guide

When your child is sick or hurt, you naturally want to act quickly to help. That's where this action guide comes in. The guide begins with step-by-step instructions for mouth-to-mouth resuscitation in the event that your child stops breathing. (As mentioned in the previous section, you will be most prepared to help your child in emergency situations such as this if you take a first-aid course, 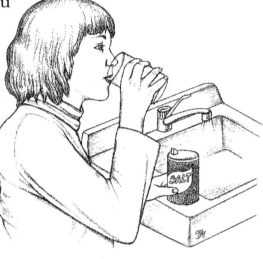 including training in cardiopulmonary resuscitation, before there's a crisis.) Next, you'll find a chart of common symptoms and the diseases or conditions that they may indicate. The chart can help you narrow down the possible causes of your child's symptoms. And finally, you'll find quick-reference pages for more than 150 childhood conditions. The quick-reference page for each condition lists the symptoms of the condition; describes any emergency action that is necessary; and indicates when and if the child should be seen by a physician and what steps, if any, you can take to care for your child at home. These pages are designed to give you a quick overview that you can use to assess your child's condition. For more in-depth information on each of these conditions, you can turn to the section entitled "Understanding Your Child's Condition."

Mouth-to-mouth resuscitation

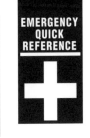

IMPORTANT

■ If the child stops breathing, begin mouth-to-mouth resuscitation immediately and send someone to call for emergency medical assistance. If you are alone, perform mouth-to-mouth resuscitation for one minute (or less if child begins breathing) before leaving child to call for medical assistance. Then, if child is still not breathing, resume mouth-to-mouth resuscitation. If you know or suspect that the child is choking on an object, follow the instructions for *Choking* on pages 71–72. Do not give mouth-to-mouth resuscitation until the object has been dislodged. Otherwise, you may force the object farther down the child's throat.

EMERGENCY TREATMENT

1. Tap child on shoulder and shout, "Are you OK?" If child does not respond, yell "help" to get attention of others.

2. **IF NO HEAD, NECK, OR BACK INJURY SUSPECTED,** tilt child's head back to open airway:

A. Kneel by child's side and place one of your hands on the child's forehead. Gently tilt the child's head back.

B. Place fingers of your other hand on bony part of child's chin—not on throat.

C. Gently lift child's chin straight up without closing child's mouth.

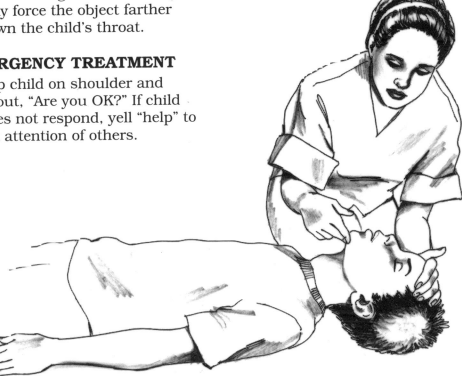

Step 2 if no head, back, or neck injury suspected

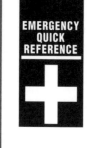

EMERGENCY QUICK REFERENCE

Mouth-to-mouth resuscitation

2. IF HEAD, BACK, OR NECK INJURY SUSPECTED, open child's airway using jaw thrust:

A. DO NOT tilt or reposition child's head or torso.

B. Place tips of your index and middle fingers at corners of

child's jaw (near ears) and your thumbs on bony portion of child's chin.

C. Gently lift jaw forward and open child's mouth without moving child's head.

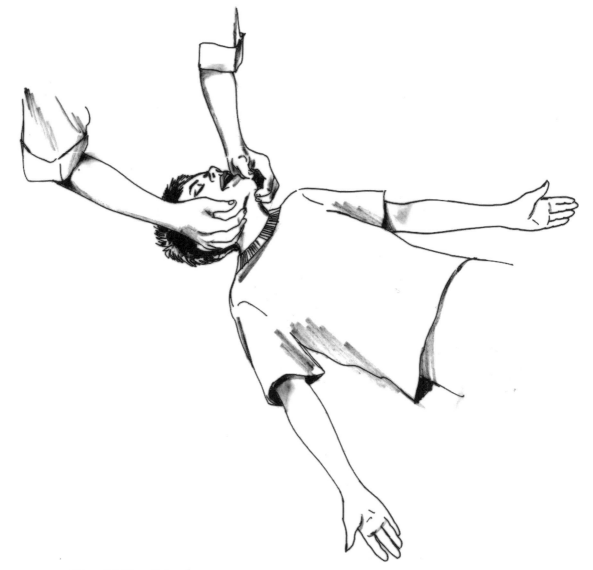

Step 2 if head, back, or neck injury suspected

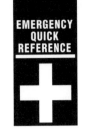

3. Look, listen, and feel for breathing for three to five seconds by placing your cheek near child's mouth and watching for chest to rise and fall.

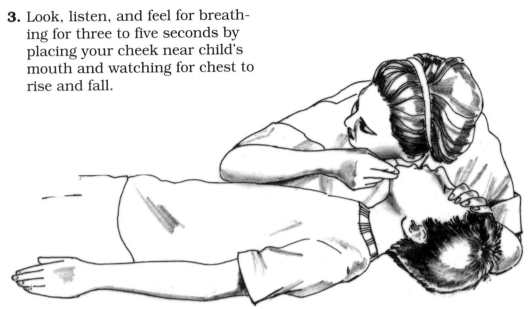

Step 3

4. INFANT:

    A. Maintain head-tilt position, but DO NOT tip head too far back.

    B. Place your mouth over infant's mouth and nose.

    C. Give two gentle puffs.

    D. Pull your mouth away and allow child's lungs to deflate.

    E. If no exchange of air, reposition infant's head and try again.

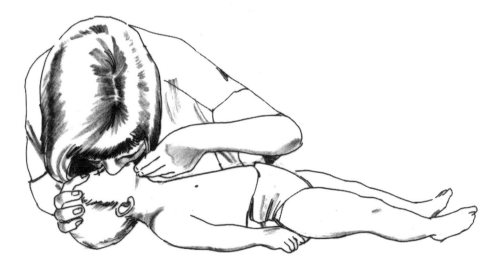

Step 4 for infant

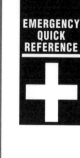
Mouth-to-mouth resuscitation

4. CHILD:

A. Maintain head-tilt position.

B. Pinch child's nose closed with your fingers and place your mouth over child's mouth.

C. Give two full, slow breaths, each lasting 1 to 1½ seconds.

D. After each breath, pull your mouth away and allow child's lungs to deflate.

E. If no exchange of air, reposition child's head and try again.

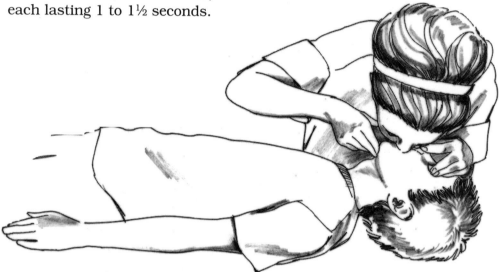

Step 4 for child

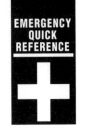

5. Check child's breathing and pulse. To check pulse:

A. Keep child's head tipped back by keeping your hand on child's forehead.

B. Place fingertips of your other hand on child's Adam's apple. Slide fingers into groove at either side of Adam's apple.

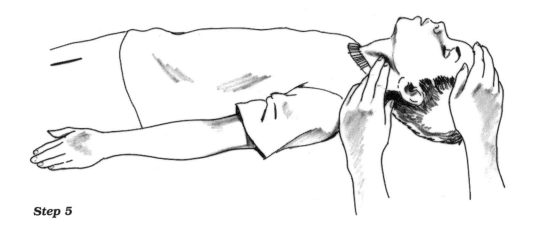

Step 5

6. Call 911 or operator if no one else has done so.

7. If victim remains unconscious and:

A. There is a pulse but no breathing, continue giving one breath every four seconds for child or one gentle puff every three seconds for infant.

B. There is no pulse and no breathing and you have not been trained in CPR, continue to give one breath every four seconds for child or one gentle puff every three seconds for infant (in case there may be a very faint pulse that you did not detect).

Cardiopulmonary resuscitation (CPR) is a life-support technique used when a person is not breathing and when the heart may have stopped beating. CPR must be learned through classroom instruction taught by qualified instructors, and it must be administered by someone trained in the technique. All parents should take a course in CPR.

Chart of symptoms

Here are some common childhood disorders (far left column on each page) and their signs and symptoms (across the top). Key symptoms are indicated by a solid circle; possible symptoms by an open circle. To use this chart, run your finger down the column on each page that corresponds to your child's symptom, and find the disorders (along the side) that may cause it; do this for each of your child's symptoms. By a process of elimination, you should be able to zero in on the possible causes of your child's illness. Then turn to the section of the book relating to the various diseases. There you'll find both the information you need to further narrow down the diagnosis and the treatment recommended.

Signs and Symptoms

Diseases	Abnormal behavior	Abnormal discharge	Blueness	Cough	Diarrhea	Difficulty breathing	Fever	Headache	Itching	Loss of function	Noisy breathing	Pain	Rash	Tenderness	Unconsciousness	Visible deformity	Vomiting
Appendicitis					○		●					●		●			○
Arthritis							○			●		●	○	○		○	
Asthma				●		●					●						
Blood poisoning							●							●			
Boils		●										●		●			
Botulism				●	●					●		●					●
Bronchiolitis		○		●		●	●				●						
Bronchitis				●			●				○	○					
Chicken pox							●		●				●				
Common cold	●			●			○	○		○	○			○			
Concussion	●	○						●		○					●	○	●
Convulsions with fever	●		●				●			○					●		○
Convulsions without fever	●									○					●		
Croup				●		●	○				●						
Cystic fibrosis				●	●											●	
Diphtheria				●		●	●				○						
Dysentery					●		●										
Earaches	○						○			○		●					
Encephalitis	●						○	○				●			○		●
Food allergies	○				●	○			○			●	●				●
Food poisoning					●		○					●					●
Fractures										●		●		●		●	
Gastroenteritis, acute					●		○					●					●
Glands, swollen												○		●		●	

● Key symptoms   ○ Possible symptoms

Signs and Symptoms

Diseases	Abnormal behavior	Abnormal discharge	Blueness	Cough	Diarrhea	Difficulty breathing	Fever	Headache	Itching	Loss of function	Noisy breathing	Pain	Rash	Tenderness	Unconsciousness	Visible deformity	Vomiting
Gonorrhea		○										●					
Hay fever		●				○		○	●								
Hepatitis							●	●				●					●
Hernia												○		○		●	
Herpes simplex						○						●	○				
High blood pressure						○		○									
Impetigo		●							○			●					
Infectious mononucleosis							●					●	○	○			
Influenza				●	○		●	●				●					○
Laryngitis				●			○										
Leukemia		○					●					○					
Measles	●	●		●			●						●				
Meningitis							●	●					○		○		●
Mumps							●	●				●		●		●	
Nephritis		●					●	○							○		○
Pinworms									●			○					
Pneumonia				●		●	●	○		○		○					
Poisoning	○					○						○			○		○
Polio							●			●		●					○
Reye's syndrome	●														○		●
Rocky Mountain spotted fever							●	●				●	●				
Roseola		○					●					●		○			
Rubella							●						●	●			
Scabies									●			●					
Sinusitis		●		●		●	●	●				●					
Sore throat							○					●					
Stomachache, acute					●							●					●
Stomachache, chronic												●					
Strep infections							●	●				●	○	○			●
Swimmer's ear		●					○		●	○		●		●			
Tetanus										●		●			○		
Tonsillitis							●			○		●		○		●	
Ulcers		●										●					○
Urinary tract infections		○			○		○					○					○
Viral infections		○	○	○	○	○	○	○	○		○	○	○				○
Whooping cough		●		●			●				●						●

● Key symptoms   ○ Possible symptoms

Acne

SYMPTOMS

- Blackheads

- Whiteheads

- Pimples

HOME CARE

- Wash with mild soap twice a day.

- Apply an over-the-counter acne preparation that contains sulfur, resorcinol, salicylic acid, or mild benzoyl peroxide.

PRECAUTIONS

- Never allow X-ray treatment of acne.

- Avoid cosmetics that contain oil.

- Do not squeeze or pick pimples.

- See your doctor if acne does not improve or if cysts develop.

- Acne in young infants should not be treated with any medication.

Anemia

SYMPTOMS

- Paleness of nail beds

- Paleness inside eyelids

- Paleness of membranes inside mouth

- Tiredness

- Shortness of breath

- Rapid pulse

- Jaundice

HOME CARE

- None. See your doctor.

PRECAUTIONS

- Never attempt to treat anemia without your doctor's advice.

- Give your children a balanced diet that includes all the necessary nutrients. Consult your doctor for advice on providing a balanced diet.

- Keep iron supplements out of the reach of children. An overdose of iron can be dangerous.

- Detecting anemia early is important. See your doctor if you suspect that your child is anemic. Be sure children have regular physical examinations.

Animal bites

SYMPTOMS
- Bite marks
- Claw marks
- Bruises

IMPORTANT
- Animal bites that break the skin may cause infection, tetanus, or rabies. Report all animal bites or claw wounds to your doctor immediately.

HOME CARE
- Scrub wound with soap and water for five to ten minutes and flush with water.
- Apply antiseptic to minor wounds.
- Report the wound to your doctor immediately.
- Call police or health authorities to deal with the animal.

PRECAUTIONS
- If redness spreads out from the wound or if the wound becomes tender, call your doctor.
- Make sure your child's tetanus immunization status is current.
- Teach your child to be careful around domestic pets and to stay away from wild animals.
- Be sure your own pets have been vaccinated against rabies.

Anorexia nervosa

SYMPTOMS

■ Aversion to food

■ Excessive dieting

■ Excessive exercise

■ Obsession with subject of food

■ Distorted body image

■ Overeating followed by self-induced vomiting

■ Absence of menstruation

■ Downy hair on body

HOME CARE

■ Anorexia nervosa requires medical care.

PRECAUTIONS

■ If the condition is not treated, the anorexic may starve to death.

■ Obedient and successful children who try hard to fulfill the expectations of others are at higher risk of becoming anorexic.

Appendicitis

KEY SYMPTOM

■ Persistent pain in the abdomen, usually starting in the area of the belly button and moving quickly to the lower right quarter of the abdomen

POSSIBLE SYMPTOMS

■ Tenderness in the abdomen

■ Nausea and vomiting

■ Fever

IMPORTANT

■ Call your doctor as soon as you suspect appendicitis. The condition can worsen rapidly and can be fatal if it is not treated by a doctor.

HOME CARE

■ Allow only clear liquids by mouth. If you strongly suspect appendicitis, do not give the child any food or drink until you have consulted your doctor.

■ Do not apply cold to the abdomen. Gentle heat may ease a stomachache. If pain continues or gets worse despite home treatment, call your doctor.

PRECAUTIONS

■ Do not give painkillers (including aspirin).

■ Do not give a laxative or an enema.

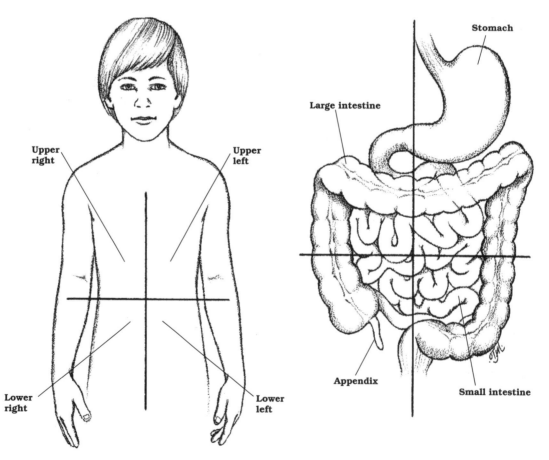

The key symptom of appendicitis is pain in the lower right quarter of the abdomen.

Arthritis

KEY SYMPTOMS
- Swelling of joints
- Stiffness or difficulty in moving joints

SYMPTOMS
- Pain or tenderness in joints
- Warmth in joints

POSSIBLE SYMPTOMS
- Redness of joints
- Fever

HOME CARE
- Do not treat at home until a doctor has diagnosed the cause.

- If a doctor is not immediately available, give aspirin or acetaminophen and rest the affected joints.

PRECAUTIONS
- Infectious arthritis is an emergency. Unless a doctor is seen within 24 hours, permanent damage may occur.

- Rheumatoid arthritis and rheumatic fever require prompt treatment.

- If a child has prolonged unexplained fever and stiffness in the joints and the neck, rheumatoid arthritis may be the cause.

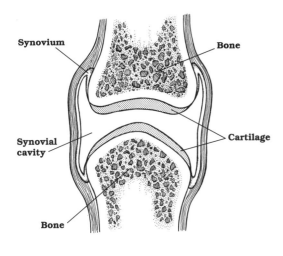

Normal joint

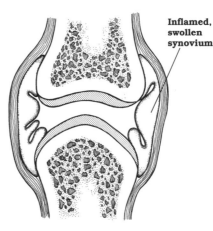

Rheumatoid arthritis

The joint is the juncture where the ends of two or more bones meet. Cartilage (elastic tissue) cushions and protects the bones with the aid of various joint fluids in the synovial cavity, which is lined and lubricated by a thin membrane called the synovium. In rheumatoid arthritis, the synovium becomes swollen and inflamed. The inflammation eventually destroys the cartilage. As scar tissue gradually replaces the damaged cartilage, the joint becomes misshapen and rigid.

Asthma

KEY SYMPTOMS
- Wheezing
- Difficulty in exhaling

SYMPTOMS
- Shortness of breath
- Cough
- Sensation of "air hunger"

HOME CARE
- Do not attempt to treat the first attack at home. Contact your doctor immediately.
- If further attacks occur, follow your doctor's prescribed home treatment.
- If an allergy has been identified as the cause of asthma, attempt to remove any offending substances from your home.

PRECAUTIONS
- Not all wheezing indicates asthma. A doctor must diagnose the cause.
- Do not use over-the-counter (nonprescription) aerosol medications on young children.
- Avoid rectal medications for asthma.
- Do not let any asthma attack go untreated.
- Avoid exposing the child to irritants such as smoke, insecticides, and paint fumes.

Athlete's foot

SYMPTOMS

■ Itching

■ Scaling and cracking skin

HOME CARE

■ Apply over-the-counter fungicidal ointment once or twice a day (half strength for delicate skin) or use ointments containing undecylenic acid or tolnaftate.

■ Avoid rubber-soled or plastic-soled shoes.

■ Have the child wear cotton socks, preferably ones that have not been dyed.

■ If treatment for athlete's foot does not promptly relieve the symptoms or if symptoms reappear, see your doctor.

PRECAUTIONS

■ Continue treatment until the skin is completely clear; otherwise, the condition may flare up again.

■ Many medications for athlete's foot may cause skin irritation.

■ Try to keep the child from scratching the affected area; scratching can cause additional infections.

Backaches

SYMPTOMS

- Back pain

- Tender or sore muscles

- Stiffness

HOME CARE

- Have the child rest in bed, or limit the child's physical activities.

- Give aspirin or acetaminophen for pain.

- Give lukewarm baths, or apply gentle heat with a heating pad.

- Use an extra-firm mattress, or place a bed board or piece of plywood under the mattress.

- Do not allow strenuous physical activity until the pain has been gone for at least a week.

PRECAUTIONS

- If the back pain is accompanied by fever, problems in urination, severe pain, or a sharp pain in one spot, see your doctor.

- Do not use muscle-relaxant medications on children unless your doctor has prescribed them.

- If there is a visible curve in the spine, see your doctor.

- Any back pain without an obvious cause, such as an injury or fall, needs to be evaluated by a doctor.

Baldness

SYMPTOMS

- Bare spots on head

- Total baldness

- Scaliness of skin on scalp

- Broken-off stubbles of hair

HOME CARE

- Alopecia areata cannot be treated at home, except with patience until the hair grows back in.

- Hereditary and congenital baldness cannot be treated, except with understanding. A hairpiece may be helpful.

PRECAUTIONS

- Do not use over-the-counter (nonprescription) preparations that promise hair growth.

- Do not consult cosmetologists for baldness. See a qualified dermatologist.

Bed-wetting

SYMPTOM

■ Frequent bed-wetting after the age of five years

HOME CARE

■ First see your doctor to find out if the cause of the bed-wetting is a physical disorder.

■ If there is no physical cause, the best home care is patience, calmness, and understanding. Try to ignore and avoid the problem as much as possible.

■ Rubber sheets and plastic pants will make housekeeping easier until the child stops bed-wetting.

PRECAUTIONS

■ If a toilet-trained child suddenly begins bed-wetting, suspect a physical illness.

■ Do not take a child out of night diapers until he or she consistently remains dry.

■ Do not make a big fuss over daytime toilet training.

■ Do not try to shame children into remaining dry at night.

■ Do not let bed-wetting bring anger and frustration into your relationship with your child.

■ Do not let other children taunt a bed wetter.

Birthmarks

SYMPTOMS

- Red, purple, or salmon-colored marks

- Blue-black marks on back or buttocks

- Brown or black moles

HOME CARE

- In most cases, birthmarks need no treatment.

- Protect strawberry marks from rubbing or scratching. If a strawberry mark bleeds, press lightly with gauze to stop the bleeding.

PRECAUTIONS

- If there is discharge, odor, or redness of the skin around a strawberry mark, call your doctor.

- In rare cases, strawberry marks may cause anemia or bleeding that needs a doctor's attention.

Blisters

SYMPTOM

■ A raised bubble of skin containing clear liquid

HOME CARE

■ Protect blisters with gauze or bandages.

■ If accidentally opened, trim away loose skin, clean with soap and water, and bandage.

■ If a blister becomes infected (red or tender), soak it in an Epsom-salts solution or Burow's solution. Have infected blisters checked by a doctor.

PRECAUTIONS

■ Do not break open blisters caused by rubbing or burns.

■ If red streaks start spreading out from a blister, see your doctor.

■ If an Epsom-salts solution is too weak, the soaking makes blisters larger. Use at least one-half cup of Epsom salts in a quart of water.

Blood poisoning

SYMPTOMS

- Wavy pink or red streaks under the skin

- Sudden, quickly rising high fever

- Swollen or tender lymph nodes

HOME CARE

- Call your doctor. Elevate the affected part of the body.

- Apply warm soaks of Epsom-salts solution (one-half cup of Epsom salts in a quart of water). If there is an infected blister, soak it as well. Give aspirin or acetaminophen for pain and fever.

PRECAUTIONS

- Always contact your doctor, since blood poisoning should usually be treated with antibiotics.

- If a child has a high fever or is prostrate (in a state of collapse), **call a medical facility immediately**.

Apply warm soaks of Epsom salts to an infected wound or blister with red streaks extending from it.

Boils

SYMPTOMS

- Redness
- Pain
- Pus

HOME CARE

- Soak with warm Epsom-salts solution (one-half cup of Epsom salts per quart of water).
- When a boil drains, catch the drainage on a clean cloth or gauze pad to avoid spreading infection.
- Frequently clean surrounding skin with soap and water.

PRECAUTIONS

- If boils develop on the face, see your doctor.
- Do not let drainage from a boil come in contact with the eyes.
- Do not squeeze boils.
- Treat all minor wounds and insect bites properly to avoid boils or other infections.

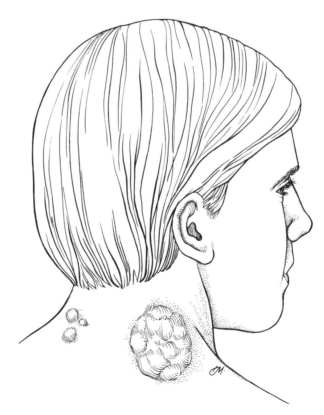

Boils are identified by the accompanying redness and pain and the formation of pus in the center. A large boil with several heads is called a carbuncle.

Botulism

SYMPTOMS

- Nausea
- Vomiting
- Diarrhea
- Abdominal pain
- Double vision (12 to 48 hours after start of pain)
- Dilated pupils
- Difficulty in speaking, swallowing, and breathing
- Paralysis

IMPORTANT

- Botulism poisoning can be fatal. If you suspect botulism, **get medical help immediately**.

HOME CARE

- None. **Call your doctor immediately**.

PRECAUTIONS

- Do not give infants unwashed, unpeeled raw foods or improperly cooked foods.
- Do not give infants honey.
- Do not use food from damaged or dented store-bought cans.
- Certain home-preserved foods (for example, vegetables and meats) should be reheated for ten minutes at a temperature of at least 180°F before eating because of the danger of botulism.
- Remember that foods contaminated with botulism look, taste, and smell normal.
- When canning and preserving food at home, follow directions for preparing and sterilizing exactly.

Bowlegs and knock-knees

SYMPTOMS

■ Legs bent outward at knees (bowlegs)

■ Legs bent inward at knees (knock-knees)

HOME CARE

■ Usually no home care is needed.

■ If you think your child has bowlegs or knock-knees, consult your doctor.

PRECAUTIONS

■ Do not use orthopedic shoes unless prescribed by your doctor.

■ To prevent rickets (a deficiency of vitamin D, which may cause bowlegs and knock-knees), all children should receive recommended amounts of vitamin D. (Milk is a good dietary source of vitamin D.)

■ Do not give your child supplements of vitamin D unless your doctor has prescribed them. Overdoses of vitamin D are harmful.

Bronchiolitis

SYMPTOMS

- Nasal congestion

- Fever

- Loss of appetite

- Cough (mild to severe)

- Rapid, sometimes difficult breathing

- Wheezing

- Irritability

- Bluish skin

HOME CARE

- None. See your doctor.

PRECAUTIONS

- Bronchiolitis can be a serious illness. See your doctor.

- Do not give cough medicines to a child who is having difficulty in breathing.

- Give the child extra liquids to prevent dehydration (serious loss of body fluids).

- Dehydration in infants can be dangerous.

- If your infant frequently has a cough, see your doctor.

- If your infant has difficulty in breathing, see your doctor.

Bronchitis

SYMPTOMS

- Dry, hacking cough

- Fever

- Tightness and pain in center of chest

- Loss of appetite

- General weakness and discomfort

- Rattling sound to breathing

HOME CARE

- The child should rest during the fever stage and the period when the cough is the worst.

- Give acetaminophen for aches and fever.

- Phenylephrine or oxymetazoline nose drops may be used.

- A humidifier or vaporizer will make breathing easier.

- Give your child extra liquids.

PRECAUTIONS

- If there is pain on the side of the chest, see your doctor.

- If there is blood in the discharge coughed up, see your doctor.

- If the condition worsens after three or four days, see your doctor.

- Do not give oral decongestants to a child with bronchitis.

- If bronchitis occurs more than once a year, see your doctor.

Bruises

SYMPTOM

■ Discolored areas of the skin (black, blue, purple, red, yellow, or green)

HOME CARE

■ Immediately after an injury, apply *cold* to decrease bleeding and bruising.

■ Twenty-four hours or more after an injury, apply *warmth* to help the body absorb the bruise.

PRECAUTIONS

■ If bruises suddenly appear without injury, see your doctor.

■ The appearance of petechiae (small, dark red or maroon bruises) scattered over the body may indicate an emergency. If there is also fever or collapse, **get medical treatment immediately**.

Burns

SYMPTOMS

- Pain

- Reddened skin

- Blisters

- Scorched or blackened skin

- Dead white skin

HOME CARE

Burns that are blistered, charred, or scorched:

- Do not treat at home.

- Cover with a clean, wet cloth. Do not apply ointments.

- Keep the child warm.

- See your doctor at once.

Burns with reddened skin only:

- Immediately apply cold compresses or hold under cold running water until the pain lessens.

- Cover the burn with a light layer of antibiotic ointment.

- Cover with several layers of gauze.

- Change the dressing every 24 to 48 hours until the burn is completely healed.

Sunburn:

- Apply over-the-counter sunburn products, if needed, and leave uncovered.

PRECAUTIONS

- A severely burned child may go into a state of shock. See *Shock* on page 184.

- Never leave young children home alone—not even for a moment.

- Keep the thermostat on the water heater turned low, and watch children closely when they are around the stove.

- Keep matches and cigarette lighters out of children's reach.

- Keep gasoline and other flammables under lock and key outside the house.

- Keep young children away from electrical wires and extension cords, and keep childproof plugs in electrical outlets.

- Keep your child's tetanus immunization status up to date.

Cat scratch fever

SYMPTOMS

- Cat scratch or bite that does not heal

- Redness

- Pus

- Swollen, tender, or red lymph nodes

- Low-grade fever

HOME CARE

- Immediately scrub cat scratches or bites with soap and water for ten minutes.

- Apply an antiseptic.

- If the wound becomes infected, see your doctor.

PRECAUTIONS

- Do not allow young children to play with cats without supervision.

- Warn children not to tease cats or any other animals.

Chest pain

SYMPTOM
- Pain anywhere in the chest

HOME CARE
- Give aspirin or acetaminophen.

- Apply gentle heat with a heating pad.

- If chest pain or soreness is caused by hard or frequent coughing, cough medicine may help.

PRECAUTIONS
- If chest pain is accompanied by shortness of breath, high fever, a cough producing blood flecks, or prostration (collapse), **get medical help immediately**.

- If there is persistent pain beneath either armpit that is made worse by breathing, see your doctor.

- Do not give cough medicine if the child is having difficulty in breathing.

Chicken pox

SYMPTOMS

- Rash with blisters (pocks)
- Fever
- Mild cold symptoms

HOME CARE

- Isolate the child.
- Cut the child's fingernails to lessen scratching.
- Bathe the child in lukewarm water with cornstarch added.
- Apply calamine lotion without phenol to the skin using a soft cloth.
- Give acetaminophen—**not aspirin**—for fever or pain.

PRECAUTIONS

- Do not give aspirin to a child with chicken pox.
- Do not apply calamine lotion that contains phenol.
- If a high fever, prostration (collapse), headache, vomiting, or convulsions develop, **see your doctor immediately**.
- If an infant is exposed to chicken pox or develops it, call your doctor.
- If a child who is taking steroids or similar drugs or who has unusually low resistance to disease is exposed to or develops chicken pox, call your doctor.
- If the pocks become infected (show increasing redness, soreness, and pus), call your doctor.
- If lymph nodes become red and tender, call your doctor.
- If bruises or broken blood vessels appear under the skin (but there has been no injury), see your doctor.
- Avoid breaking the blisters or disturbing the scabs, since scarring can occur.

Child abuse and neglect

SYMPTOMS

■ Bruises, burns, fractures, and similar injuries

■ Behavioral changes

■ Withdrawal from friends, family, and teachers

■ Unexplained weight loss or, in a young child, failure to grow

■ Stealing of food

HOME CARE

■ If the child is in immediate danger, get the child out of the abusing situation and to a safe place.

■ Depending on laws in your state, you may be required to report your suspicions of child abuse or neglect to the state agency responsible for protecting children from abuse.

■ If you are the abuser, get help immediately.

PRECAUTION

■ If you have concerns that you are or have the potential to be a child abuser, get help before it happens.

Choking

SYMPTOMS

■ Inability to breathe

■ Inability to cry out or speak

■ Skin turns blue

IMPORTANT

■ If an object completely blocks the air passage, you have only a few minutes to reestablish an airway before brain damage or death occurs.

EMERGENCY TREATMENT FOR AN INFANT

1. Immediately call the police or paramedic squad for help.

2. Give the child **one minute** to cough up the object. If unsuccessful...

3. Lay the baby facedown on your forearm, with your hand supporting his head. The baby's head should be lower than his chest.

4. Using the heel of your hand, give four quick blows to the baby's back between the shoulder blades.

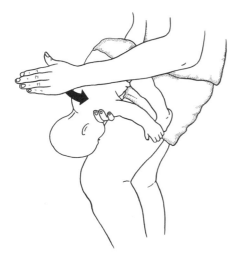

5. Place your free hand on the back of his head and, holding him between your forearms, turn him faceup, with his head still lower than his body.

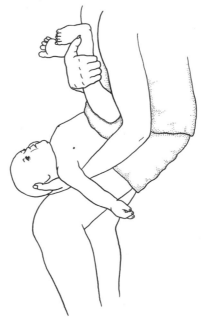

6. Put two fingertips on the baby's chest between the nipples. Press quickly and fairly hard four times.

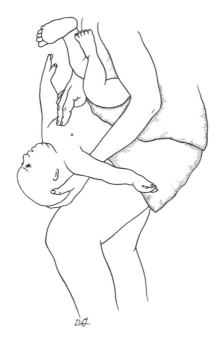

Choking

7. Repeat the cycle of four blows and four presses for as long as the baby is still choking. *Don't give up.*

8. If breathing stops, begin mouth-to-mouth resuscitation once the airway is clear. See the section on *Mouth-to-mouth resuscitation* (page 39).

EMERGENCY TREATMENT FOR AN OLDER CHILD

1. Immediately call the police or paramedic squad for help.

2. Give the child **one minute** to cough up the object. If unsuccessful ...

3. Stand behind the child.

4. Reach around the child, lock your hands together, and place them just below her breastbone.

5. Use a quick upward motion while pulling her stomach in.

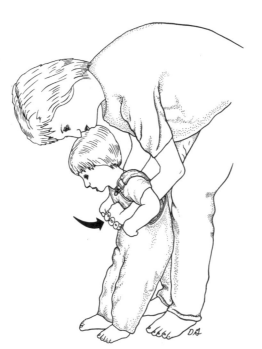

6. Repeat if necessary.

7. If breathing stops, begin mouth-to-mouth resuscitation once the airway is clear. See the section on *Mouth-to-mouth resuscitation* (page 39).

PRECAUTIONS

■ **Do not** abandon your efforts to help a choking child until medical help arrives. The obstructing object may be only partially blocking the airway, even though you may not think so.

■ **Do not** give mouth-to-mouth resuscitation until after the object has been removed.

■ **Do not** try to reach into the throat to remove the object unless all other, safer methods have failed.

■ Prevent choking. Examine all toys for loose eyes, beads, and small parts. Keep tablets under lock and key. Do not give peanuts, popcorn, or hard candies to toddlers, and keep such foods out of their reach.

■ A baby who has been vomiting should be placed on his or her stomach to lessen the chance of choking on the vomit.

Circumcision

INDICATIONS

- No opening in the foreskin

- Opening too small to allow urine through

- Pulled-back foreskin cannot be drawn forward

HOME CARE

- Cover a circumcision with gauze coated with petroleum jelly and a nonstick bandage until it has healed.

- Do not submerge the circumcision in bathwater until it has healed.

PRECAUTIONS

- If a circumcision bleeds more than a few drops, call your doctor.

- If there are signs of infection (pus, spreading redness, swelling of the penis), see your doctor.

- During bathing, any part of the foreskin remaining after healing of the circumcision should be pulled back to expose the base of the glans (the head of the penis) for cleansing.

- Boy babies born with any malformations of the penis usually should not be circumcised.

Colic

SYMPTOMS

- Crying for hours at a time

- No other obvious cause of crying

HOME CARE

- Look for possible signs of illness or other causes of discomfort.

- Offer a feeding to see if the baby is simply hungry.

- If colic seems to be the problem, apply gentle heat to the baby's abdomen.

- Sometimes a ride in a car (in the safety seat) helps. Another method to try is to attach a safety seat to the top of a clothes dryer, strap the baby in the seat, and run the dryer. The gentle vibration often settles down babies with colic.

- A pacifier may calm the child.

- Try inserting a glycerine suppository or lubricated thermometer to help the child pass a bowel movement.

PRECAUTIONS

- If the baby is being bottle-fed, make sure that the formula is prepared properly.

- Keep the bottle's nipple full to keep the baby from swallowing too much air.

- Make sure that the bottle's nipple hole is large enough to allow the baby to finish feeding in less than 20 to 25 minutes.

- After each feeding, carefully burp the baby in different positions.

- If the baby is being breast-fed, be sure that the mother's nipples are not bleeding. Swallowed blood causes cramps.

- Between feedings, try keeping the baby partly upright in an infant carrier to avoid regurgitation of food into the esophagus (food tube).

Common cold

SYMPTOMS

- Nasal congestion
- Sneezing
- Clear nasal discharge
- Scratchy sore throat
- Fever
- Red, watery eyes
- Dry cough
- Swollen, tender lymph nodes in the neck
- Mild pain in the ears

HOME CARE

- Give the child plenty of liquids.
- Do not permit strenuous activities while the child has a fever.
- Increase room humidity with a vaporizer or humidifier.
- Give acetaminophen for fever or pain.
- Use nose drops or oral decongestants and a nasal aspirator to relieve nasal congestion.
- Use cough medicine if the cough is severe.

PRECAUTIONS

- Do not overuse cold medications. Overuse can cause more harm than good. There are questions about the effectiveness of any over-the-counter medicines used for treating colds.
- Do not expose young infants to anyone with a cold, even a mild one.

- The following are usually *not* cold symptoms but signs of another illness: fever lasting more than two or three days; puslike discharge from the eyes, nose, or ears; redness or extreme tenderness of the lymph nodes in the neck; breathing difficulties; chest pain; severe headache; stiff neck; vomiting; chills accompanied by shaking; prostration (collapse). If any of these symptoms occurs, call your doctor.

Concussion

SYMPTOMS

- Unconsciousness at the instant of injury

- No memory of the accident

- No memory of events before the accident

- Confusion

- Persistent vomiting

- Inability to walk

- Eyes not parallel

- Pupils of different sizes

- Pupils that do not become smaller when a bright light is shined in the eyes

- Blood coming from the ear

- Bloody fluid that does not clot coming from the nose

- Increasingly severe headache

- Stiff neck

- Increasing drowsiness

- Slow pulse

- Abnormal breathing

HOME CARE

- If there are any signs of concussion, see your doctor. While waiting to see the doctor, have the child rest lying down with the head on a pillow.

- If there is a head injury with no signs of concussion, have the child rest in bed with the head on a pillow.

- The child may sleep but must be wakened every hour so that you can check on the child's condition.

- Continue bed rest until at least one day after the child seems fully recovered.

- Give only aspirin or acetaminophen for headache.

PRECAUTIONS

- **Do not** try to treat the child at home if there are any signs of concussion.

- **Do not** give painkillers, sedatives, or any medicine stronger than aspirin or acetaminophen to a child with a head injury.

- If the scalp is depressed (pushed in) at the site of the injury, see your doctor.

- If gentle tapping of the skull produces the dull sound of a broken melon, see your doctor.

Conjunctivitis

SYMPTOMS

- Redness of the entire white of the eye

- Yellow pus coming from the eye

- Swollen, red eyelids

- Burning sensation in the eye

- Eyelids that are "glued" shut in the morning

HOME CARE

- If you think your child has conjunctivitis, call your doctor.

- Your doctor may see the child or may prescribe antibiotic eyedrops or ointment over the telephone. Place the prescribed eyedrops or ointment into the eyes as frequently as directed.

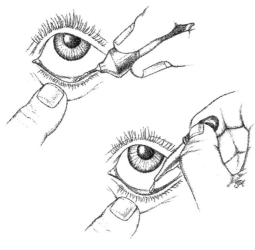

To place eyedrops or ointment into the eye, gently pull down the lower lid to form a pouch. Place the prescribed amount of medication into the pouch. Do not touch the eyedropper or ointment tube to the eye. Direct the child to close the eyes, but not to rub them. Wipe away excess medication around the eye with a clean tissue.

- Treat both eyes, even if only one eye seems infected. Continue treatment for 24 hours after the eyes seem normal.

- Warm compresses placed on the eyelids may relieve some of the discomfort. Use paper towels for the compresses, and throw them away after a single use. Some children find warm tea-bag compresses comforting.

- Isolate your child from other people.

- Watch other family members for symptoms.

PRECAUTIONS

- If the eyes don't begin clearing within 24 hours after beginning the medication, call your doctor.

- Eye ointments will cause blurred vision for a few minutes after each application. If there are any other vision problems, call your doctor.

- Notify your doctor if a child with conjunctivitis shows any other signs of illness (a head cold; nasal discharge; sore throat; earache; fever; or swollen, tender lymph nodes).

Constipation

SYMPTOMS

- Hard, dry stools

- Stools larger in diameter than usual

- Pain during bowel movements

- Red blood on or around stools

- Abdominal cramps

- Loss of appetite

HOME CARE

For immediate, temporary relief:

- Use a glycerine suppository or give an enema.

For long-term cure:

- Include more roughage in your child's diet (fruits, vegetables, and unrefined grains).

- Give your child fewer constipating foods, such as milk and milk products. (Check with your physician to ensure that your child's diet is nutritionally adequate, though.)

PRECAUTIONS

- **Do not** give laxatives to a child unless recommended by your doctor.

- **Do not** use enemas, suppositories, or laxatives on a regular basis. They are habit-forming.

- **Do not** assume that a child is constipated if bowel movements do not occur daily. Constipation is hardness of the stools; it has nothing to do with the number of bowel movements. Normal, healthy children may have several bowel movements a day or only several a week.

- If a child becomes constipated during toilet training, stop training efforts.

- Remember that breast-fed babies don't have as many bowel movements as babies fed formula.

Convulsions with fever

SYMPTOMS

■ Fever

■ Unconsciousness

■ Uncontrollable jerking movements

■ Muscle spasms

■ Brief cessation of breathing

■ Bluish skin

■ Loss of control of bladder or bowels

HOME CARE

■ Protect the child from injury during the thrashing or jerking movements.

■ Call your doctor immediately.

■ Do not put your fingers into the child's mouth.

PRECAUTIONS

■ Do not give aspirin or any other medication by mouth to an unconscious child.

■ Do not give mouth-to-mouth resuscitation to a child having convulsions.

■ Do not place a convulsing child in a tub of water to reduce the child's temperature.

■ If the child cannot bend the neck forward after convulsions have ended, or if the child has collapsed or is exhausted, report this to your doctor.

■ If a child tends to have convulsions with a fever, sponge the child's body with a damp (lukewarm) sponge at the first sign of fever.

Convulsions without fever

SYMPTOMS

- Unconsciousness
- Stiffened body
- Jerking or thrashing movements
- Muscle spasms
- Loss of control of bladder or bowels
- Deep sleep after spasms end
- Confusion and sleepiness after awakening

HOME CARE

- Protect the child from injury during jerking or thrashing movements.
- Do not put your fingers into the child's mouth in an attempt to grab the tongue during a convulsion.
- Call your doctor.

PRECAUTIONS

- Call your doctor any time a child has convulsions. The cause and treatment must be determined by a doctor.
- Convulsions without fever may be caused by a variety of illnesses. Epilepsy is not always the cause.
- If you find your child unconscious, consider the possibility that epilepsy or another illness has led to a fall and unconsciousness.

- Do not give mouth-to-mouth resuscitation to a child having convulsions.
- See your doctor if your child has any signs of epileptic seizures without convulsions.

SYMPTOMS OF EPILEPTIC SEIZURES WITHOUT CONVULSIONS

Staring into space

Rapidly blinking or fluttering eyelids

Sitting motionless

Making repeated or unusual movements

Feeling tingling in the hands and feet

Perceiving bad odors

Seeing flashing lights

Speaking unintelligibly

Coughs

NOTE

■ Coughing is not an illness itself, but rather a symptom of illness (such as asthma, bronchiolitis, bronchitis, the common cold, croup, pneumonia, sinusitis, viral infection, or whooping cough) or irritation (such as may be caused by inhaling irritating particles or a foreign body).

HOME CARE

■ Give the child plenty of liquids.

■ Use a vaporizer or humidifier to add moisture to the air.

■ Ask your doctor if cough medicine should be given for the illness your child has. If so, ask what type of cough medicine should be used.

■ Treat the whole illness, not just the cough.

PRECAUTIONS

■ Do not give cough medicine if the child has croup.

■ Do not give cough medicine if the child has any breathing difficulty.

■ Do not give cough medicine if the child may have inhaled a foreign body.

■ For some illnesses (especially asthma and pneumonia), coughing is useful and should not always be suppressed.

Cradle cap

SYMPTOMS

- Yellow, scaly, or crusty patches on the scalp

- Loss of hair in patches

HOME CARE

- Mild cases can usually be cleared by daily, vigorous shampooing. Use soap on a wet, rough washcloth wrapped around your hand.

- If regular shampooing doesn't work, try special shampoos that contain coal tar or salicylic acid; read and follow directions carefully.

- If necessary, apply ointments that contain sulfur, salicylic acid, or coal tar to the scalp daily; read and follow directions carefully.

PRECAUTIONS

- Keep medicated shampoos and ointments out of the child's eyes.

- Stop using medicated shampoos or ointments if the scalp or skin becomes irritated or red.

Crossed eyes

SYMPTOMS

■ One or both eyes are turned abnormally inward toward the nose.

HOME CARE

■ None. See your doctor.

PRECAUTIONS

■ If the pupils of the child's eyes are not equally black, smoothly round, and the same size, see your doctor.

■ If your child's eyes are not parallel, see your doctor to avoid development of a lazy eye.

■ All children should have their vision checked annually beginning at the age of four or five years.

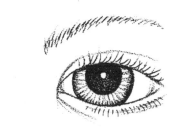

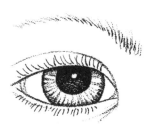 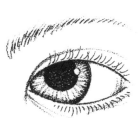

To judge the straightness of a child's eyes, shine a light into the eyes while the child is looking straight ahead. The highlight should be at the same spot in each eye (as shown at top). If the highlight is at different spots (as shown at bottom), one eye may be crossed.

Croup

SYMPTOMS

Croup:

- Barking cough

- Hoarseness

- Difficulty in breathing, especially inhaling

- Crowing sound when inhaling

Epiglottitis:

- Fever (as high as 105°F)

- Difficulty in breathing

- Difficulty in swallowing

- Sore throat

- Drooling

- Sitting with head forward, mouth open, and tongue hanging out

HOME CARE

- **If a child has serious difficulty in breathing, do not treat at home.** Notify your doctor, and go immediately to the nearest hospital emergency room.

- For mild, repeated attacks of croup (if there is no serious breathing problem), add moisture to the air to make breathing easier. Use a vaporizer or humidifier. Sit with the child in a closed bathroom with a hot shower running to build steam. If steam does not relieve the symptoms, call your doctor. Some children respond better to exposure to the cool night air.

- The first time you suspect that your child has croup (even a mild case), call your doctor.

PRECAUTIONS

- If your child has a high fever, has difficulty in breathing and swallowing, is drooling, or sits with the head forward, mouth open, and tongue hanging out, **get medical help immediately**.

- **Do not** give cough medicine to a child who has croup or any difficulty in breathing.

- **Do not** give ipecac to a child with croup.

Cuts

SYMPTOMS
- Break in the skin
- Bleeding

HOME CARE
- First, stop the bleeding. Apply firm pressure directly on the cut for ten minutes with sterile gauze or a clean cloth.
- If the bleeding will not stop, get medical help immediately.
- If the bleeding has stopped, wash the area with soap and water. Examine the cut to decide if a doctor should treat the wound. If the wound is more than skin deep, if it has ragged edges or deeply imbedded dirt, or if the cut is on an area that moves frequently (such as near a joint or on some parts of the face), call your doctor. If you are unsure about the severity of the wound, call your doctor.

If the cut can be cared for at home:
- Apply a nonstinging antiseptic.
- Draw the edges of the wound together with adhesive "butterfly" bandages.

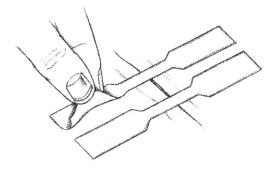

If a cut can be treated at home, draw the edges of the cut together with adhesive butterfly bandages.

- Cover the wound with sterile gauze and a bandage to prevent infection.
- Inspect the wound daily for signs of infection.
- Remove the butterfly bandages only after the cut has completely healed (seven to ten days).

PRECAUTIONS
- **Do not** use a tourniquet to stop bleeding from a cut.
- Any cut that needs stitches should be seen by a doctor as soon as possible, preferably within eight hours. Although some lacerations can be stitched up to 24 hours after they occur, the sooner the cut is stitched, the better.
- If a wound shows signs of infection (tenderness, swelling, discharge of pus, or red streaks spreading out from the wound), see your doctor.
- Be sure your child receives tetanus boosters as recommended by your doctor.

Cystic fibrosis

SYMPTOMS

- Frequent respiratory infections

- Frequent episodes of bronchitis or pneumonia

- Chronic cough

- Failure to gain weight

- Frequent constipation or diarrhea with foul-smelling stools

- Protrusion of the rectum

- Broadening of the fingertips and toes

- Salty taste to the skin when kissed

HOME CARE

- If you suspect cystic fibrosis, see your doctor. If cystic fibrosis is diagnosed, follow the doctor's instructions for home care.

PRECAUTIONS

- If your child shows any symptoms of cystic fibrosis, ask your doctor to perform a sweat test.

- If there is any history of cystic fibrosis in your family, a sweat test should be considered for all children (even if they appear healthy). The sweat test is not reliable before the age of one month and is less reliable during adolescence. Cystic fibrosis is the most common serious inherited disease in the United States.

- The earlier cystic fibrosis is diagnosed and treated, the better the outcome.

Deafness

SYMPTOMS

- Three-month-old infant ignores sounds or does not turn head toward sound.

- One-year-old does not speak a few words or babble.

- Two-year-old does not speak two-word or three-word sentences.

- Five-year-old does not speak so that strangers can understand.

- Child has learning problems in school.

- Child simply does not seem to hear well.

HOME CARE

- Home care depends on the cause and type of hearing loss. See your doctor to determine cause and treatment.

- If the child has an earache, call your doctor.

PRECAUTIONS

- Every child should be given a professional hearing test before starting kindergarten.

- A deaf or hearing-impaired child should start special training as soon as possible.

- Do not put any object (including cotton swabs) into your child's ear canal for any reason.

- Every woman of childbearing age should consult her doctor about rubella (German measles) immunization. If a pregnant woman contracts rubella, her child may be born deaf.

Dehydration

SYMPTOMS

- Infrequent urination

- Smaller amounts of urine than usual (except in a diabetic child)

- Urine that is dark colored and has a strong odor

- Sunken eyes

- Drowsiness

- Rapid or slow breathing

- Tearless crying

- Sunken soft spot on the top of an infant's head

- Dryness in the membranes of the mouth

- Loss of resilience of the skin

HOME CARE

- If there are any symptoms of dehydration, call your doctor.

- If a child is vomiting, stop the vomiting first. Do not give solid foods. Give clear liquids.

- If a child is losing fluids, give plenty of extra liquids. Commercial electrolyte solutions (available from your pharmacist) are best. Also give gelatin desserts (liquid or gelled), weak tea with sugar, carbonated drinks, and fruit juices.

PRECAUTIONS

- Do not give milk or milk products.

- The younger the child, the more serious dehydration can be.

- Dehydration in infants is especially serious. Infants can become dehydrated as quickly as 12 to 24 hours after the start of diarrhea, vomiting, or breathing problems.

- The amount of urine output is *not* a clue to dehydration in a diabetic child.

- Common causes of dehydration include the following: diarrhea, vomiting, excessive sweating, rapid breathing from an illness, diabetes mellitus.

Diabetes mellitus

SYMPTOMS

- Increased hunger

- Increased thirst

- Frequent urination

- Greater amounts of urine than usual

- Sudden onset of bed-wetting

- Weight loss

- Fatigue

- Irritability

- Deep, rapid breathing and unconsciousness (diabetic coma)

HOME CARE

- Do not try to treat on your own. See your doctor for diagnosis and instructions for home care.

PRECAUTIONS

- See your doctor if a toilet-trained child suddenly begins regular bed-wetting.

- If there is diabetes in your family background, your child should be regularly screened for diabetes.

- Untreated or uncontrolled diabetes can lead to dehydration.

Diaper rash

SYMPTOMS

- Reddened skin
- Rough, scaly skin
- Ammonia odor
- Red, scaly spots

HOME CARE

- Keep the baby as dry as possible. Change diapers often.
- Do not use an airtight outer covering over diapers.
- Try changing the products used to launder diapers.
- *For simple diaper rash:* Apply petroleum jelly, zinc oxide, vitamin A & D ointment, or an ointment combining zinc oxide, cod liver oil, petrolatum, and lanolin.
- *For ammonia rash:* Do not use an airtight outer covering over the diapers. Wash the diaper area frequently with clear water.
- *For allergic rashes:* Stop giving the child any new foods or beverages started in the previous month. Ask your doctor if you should discontinue a recently prescribed medication.
- *For rash from an infection:* Wash the area with soap and water. Apply antibiotic ointment often.
- *For rash from yeast:* Wash the area with soap and water. Exposing the area to air and keeping the area dry help. Ask your doctor about antiyeast creams.

PRECAUTIONS

- If the rash is spreading or severe or worsens after two days of home treatment, see your doctor.
- If the child has a fever, irritability, loss of appetite, or any other signs of illness, see your doctor.
- Do not use more than one type of ointment at any one time (unless both were prescribed by your doctor).

Diarrhea in older children

SYMPTOMS

- Loose, watery stools
- Mucus in stools
- Red flecks of blood in stools
- Cramps
- Fever
- Loss of appetite
- Weight loss

HOME CARE

- If the child is also vomiting, stop the vomiting first. Restrict the child's diet to clear liquids only. When the vomiting has stopped, treat the diarrhea. Limit or do not reintroduce solid foods. Avoid butter, fatty meats, peanut butter, whole-grain cereals, vegetables, and most fruits (bananas and apples are OK).

- Do not give milk.

- Give the child extra liquids—tea, water, flavored gelatin water, and commercial electrolyte solutions (available from your pharmacist) are best.

PRECAUTIONS

- Do not give antidiarrheal medications to children.

- Isolate infants from children who are vomiting or who have diarrhea.

- If there is blood in the stools, high fever, extreme weakness, or severe or prolonged diarrhea (lasting more than two to three days), call your doctor.

- Call your doctor if your child frequently has diarrhea (especially if the child is losing weight).

- A child with diarrhea needs extra liquids to avoid dehydration (serious loss of body fluids).

DIETARY TREATMENT OF DIARRHEA (IN SUGGESTED ORDER OF INTRODUCTION)

Commercial electrolyte solutions (available from your pharmacist)

Sweetened tea

Flavored gelatin water

Diluted beef bouillon

Flavored gelatin

Lean beef or lamb

Boiled chicken

Cooked rice

Baked or boiled potato, dry

Banana

Apple

Toast or crackers and jelly (no butter or margarine)

Soft- or hard-boiled egg

Diarrhea in young children

SYMPTOMS

- Loose, watery stools
- Mucus in stools
- Red blood flecks in stools
- Cramps
- Fever
- Loss of appetite
- Weight loss

HOME CARE

- If the child is also vomiting, treat the vomiting first. Restrict the child's diet to clear liquids only. When vomiting has stopped, treat the diarrhea. Stop all foods with roughage, including vegetables and most fruits (bananas and apples are OK). Do not give cow's milk or cow's-milk-based formula.

- Stop any foods and beverages that have recently been added to the child's diet. Such additions sometimes cause diarrhea in infants.

- To avoid dehydration (serious loss of body fluids), give the child plenty of clear liquids; tea, water, flavored gelatin water, and commercial electrolyte solutions (available from your pharmacist) are best.

- Continue treating the diarrhea until the child has no stools or normal stools for 24 to 48 hours.

PRECAUTIONS

- Do not give antidiarrheal medications to infants and children.

- Diarrhea and vomiting can cause dehydration. Be alert for the symptoms of dehydration (see list of symptoms on page 88). Dehydration can be especially serious in infants and children under the age of five.

- In infants, dehydration can occur as rapidly as 12 to 24 hours after the start of diarrhea or vomiting.

- If an infant or young child shows any symptoms of dehydration, call your doctor.

- Solid foods aggravate diarrhea. If the child is drinking plenty of liquids, solid foods can be avoided for several days without any danger to the child's health.

- Improperly prepared and improperly refrigerated formulas commonly cause serious diarrhea in infants. Be careful when normal refrigeration and cooking facilities are not available (picnics, camping, traveling, power outages).

- Many antibiotics cause diarrhea in some infants. If your child is taking an antibiotic, ask your doctor if the medication may be causing diarrhea in your child. (However, do not discontinue giving an antibiotic without your doctor's permission.)

Diphtheria

SYMPTOMS

- Persistent, severe sore throat
- Pus in throat
- Gray membrane in throat
- Fever
- Cough
- Difficulty in breathing

HOME CARE

- None. Diagnosis and treatment must be handled by a doctor.
- If your child has a severe sore throat, see your doctor.
- If a child with a sore throat has not been immunized against diphtheria or has not had the appropriate diphtheria boosters, tell your doctor. Otherwise, the doctor may not look for diphtheria.

PRECAUTIONS

- Diphtheria is a serious (possibly fatal) illness.
- Prevent diphtheria by getting your children immunized and by getting required booster shots.
- If your child has not been immunized, every cough, sore throat, or case of croup could be diphtheria.
- If a child is having any trouble breathing, **do not** attempt to look in the child's throat.
- Do not give cough medicine to a child who is having any trouble breathing.

- Throat cultures to detect strep throat do not show diphtheria bacteria. A separate culture for diphtheria must be taken.
- A child may have both strep throat and diphtheria at the same time.
- A child who has not been immunized can catch diphtheria from a healthy person who is a carrier of diphtheria bacteria.
- Do not travel to an underdeveloped country where diphtheria is common without immunization and appropriate booster shots.

Dislocated elbow

SYMPTOMS

■ Pain in the arm (anywhere from the elbow to the wrist), particularly if it is known that the arm was yanked or pulled

■ Holding the arm against the side with the palm facing back

■ Pain when trying to turn the palm forward

■ Swelling of wrist and hand

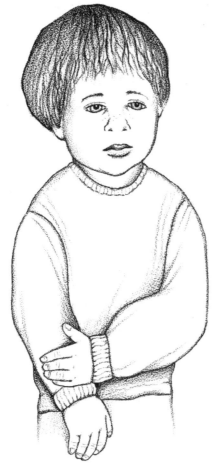

A child with a dislocated elbow will hold the arm to the side with the palm facing backward.

HOME CARE

■ The first time you suspect a dislocated elbow, see your doctor for proper treatment.

■ If the elbow becomes dislocated often, your doctor may teach you how to correct a dislocated elbow at home.

PRECAUTIONS

■ Do not try to correct a dislocated elbow unless you have been taught the proper procedure by a doctor.

■ Do not use the procedure for correcting a dislocated elbow unless the symptoms exactly match the description and you are sure the arm has been yanked. A fracture of a forearm bone can cause similar symptoms.

■ A dislocated elbow should be treated as soon as possible (within a few hours).

■ Be especially careful for three to four weeks after dislocation. A dislocation can easily recur during the healing period.

■ Do not lift children by pulling on their hands, wrists, or arms.

Dislocated hips

SYMPTOMS

- Child moves one leg more than the other

- Folds of the buttocks do not match

- Creases on sides of groin do not match

- Child limps

- Child waddles

HOME CARE

- None. See your doctor.

PRECAUTIONS

- Dislocation of the hip is a disabling condition if not treated early and properly.

- Be sure that your baby's hips are carefully examined during regular visits to the doctor until the child is older than one year.

- If your child's legs are not the same (in length, size, shape, position, or movement), tell your doctor.

Dizziness

SYMPTOMS

■ Spinning sensation

■ Loss of balance

■ Jerking movements of the eyes

■ Nausea

■ Vomiting

HOME CARE

■ Have the child sit with the head lowered to the knees. Place your hand on the back of the child's head and have the child push up slightly against your hand. If the dizziness is not relieved, have the child lie down to rest, with the feet raised higher than the head.

■ If rest does not relieve dizziness, see your doctor.

PRECAUTIONS

■ See your doctor if dizziness occurs often.

■ See your doctor if dizziness lasts more than one or two hours.

■ Before calling your doctor, be sure the child is describing a sense of rotating.

■ Children sometimes confuse dizziness with faintness, light-headedness, nausea, or vision problems.

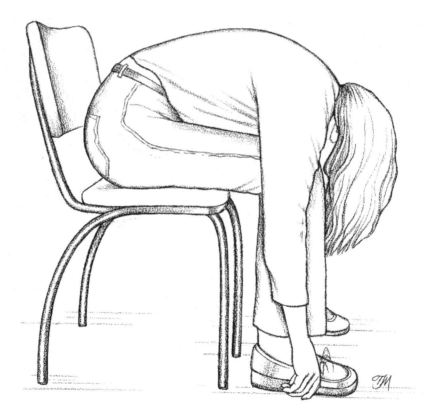

Simple dizziness may be helped by having the child sit down with her head lowered to her knees.

Draining ear

SYMPTOM

■ Any discharge from the ear (other than normal earwax)

HOME CARE

■ Do not treat at home. See your doctor promptly.

■ While waiting to see the doctor, give the child acetaminophen if there is pain.

PRECAUTIONS

■ A doctor should examine a draining ear within 12 to 24 hours.

■ Do not pack cotton into a draining ear.

■ Do not use a cotton swab or any other object to remove material still in the ear canal.

■ Do not wash out a draining ear, since the eardrum may be broken.

Drug and alcohol use

SYMPTOMS

- Behavioral changes

- Excessive time spent alone

- Changes in friends

- Lack of motivation

- Deterioration in academic or job performance

HOME CARE

- Have frank and open discussions about drugs and alcohol with your child.

- Be a good role model by not smoking or using recreational drugs and by consuming alcohol responsibly and only in moderation.

- Foster a close and nonjudgmental relationship with your child.

PRECAUTIONS

- If you suspect your child is using drugs or alcohol, get help right away.

- Know the warning signs of alcohol or drug use.

Dysentery

SYMPTOMS
- Severe or bloody diarrhea
- Prolonged high fever
- Extreme weakness

HOME CARE
- Do not treat on your own. See a doctor.
- While waiting to see the doctor, give the child plenty of clear liquids; tea, flavored gelatin water, and commercial electrolyte solutions (available from your pharmacist) are best.
- Limit or stop giving solid foods. Avoid giving foods with roughage (including vegetables and fruits, except bananas and apples), butter, fatty meats, and peanut butter.
- Do not give the child cow's milk or cow's-milk-based formula.

PRECAUTIONS
- Always report severe or bloody diarrhea to your doctor.
- A child with diarrhea needs extra liquids to avoid dehydration (a serious loss of body fluids).
- Dehydration is more likely in younger children. Infants can become dehydrated rapidly (within 12 to 24 hours after diarrhea begins).
- Do not give antidiarrheal medications to children.
- When traveling, beware of unsanitary sources of food and water.

- If you suspect dysentery, isolate the child and dispose of stools carefully.
- Practice good hygiene at home.

Dyslexia

SYMPTOMS

- Confusion about being right-handed or left-handed

- Difficulty in telling time or remembering sequences

- Hyperactivity

- Language problems

- Lack of coordination

- Poor memory

- Lack of balance

- Seeing letters or numbers reversed

HOME CARE

- The dyslexic child needs to be encouraged and supported, but not overprotected, by the family.

- Work with the child's doctor and teachers to help the child.

- Be sensitive to the effect the child's dyslexia may have on other family members.

PRECAUTIONS

- Professional help for the dyslexic child should be sought as soon as possible.

- Be aware that an intelligent child who experiences unexpected reading problems may be dyslexic.

- The brothers and sisters of a dyslexic child may need special attention or professional counseling. Parents also may find counseling helpful in meeting the dyslexic child's needs.

- Remember that dyslexia is not caused by, or a sign of, mental retardation, nor is it related to low intelligence, physical disability, cultural disadvantages, social or economic position, or brain damage.

- The possibility of a physical or psychological cause for the child's problems must be ruled out before a diagnosis of dyslexia is made.

Earaches

SYMPTOM
- Mild to severe pain in the ear

POSSIBLE SYMPTOMS
- Fever
- Nasal congestion
- Hearing problems

HOME CARE
- Give acetaminophen to relieve pain.
- Applying gentle heat to the ear may relieve pain but sometimes worsens pain.
- Check with your doctor before using anesthetic eardrops.
- If earache may be caused by nasal congestion, use nose drops and oral decongestants to relieve congestion.

PRECAUTIONS
- If an earache is severe, see your doctor.
- If an earache lasts more than a few hours, see your doctor.
- Never put any object (including a cotton swab) in your child's ear canal for any reason.
- A child with a congested nose should not go swimming or fly in an airplane unless absolutely necessary.
- Early treatment of nasal congestion with nose drops and oral decongestants may prevent some ear problems.
- Preventive eardrops should be applied at the end of each swimming day in children who tend to get swimmer's ear.

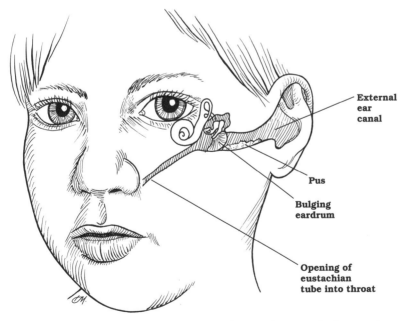

External ear canal

Pus

Bulging eardrum

Opening of eustachian tube into throat

A middle ear infection may cause the eardrum to bulge and rupture, discharging pus into the external ear canal. Such an infection may follow a nose or throat infection that migrates to the middle ear through the eustachian tube.

Earring problems

SYMPTOMS

- Redness of the earlobe

- Itchy, scaly skin on earlobe

- Swelling of earlobe

- Lumps in earlobe

- Tenderness of earlobe

- Discharge from earlobe

- Rawness around pierced openings

- Tear in earlobe from injury

HOME CARE

- At the first sign of an earlobe problem, remove pierced earrings and leave them out until the condition has healed.

- Soak the earlobe in warm water, and then apply antibiotic ointment to the front and the back of the earlobe.

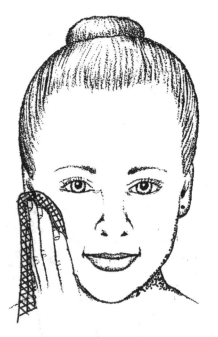

At the first sign of any earlobe problem, remove the earring, soak the earlobe in warm water, and apply an antibiotic ointment to both sides of the lobe.

PRECAUTIONS

- If the irritation is severe, see your doctor.

- If the irritation does not clear up with home treatment, see your doctor.

- If there are any signs of infection (swelling, redness, lumps, tenderness, discharge, rawness), see your doctor.

- Leave training earrings in place for one month after piercing. Turn them daily, and splash the fronts and backs with alcohol.

- Do not use earrings with posts that are too short for the earlobes.

- Do not push guards in too far along the posts so that earrings are too tight.

- Do not pull down on the earlobe when inserting earrings.

- Do not permit your child to wear earrings containing metals to which the child has a sensitivity.

- Do not permit your child to wear large earrings or hoop earrings during athletic activities or dancing.

- Do not pierce the ears of any child too young to understand the procedure or how to care for the pierced ears.

Eczema

SYMPTOMS

- Dry, scaly, pink rash
- Itching skin

HOME CARE

- Stop giving the child any new foods and beverages that were added to the diet in the month before the rash broke out.

- If discontinuing new foods and beverages does not improve the rash within four to seven days, ask your doctor if you should stop giving foods and beverages that are most likely to cause eczema (see box).

- Look for and remove irritating substances that may be coming in contact with the child's skin (see box).

- Ask your physician if any medication your child has recently received could be causing the problem. (Do not discontinue any medication without your doctor's permission.)

- To avoid further drying of the skin, use a humidifier to moisten dry air.

- Bathe the child sparingly, using a mild soap.

- If eczema clears up, try gradually returning discontinued foods to the child's diet. Reintroducing only one food per week may help you to detect foods that cause a reaction. Avoid those foods.

PRECAUTIONS

- If the rash is severe or infected, see your doctor.

- If the rash does not improve after one week of home treatment, see your doctor.

- As you add new foods to your infant's diet, watch for signs of a rash.

- If your infant is allergic to both cow's milk and soy formula, your doctor can recommend a nonsoy, nonmilk formula.

- Keep a child using coal-tar ointments out of the sun as much as possible. Coal-tar ointments increase sensitivity to sunburn.

FOODS LIKELY TO CAUSE ECZEMA IN INFANTS UNDER ONE YEAR OF AGE

Cow's milk • milk products • wheat flour • eggs • citrus fruits and juices • chocolate • nuts • peanut butter • fish • shellfish • tomatoes and tomato juice • tropical fruit drinks and desserts

FOODS LIKELY TO CAUSE ECZEMA IN CHILDREN ONE YEAR OF AGE AND OLDER

Citrus fruits and juices • chocolate • nuts • peanut butter • fish • shellfish • tomatoes and tomato juice • tropical fruit drinks and desserts • candies • ice cream • spices (except salt) • corn • berries

SUBSTANCES LIKELY TO CAUSE ECZEMA

Soaps • detergents • fabric softeners (especially sheets for the dryer) • wool • synthetic fabrics • stretch-cotton fabrics • fabric dyes (particularly red and blue) • water softeners • cosmetics • metals • plastics

---

Encephalitis

KEY SYMPTOMS

■ Stiff neck

■ Inability to sit up unassisted

OTHER SYMPTOMS

■ Headache

■ Vomiting

■ Sleepiness

■ Disorientation (confusion)

■ Mild to high fever

■ Convulsions or loss of consciousness

IMPORTANT

■ Encephalitis is a life-threatening disease. See your doctor immediately if key symptoms appear.

HOME CARE

■ None. See your doctor immediately.

PRECAUTIONS

■ If there are symptoms of encephalitis, let your doctor know if the child has been exposed to any poisons (including lead and mercury).

■ If your child has had a severe reaction to any vaccines, tell your doctor before the child gets booster shots.

Eye allergies

KEY SYMPTOMS

- Red, itchy eyes
- Watering eyes
- Swollen whites of the eyes

OTHER SYMPTOMS

- Swollen, red eyelids
- Rough, scaly skin on the eyelids
- Swollen, bluish pouches beneath the eyes

HOME CARE

- Give the child antihistamines by mouth.
- Apply cold compresses to the eyes.
- Try to identify and avoid substances that cause allergic reactions.

PRECAUTIONS

- If there is pus or pain in the eyes, the condition is almost certainly not an allergy.
- If the pupils of the eyes are enlarged and slow to respond to light, see your doctor.
- If home treatment does not improve the eyes within 24 hours, see your doctor.
- If vision is affected, see your doctor.
- Check with your doctor before using any eyedrops.

Eye, blocked tear duct

SYMPTOMS

■ Watering eyes

■ Green or yellow pus in the eyes

■ Red, raw skin at the outer corners of the eyelids

■ Swollen tear sac at the side of the nose

HOME CARE

■ Simple tearing needs no treatment. Wipe away tears and clean eyelids with sterile water on a cotton ball.

■ If the skin is red at the outer corners of the eyes, if the eyes themselves are red, or if there is pus, call your doctor. The doctor may prescribe antibiotic eyedrops over the telephone.

■ If the tear sac at the side of the nose is swollen, see your doctor.

PRECAUTIONS

■ With home treatment, the eyes should improve within 24 hours. If there is no improvement, call your doctor.

■ If improvement is prompt, continue home treatment until the eye has been clear for at least two days.

■ Repeated problems of tearing from obstructed tear ducts are common in infants.

Eye injuries

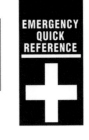
SYMPTOMS

- Pain in the eye

- Inability to open the eye

- Bleeding from or in the eyeball

- Differences in the color or position of the irises (the colored portions of the eyes)

- Differences in the size or color of the pupils

- Collapse of the eyeball

- Blurring of vision

- Visible foreign object on the eye surface or under the eyelid

- Harmful liquid or powder has come in contact with the eye

HOME CARE

If harmful liquid or powder has entered eye:

- Act immediately! Seconds count! Hold the eye open, and flush it with several pints of cool water. Pour the water from the inner corner of the eye toward the outer corner; do not let the water flow into the unaffected eye. If possible, put the child into a cool shower, clothes and all, and wash out the eye. Then immediately take the child to a doctor.

If object has penetrated eye:

- **Do not** try to remove the object. Go directly to the nearest emergency room.

If child cannot easily open eye:

- **Do not** try to force the eye open.

- **Do not** try to treat the injury at home. Place a soft bandage over the eye, and go to the doctor.

If child can easily open eye:

- Look for the following signs of damage: bleeding from or in the eyeball; differences in the size or color of the pupils; differences in the color or position of the irises; any collapse of the eyeball; blurring of vision. If any of these symptoms appears, **do not** try to treat at home. Place a soft bandage over the eye, and see your doctor promptly.

If child can easily open eye and none of above signs appears:

- Look for a speck on the eyeball or under the eyelid. If the child is cooperative, you may try to remove a speck with gentle strokes with a cotton swab. If the speck does not immediately come off, **stop**. The object may be embedded. See a doctor.

PRECAUTIONS

- Be cautious about treating eye injuries yourself.

- Do not let young children play with golf balls. Do not let anyone unwind a golf ball. If unwound, some golf balls explode and cause eye injuries.

- Aerosol spray cans and carbon dioxide cartridges explode violently in fires. Be sure that your child knows this.

- Keep children far away from areas where machine sanders, paint removers, grindstones, and similar types of equipment are being used. These machines throw off particles that can injure the eyes. Anyone around these machines should use protective eyewear.

Fainting

SYMPTOMS

- Light-headedness
- "Dizziness"
- Blurred vision
- Cold, moist skin
- Mild nausea
- Pale or greenish skin
- Glazed look in the eyes
- Loss of consciousness
- Rapid, complete recovery

HOME CARE

- Protect a fainting child from being injured by a fall. Try to catch the child.
- Place the child flat on his or her back, with the feet raised higher than the head.
- Cool air from a window or air conditioner may help.
- Keep the child lying down for five to ten minutes after regaining consciousness.
- If the child feels faint but is still conscious, have the child sit with the head between the knees. Place your hand on the back of the child's head, and have the child push up slightly against your hand.

PRECAUTIONS

- If fainting occurs often, or if there are any signs of epilepsy, see your doctor. See *Convulsions without fever* on page 80 for information on the symptoms of epileptic seizures both with and without convulsions.

- If the child's skin turns bluish during an apparent faint, or if the child is not completely well before and after fainting, see your doctor.

- Smelling salts are not necessary and are not always helpful. There is also a danger of burning the membranes inside the nose if they are held too near the nose for too long.

Fifth disease

KEY SYMPTOMS

■ Bright red rash on cheeks

■ Pink rash (forming a lacelike pattern) on trunk and limbs

■ Slight fever or no fever

■ Itching

POSSIBLE SYMPTOMS (OLDER CHILDREN ONLY)

■ Headache

■ Sore throat

■ Runny nose

■ Loss of appetite

■ Nausea

HOME CARE

■ No treatment is required.

■ Itching may be treated with antihistamines.

PRECAUTIONS

■ None

Flatfoot

SYMPTOMS

- No arches in the feet

- Entire soles of the feet rest on the ground

- Walking on the inner edges of the feet

- Worn inner edges of the heels and soles of shoes

- Pain in the feet after brief exercise

PRECAUTIONS

- Don't be concerned if your young child seems flat-footed. All infants and toddlers have flatfoot to some degree. The arches are not fully developed until children are three or four years old.

- If a child under three or four years old wears out the inner edges of shoes before the shoes are outgrown, buy shoes of a style with a strong counter (the part of the shoe that curves around the back of the heel).

- Do not use orthopedic shoes or devices without competent professional advice. Orthopedic shoes and devices may actually harm normal feet.

- Pain in the feet after excessive use and exercise is normal.

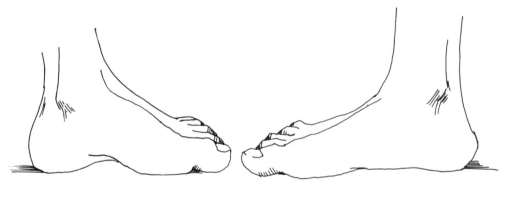

Normal foot   **Flatfoot**

Flatfoot is a condition in which the arches of the feet are flattened, so that the entire sole of the foot touches the ground.

Food allergies

SYMPTOMS

- Abdominal cramps
- Vomiting
- Diarrhea
- Blood in stool
- Hives
- Eczema
- Runny nose
- Asthma

HOME CARE

- Introduce new foods slowly, one at a time.
- If you suspect that an unfamiliar food is causing stomach cramps, diarrhea, or vomiting, withdraw that food from your child's diet. If a child continues to have symptoms or seems generally unwell, call your doctor.

PRECAUTIONS

- An enzyme deficiency can cause a malabsorption syndrome, with symptoms similar to those of a food allergy. A child who is generally not doing well should be seen by a doctor.
- Persistent diarrhea may indicate an allergic reaction or a malabsorption problem.
- When you introduce new foods into a child's diet, watch for reactions that may indicate an allergy or other problem.

Food poisoning

SYMPTOMS

- Vomiting

- Abdominal cramps

- Diarrhea

- Fever or no fever

HOME CARE

- Treat vomiting first by restricting the child's diet to clear liquids only.

- When vomiting has stopped, treat diarrhea by limiting or not reintroducing solid foods. Especially avoid butter, fatty meats, peanut butter, whole-grain cereals, vegetables, and most fruits (apples and bananas are OK).

- Do not give the child cow's milk or cow's-milk-based formula.

- Give the child plenty of clear liquids, such as tea, water, flavored gelatin water, and commercial electrolyte solutions (available from your pharmacist).

PRECAUTIONS

- Do not prepare food that needs refrigeration for a child's lunch box or for a picnic if refrigeration will not be available.

- A child with diarrhea and vomiting needs plenty of clear liquids to avoid dehydration (a serious loss of body fluids). Watch for symptoms of dehydration (see page 88). If you notice any symptoms of dehydration, call your doctor.

- Do not give antidiarrheal medications to children.

- Isolate an infant from children who are ill with vomiting and diarrhea.

- If there is blood in the stools, high fever, extreme weakness, or severe or prolonged diarrhea (more than 12 to 24 hours for a young infant or more than two to three days for an older child), call your doctor.

Fractures

SYMPTOMS

- Deformity of a bone that can be seen or felt

- Pain that is worsened by moving the bone

- Tenderness to pressure

- Inability to move a bone normally

- Swelling

- Bruising

IMPORTANT

- Do not move the child if there is any possibility of a spine or neck fracture. Call an ambulance to take the child to an emergency room.

HOME CARE

- Whenever you suspect a broken bone, see your doctor.

- When a possible fracture occurs, protect the injured part of the body and keep the injured bone from moving. If in doubt, it's best to splint a possible fracture.

- Use a thick newspaper to splint a possibly fractured arm or leg.

- Keep the child from putting weight on a possibly fractured leg, foot, or toe.

- Once the injured area has been immobilized in a comfortable position, take the child to a doctor.

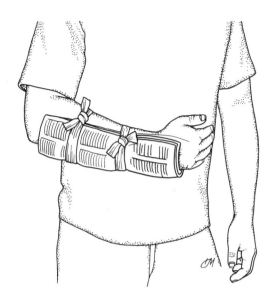

If you think your child may have a fractured bone, protect the injured part of the body and keep it from moving. Splint a possible fracture in the position in which you found it. A thick newspaper tied around the affected area is often the best splint.

PRECAUTIONS

- Have a doctor treat all possibly fractured bones. A fractured bone that is not properly positioned during healing can affect growth or cause bone deformity in children.

- Do not move an injured limb when applying a splint. Splint a possible fracture in the position in which you found it.

Frequent illness

SYMPTOMS

- Frequent attacks of the same illness

- Frequent different minor illnesses

- Frequent complications of minor illnesses

- Frequent major illnesses

HOME CARE

- Consider whether your child is actually ill more often than most other children.

- Keep older children who are ill away from infants.

- Keep an ill child away from your other children as much as is practical.

- Isolating your healthy child from other children in an attempt to prevent illness can do more harm than good.

PRECAUTIONS

- Frequent illnesses are not necessarily a sign of an underlying medical problem.

- The average, normal child between 1 and 12 years of age may have as many as eight illnesses per year.

- If a child has frequent attacks of the same illness, discuss this with your doctor.

- Frequent illnesses that could interfere with normal growth must be investigated.

- Repeated pneumonia in the same part of a lung must be evaluated by your doctor.

- Frequent lower respiratory tract infections with a prolonged cough can be a sign of cystic fibrosis or asthma.

Frostbite

SYMPTOMS

First-degree:

- Whitish or slightly yellow skin

- Burning or itching sensation

Second-degree:

- Loss of sensation

- Reddening and swelling of tissues

- Blistering and peeling of rewarmed skin

Third-degree:

- Waxy white, hard skin

- Swelling

HOME CARE

- Prevent frostbite by having your child wear adequate and appropriate clothing.

- If frostbite does occur, warm the affected area by immersing in lukewarm (not hot or cold) water and then carefully patting the skin dry.

- If you are outdoors, have the child warm the frostbitten areas by placing them in contact with warm parts of your body or the child's own body (for example, under the arms or between the thighs) until shelter can be reached.

- Give the child warm drinks, and keep the frostbitten areas clean.

- After the frozen areas have thawed, elevate them to improve blood circulation, and keep the skin at room temperature.

- Consult your doctor about all cases of frostbite.

PRECAUTIONS

- In administering first aid for frostbite, **do not** rub the affected areas.

- Do not let the child walk on frostbitten feet or exercise frostbitten parts of the body.

- Do not expose frostbitten areas to the direct heat of a radiator, stove, or fire.

- Loss of sensation in the affected areas is a danger signal.

- Frostbite can have serious consequences, including gangrene, which may necessitate amputation of the affected part.

Funnel chest

SYMPTOMS

■ Breastbone sinks in when the child breathes out

■ Hollow appears in the center of the chest

HOME CARE

■ True funnel chest cannot be treated at home. Bring it to your doctor's attention at a routine checkup.

PRECAUTIONS

■ Do not be alarmed if the breastbone is only mildly sunken in an infant or young child.

■ A mild funnel chest usually causes no harm and will gradually correct itself as the child's ribs grow heavier and stronger.

■ Do not restrict your child's activities.

■ If the breastbone retracts (is pulled in) in a child who has shown no earlier signs of funnel chest, this may be a sign of breathing difficulty. Consult your doctor.

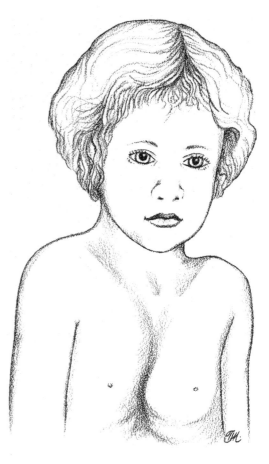

When a child with true funnel chest breathes out as well as in, the lower half of the breastbone is pulled in, creating a hollow in the center of the chest.

Gastroenteritis, acute

SYMPTOMS

- Sudden vomiting

- Sudden diarrhea

- Abdominal cramps

- High fever, low fever, or no fever

- Small amounts of blood in the vomit

HOME CARE

- Treat both vomiting and diarrhea by limiting the child's diet to clear liquids until the illness subsides. Do not give the child cow's milk or cow's-milk-based formula.

- To avoid dehydration (a serious loss of body fluids), give the child plenty of clear liquids, such as tea, flavored gelatin water, and commercial electrolyte solutions (available from your pharmacist).

- Give acetaminophen rather than aspirin for fever, since aspirin sometimes aggravates vomiting.

PRECAUTIONS

- Wash your hands carefully after contact with the child.

- The disease is usually not serious except in young babies, who may become dehydrated.

- If the disease develops in a young child, watch for signs of dehydration (infrequent urination, dryness in the mouth, sunken eyes, drowsiness, rapid or slow breathing, tearless crying, sunken soft spot at the top of the head). If any of these symptoms appears, call your doctor.

- Do not give antidiarrheal medications to children.

- If there is blood in the stools, high fever, extreme weakness, or diarrhea that is severe or prolonged (for more than 12 to 24 hours for a young infant or more than two to three days for an older child), call your doctor.

Geographic tongue

SYMPTOM

■ Smooth, bright red patches on the tongue that change size, shape, and location

HOME CARE

■ No treatment is necessary.

PRECAUTIONS

■ Geographic tongue does not indicate a vitamin deficiency, a reaction to toothpaste, or any other problem.

■ Do not try any home treatment. Geographic tongue is harmless.

■ Reassure your child that there is no need to be concerned about a geographic tongue.

Glands, swollen

SYMPTOMS

■ Swelling or tenderness of the lymph nodes

■ Unusual swelling, pain, and redness of the skin over infected lymph nodes

HOME CARE

■ Mildly swollen lymph nodes usually require treatment only for the disease or infection causing the swelling.

PRECAUTIONS

■ Because infants have limited immunity to disease, swollen lymph nodes in an infant should always be examined by a doctor.

■ Consult the doctor if a lymph node continues to increase in size or tenderness, or if the overlying skin becomes red.

■ Swollen lymph nodes are a sign of infection or illness, ranging in severity from the common cold to more serious conditions, such as leukemia. Always consult your doctor about persistent or recurring lymph-node enlargement.

■ Swollen lymph nodes in many areas of the body at once usually indicate a general illness or widespread infection.

■ When your child turns his or her head, you may notice lymph nodes the size of a pea or smaller in the sides of the neck. This is normal.

Goiter

SYMPTOM
- Swelling in the front of the neck.

HOME CARE
- Do not attempt to treat at home. Treatment depends on the cause, which must be diagnosed by a doctor.

PRECAUTIONS
- During pregnancy, do not take any medications (even over-the-counter drugs) without your doctor's approval. Some drugs taken by the mother can interfere with synthesis of thyroid hormone in the fetus, causing congenital (present at birth) goiter.

Gonorrhea

SYMPTOMS

In boys:

- Burning during urination

- Discharge from the penis

In girls:

- Vaginal discharge

- Abdominal pain

- Often, no symptoms

HOME CARE

- Gonorrhea must be diagnosed and treated by a doctor.

- The best preventive measure is to provide your children with appropriate and adequate sex education.

PRECAUTIONS

- Be aware that venereal (sexually transmitted) gonorrhea is being seen with increasing frequency among sexually active teenagers and younger children.

- Sexually abused children may contract this disease.

- A mother who has gonorrhea can transmit the disease to her baby as the child passes through the birth canal during delivery.

- A girl with gonorrhea may have no symptoms, and the infection may go undetected and untreated. Serious consequences, including sterility (inability to conceive children), may result.

- Some doctors recommend that sexually active girls be tested for gonorrhea at the time of routine school or annual medical checkups.

Growing pains

SYMPTOM

■ Pain in the legs or feet that occurs only while the child is resting or sleeping.

HOME CARE

■ Massage or apply heat to painful muscles.

■ Give aspirin or acetaminophen for pain.

■ Having the child wear sturdier shoes may reduce the frequency or severity of the pains.

■ Growing pains can be quite severe. It is important to reassure and comfort the child.

PRECAUTION

■ If your child complains of frequent pain that occurs at night in the same part of the body, take the child to a doctor.

G6PD deficiency

SYMPTOMS

- Paleness

- Jaundice

- Dark-colored urine

- Back pain

HOME CARE

- Consult your doctor if your child shows signs of having this condition, particularly if the child has an infection or has been taking medication.

PRECAUTIONS

- A child with G6PD deficiency should not be given aspirin.

- Before a child is given medication, the prescribing doctor should be told that the child has G6PD deficiency.

- The mother of a breast-fed baby who has this condition needs to be careful about what kinds of foods and medications she takes.

- Keep fava beans out of the child's diet if they cause a reaction.

Gumboils

SYMPTOMS

- Inflammation, swelling, or pain at the base of a decayed tooth

- Injury or discoloration of associated tooth

HOME CARE

- Aspirin or acetaminophen will help relieve pain.

- Have the child rinse his or her mouth with warm salt water or apply warm soaks to the affected area.

- If the tooth is about to come out naturally, the loss of the tooth will allow the pus to drain and the gumboil to heal without treatment.

- If the tooth is not loose or is a permanent tooth, consult a dentist.

PRECAUTIONS

- Do not confuse a gumboil with a canker sore, which does not protrude in the same way as a gumboil.

- If the child loses baby molar teeth prematurely, the spacing and positioning of the permanent teeth can be affected.

- Some dentists believe that a gumboil on a baby tooth can endanger the permanent tooth before it emerges. If your young child has a gumboil, see the dentist.

- **Never** apply aspirin directly on a gumboil or the surrounding area.

Gynecomastia

SYMPTOM

■ Development of breasts in a boy

HOME CARE

■ Reassure the child that the condition will disappear.

■ Try to spare the child embarrassing situations, such as undressing or showering in front of other children.

■ Be sure that the child is not subjected to teasing or taunting by other children.

PRECAUTIONS

■ Normal adolescent boys commonly develop small breasts that may persist for up to two years. It is necessary to consult a doctor only if the condition persists for an unusually long time.

■ Parents should be aware of, and sympathetic toward, the embarrassment gynecomastia can cause a boy.

■ Overweight boys may develop accumulations of fat that resemble breasts but that contain no true breast tissue.

■ If a boy tries to conceal breast development because he is embarrassed, his parents may not be aware of the condition.

Hand, foot, and mouth disease

SYMPTOMS

■ Blisters and sores inside the mouth and on the fingers, hands, toes, and feet

■ Fever

HOME CARE

■ Give acetaminophen for fever or soreness of the mouth.

■ Do not give the child foods that will sting the mouth, such as citrus juices, ginger ale, and heavily spiced foods.

■ Consult the doctor before giving nonprescription antihistamines to relieve itching.

PRECAUTIONS

■ Keep the child away from babies, in whom this disease can be dangerous.

■ If your infant contracts hand, foot, and mouth disease, call the doctor.

■ Children may become dehydrated if they refuse liquids because of mouth pain.

Hay fever and other nasal allergies

SYMPTOMS

- Nasal congestion

- Sneezing

- Clear nasal discharge

- Itchy nose

- Paleness of the membranes inside the nose

- Headache

- Slight hearing loss

- Bluish circles under the eyes

- Fatigue

HOME CARE

- Try to keep the child away from the substances responsible for the allergic reaction.

- Have the child sleep on a nonallergenic pillow.

- The use of air conditioners or dehumidifiers can help remove allergy-causing substances from your home, as can filters on hot-air ducts.

- Consult your doctor before giving the child medications for hay fever and other allergies.

PRECAUTIONS

- Antihistamines and decongestants can help relieve the allergic reaction but should be given only on a doctor's recommendation.

- Repeated use of decongestant nasal drops or sprays can have a rebound effect and cause even worse congestion.

- Mold may breed in foam-rubber pillows as they age.

- The dander of a cat or dog allowed into the house only once can remain for weeks.

- Nasal allergic reactions rarely occur as a reaction to foods, drinks, or medications.

- Dander from guinea pigs, hamsters, gerbils, or mice does not usually cause hay fever.

- A nasal allergic reaction can be followed by a bacterial infection, indicated by fever, earache, swollen lymph nodes in the neck, or thick nasal discharge.

- A child with severe hay fever or other allergies may need a series of injections to make him or her less sensitive to allergy-causing substances.

Headaches

SYMPTOM

■ Pain, ache, or throbbing in any area of the head

HOME CARE

■ Give aspirin or acetaminophen to relieve pain.

■ Apply cold compresses to the forehead.

■ Have the child lie down in a darkened room.

■ If the headache is accompanied by nasal congestion, antihistamines or nose drops may ease both conditions. Warm compresses may also help.

■ Try to identify any source of stress that may be causing the headache. Comfort and cuddle the child whose headache may be due to emotional factors.

■ See the doctor if headaches persist.

PRECAUTIONS

■ **Get medical help immediately** if the child has a sudden, severe headache, especially if it is accompanied by any of the following: fever, extreme weakness or collapse, severe vomiting, stiff neck, or confusion.

■ If the child has recurring headaches that become more frequent or severe, consult your doctor.

■ Your information about the child's headaches will be important to the doctor. Note where the pain is located, when it occurs, what circumstances seem to provoke it, how long it lasts, if there are other symptoms, and whether the headache responds to pain-relieving medication.

Head lice

SYMPTOMS

- Itching scalp

- Red, scaly rash on the back of the neck

- Sores caused by scratching

- Enlarged lymph nodes at the base of the skull

- Dandrufflike eggs (called nits) attached to hair shafts

HOME CARE

- You can distinguish the nits of head lice from dandruff because dandruff can easily be brushed away, but the nits cling to the hair shafts.

- Your doctor will prescribe a shampoo to kill the lice and the nits. Apply the shampoo exactly according to the instructions, taking care not to get it in the child's eyes or mouth.

- If necessary, apply a vinegar rinse to loosen the nits, then comb the child's hair with a fine-tooth comb until all the nits have been removed.

- Clean combs and brushes with the shampoo, launder pillow-cases, and have caps or hats washed or dry-cleaned.

PRECAUTIONS

- If one member of the family has head lice, it is often necessary to treat the rest of the family as well (except infants and pregnant women).

- The ingredient gamma benzene hexachloride prescribed in shampoo form for head lice is poisonous if swallowed or absorbed through the skin. It can also harm the eyes. Use it exactly as directed. Do not repeat the application more than twice, at the stated intervals. Do not leave the shampoo within reach of the child.

- Consult your doctor if head lice are accompanied by infected sores on the scalp or enlarged lymph nodes at the base of the skull.

- Children should be discouraged from sharing hats, combs, and other such items.

Heart murmurs, innocent

SYMPTOM

■ Extra sounds made by the heart that are known not to indicate an abnormality

HOME CARE

■ No home care is required for an innocent murmur.

PRECAUTIONS

■ Believe your doctor's assurance that innocent murmurs are normal.

■ Do not make the mistake of overprotecting a child who has an innocent murmur. It is not necessary.

■ Try not to be alarmed by the long medical names given to innocent murmurs.

■ Most innocent murmurs disappear by the time the child is a teenager.

Heat rash

SYMPTOM

- Tiny pink or red eruptions, each surrounding a skin pore on the cheeks, neck, and shoulders; in skin creases; and in the baby's diaper area

HOME CARE

- Keep the child as cool as possible, preferably in an air-conditioned room.

- Cool baths and careful dusting with cornstarch or baby powder help relieve discomfort.

- If the rash is on the face, rest the child's face on an absorbent pad placed in the crib.

- Be careful not to overdress the child.

- Use prickly heat powders during warm weather.

PRECAUTIONS

- Use baby powder carefully—if a baby inhales it, lung inflammation can occur.

- Overdressing a baby is a frequent cause of heat rash. The baby needs to be dressed no more warmly than you would dress yourself.

- Some detergents and bleaches used to launder bed linens and clothing may aggravate heat rash.

- Avoid using bubble baths, water softeners, and oily lotions.

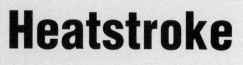

EMERGENCY
QUICK
REFERENCE

Heatstroke

SYMPTOMS

- Feeling that the lungs and muscles are "on fire"

- Dry mouth

- Breathing difficulty

- Dizziness

- Nausea

- Blurred vision

- Hot, dry skin

- High fever

- Absence of sweating

IMPORTANT

- A child with heatstroke who does not revive within minutes after treatment is in danger and requires **immediate emergency care**.

EMERGENCY TREATMENT

1. Call for emergency help.

2. Remove the child's clothing and lay the child down, with the feet higher than the head, in a shady area.

3. Pour cold water over the child's body, rub the body with ice, and then fan the child to promote evaporation.

4. When the child is conscious and the body temperature is normal, give plenty of fruit juices to replace fluids and minerals lost during dehydration.

5. Watch the child closely and repeat treatment if the symptoms recur.

PRECAUTIONS

- Heatstroke can be fatal if not treated immediately.

- Heatstroke occurs most often when both temperature and humidity are high.

- Strenuous exercise within one week of an attack of heatstroke increases the possibility of another attack.

- Susceptibility to heatstroke is increased by lack of water, excessive sweating, vomiting, and diarrhea.

- Salt tablets are not helpful in preventing heatstroke.

Henoch-Schönlein purpura

SYMPTOMS
- Rash of tiny purplish spots or a purple bruise
- Abdominal pain
- Blood in the urine
- Pain and swelling in the joints

HOME CARE
- A doctor should direct treatment of this disorder.

PRECAUTIONS
- Contact the doctor promptly if your child develops a rash of tiny purple dots or a large purple bruise.
- A purpura rash can also indicate a serious blood disease.
- If a child with Henoch-Schönlein purpura has severe abdominal pain or blood in the stool, consult the doctor at once.
- A child who has had this disorder should have checkups and kidney and urine tests for up to six months after recovery.

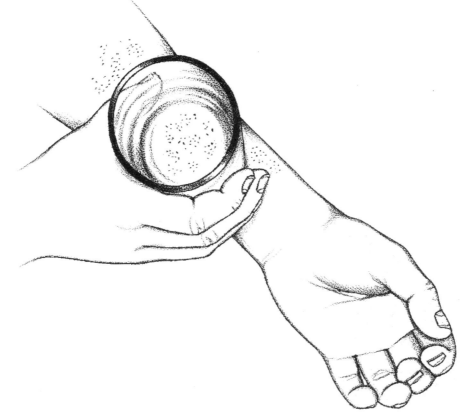

One way to tell if a rash is purpura is to press a glass against the skin. If the rash remains visible, it is purpura.

Hepatitis

SYMPTOMS

■ Loss of appetite

■ Nausea

■ Vomiting

■ Upper abdominal pain

■ Jaundice (characterized by yellowed skin and whites of eyes, dark amber urine, and light-colored stools)

■ Fever

■ Headache

■ General discomfort

HOME CARE

■ Isolate the child, and then call the doctor.

■ When a diagnosis has been made, the doctor will order a home care program that includes rest, liquids, and a low-fat diet.

PRECAUTIONS

■ Hepatitis must be diagnosed and treated by a doctor.

■ The child and other family members who have been exposed to hepatitis should be given preventive gamma globulin or hepatitis B immune globulin injections as soon as possible after exposure.

■ Hepatitis B is contagious. Isolate the child and practice good health habits to limit spread of the disease.

■ A pregnant woman can pass hepatitis B to her unborn baby.

■ Hepatitis A can be contracted from contaminated water or food, such as shellfish.

Hernia

SYMPTOM

■ A bulge just above or below the crease of the groin, just above or below the navel, or at the navel

HOME CARE

■ If you suspect a hernia, take your child to the doctor.

PRECAUTIONS

■ A strangulated hernia is a **medical emergency** that must be surgically corrected immediately (within hours). Signs that a hernia has become strangulated are swelling, severe pain, nausea, vomiting, and severe weakness or collapse. If these symptoms appear, take your child to the emergency room immediately. Never attempt home care for a strangulated hernia.

■ Trusses or belts used to reduce a hernia are useless and may be harmful or dangerous.

■ Doctors do not consider it beneficial to strap an umbilical hernia.

Herpes simplex

POSSIBLE SYMPTOMS

■ Multiple painful ulcers on the mucous membranes of the mouth or on the eyeballs

■ Painful, swollen red gums

■ Fever blisters near the lips

■ Swollen lymph nodes in the neck

■ Fever

■ Painful ulcers and blisters on the genitalia

HOME CARE

■ For oral (mouth area) herpes, give acetaminophen to relieve pain, and have the child eat bland foods.

■ An older child can rinse the mouth with a mild salt solution or be treated with triamcinolone or local anesthetic ointments.

■ Apply antibiotic ointment to fever blisters to prevent cracking and lessen the possibility of further infection.

■ Dabbing oral lesions with liquid diphenhydramine (Benadryl) helps to lessen the pain.

■ For genital herpes, warm soaks help relieve inflammation and pain.

PRECAUTIONS

■ In the case of herpes of the eyeball, consult an eye doctor promptly.

■ If a baby contracts herpes, get prompt medical attention.

■ Keep adults and children with herpes isolated from babies.

■ A pregnant woman with genital herpes can infect her child as the infant passes through the birth canal during delivery.

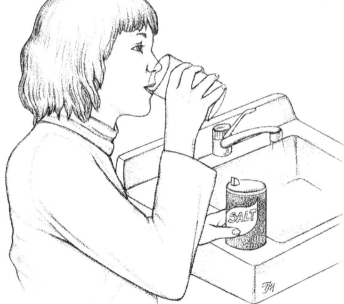

Encourage an older child with oral herpes to rinse the mouth with a mild salt-water solution.

High blood pressure

SYMPTOMS

■ Most often, there are no symptoms.

POSSIBLE SYMPTOMS

■ Headaches

■ Pounding heartbeat

■ Shortness of breath during exercise

■ Flushed face

HOME CARE

■ High blood pressure must be diagnosed and treated by a doctor.

PRECAUTIONS

■ Your child should have regular checkups, and the doctor should measure the child's blood pressure during each examination.

■ High blood pressure can be dangerous if left untreated.

Hip problems

SYMPTOMS

- Pain in hip or knee

- Limp

- Limited movement of hip joint

- Slight fever (in case of acute synovitis)

HOME CARE

- Keep the child off his or her feet for three or four days.

- Consult the doctor if the condition does not improve.

PRECAUTIONS

- Pain in the knee may be a sign of a hip problem.

- A severe form of arthritis may be signaled by hip pain and a limp accompanied by high fever. If the child appears to have a hip problem and also has a high fever, call the doctor.

- Some hip problems can cause permanent deformity if left untreated.

Hives

SYMPTOMS

■ Raised, red welts

■ Itching

■ Welts that change appearance rapidly

HOME CARE

■ Use cold-water compresses, calamine lotion, and cornstarch baths to help relieve itching.

■ If hives are caused by an allergy, medication prescribed by the doctor can be given to the child when the hives appear.

■ Diphenhydramine, an over-the-counter antihistamine, helps relieve allergic reactions and lessen the itching of hives.

PRECAUTIONS

■ **If the hives appear after an insect bite or sting, take the child to the nearest emergency room.**

■ See the doctor if hives appear on the child's tongue.

■ See the doctor immediately if the child is coughing or has difficulty in breathing or swallowing.

■ If the child has hives accompanied by fever, the doctor will order a culture to check for strep throat.

■ If an allergic child's medication does not relieve the hives, call the doctor.

Hoarseness

SYMPTOMS

■ Speaking or crying in an unusually low-pitched voice

■ Inability to speak above a whisper

■ Loss of voice

HOME CARE

■ Have the child rest his or her voice.

■ Encourage the child to inhale steam and drink warm liquids.

■ If hoarseness is caused by an allergy, antihistamines prescribed by the doctor should help.

PRECAUTIONS

■ Consult the doctor if the hoarseness is severe or persists longer than two to three days.

■ A baby is sometimes born with a soft larynx (voice box), which may give a hoarse note to the baby's cry. This is nothing to worry about and usually disappears by the time the child is a year old.

Hyperactivity

SYMPTOM

■ Inability to sit still or be quiet for more than a very short period

HOME CARE

■ Hyperactivity always requires professional evaluation and treatment.

PRECAUTIONS

■ Do not confuse a child's natural tendency to be active with true hyperactivity.

■ Never accept a diagnosis of hyperactivity from anyone except a professional.

■ Do not try to deal with hyperactivity at home. It always requires medical assessment and treatment.

■ Remember that the hyperactive child is not misbehaving; the behavior is involuntary.

■ If a child over the age of two years suddenly becomes much more active than usual, look for causes in the child's environment; true hyperactivity is present from infancy.

■ A child who is overactive with one family member but not others is not hyperactive.

■ A hyperactive child may need to take medication for extended periods. The child may also need special schooling or counseling.

Hyperventilation

SYMPTOMS

■ Feeling of difficulty in breathing, although the child is actually getting many full breaths of air

■ Tingling or numbness in the hands and feet

■ Muscle spasms

■ Fainting

HOME CARE

■ Remain calm, and reassure the child.

■ Have the child breathe into a paper bag placed loosely over the mouth and nose.

PRECAUTION

■ Rapid, deep breathing that causes fainting has become a party stunt in some circles. Discourage this kind of game.

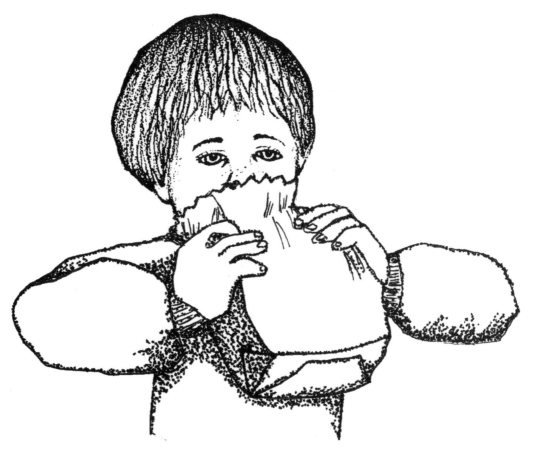

Have the child breathe into a paper bag placed loosely over the mouth and nose.

Impetigo

SYMPTOMS

- Blisters that contain thin, yellow pus

- Broken blisters that develop into open, weeping sores

- Pus that dries to the consistency of hardened honey

HOME CARE

- A mild case of impetigo can be treated by scrubbing the crusts of the sores with soap and water and then applying a nonprescription antibiotic ointment at intervals.

- Cover the affected area with gauze. This will help keep the child from scratching and spreading the condition.

PRECAUTIONS

- Impetigo is highly contagious.

- Minor scratches and scrapes on the skin may invite impetigo. To avoid infection, clean such minor wounds with soap and water and cover them with a sterile bandage.

- Keep an infected child's clothes and linens separate from those used by other family members to help prevent the disease from spreading. Launder the child's clothes frequently.

- If home treatment for impetigo is effective, continue it until all the sores have completely healed. It can take a long time to eliminate the condition.

- See the doctor if home treatment is not effective.

Infectious mononucleosis

SYMPTOMS

■ General weakness and bodily discomfort

■ Sore throat

■ Pus on the tonsils

■ Prolonged fever

■ Swollen lymph nodes, particularly in the neck

■ Prolonged fatigue

■ Mottled red rash

HOME CARE

■ Rest, acetaminophen, and a general diet (as tolerated) are the basis of home care.

■ If your doctor has found that the child's spleen is enlarged, the child's activities should be restricted.

PRECAUTIONS

■ Do not allow a child who has had mononucleosis to return to school or other activities until weakness and fatigue have disappeared.

■ Do not allow a child with an enlarged spleen to take part in contact sports or other strenuous activities until the spleen has returned to its normal size.

Influenza

SYMPTOMS

- Sudden chills
- Sharp rise in temperature
- Flushing
- Headache
- Sore throat
- Cough
- Pain in the back and limbs
- Vomiting and diarrhea (in young children)

HOME CARE

- Bed rest is necessary while the fever is high.
- Give acetaminophen, **not aspirin**, for fever and pain.
- Have the child drink plenty of fluids.
- Isolate the child from other family members.
- Keep the child home from school until he or she is completely well.

PRECAUTIONS

- Because the use of aspirin to treat influenza has been associated with Reye's syndrome, **do not give aspirin**. Use acetaminophen instead.
- Do not assume that the child is better because the fever goes away for a day. It will probably recur.
- Watch for complications and inform the doctor if they occur.
- Do not allow the child to resume everyday activities until the temperature has been normal for at least two days.
- Influenza vaccines are not generally recommended for children who do not fall into a "high risk" category.

Ingrown toenails

SYMPTOMS

- Swollen, red, and painful area near the toenail

- Thin, watery pus from the infected area

- Raw, red tissue covering part of the nail

HOME CARE

- Soak the toe frequently in warm water.

- If possible, gently cut out the ingrown part of the nail.

- If the ingrown spur cannot be removed, cover the foot with a bandage or cloth, and soak both foot and bandage in a solution of Epsom salts and encase the foot, complete with bandage, in plastic wrap or a plastic bag.

- In the case of an infant, do not try to remove the ingrown nail. Instead, wipe the toe several times daily with rubbing alcohol and then soak in warm water.

- Any time home treatment does not work, consult the doctor.

PRECAUTIONS

- Be sure your child always wears well-fitting shoes. If the shoes are too small or too pointed, they can cause ingrown toe-nails.

- Show your child how to trim his or her toenails correctly.

Insect bites and stings

EMERGENCY SYMPTOMS

■ Hives

■ Difficulty in breathing

EMERGENCY TREATMENT

■ Take the child to the nearest emergency room if he or she has an allergic reaction (such as hives or difficulty in breathing).

SYMPTOMS

■ Swelling

■ Itching

■ Stinger left in wound (honeybee)

■ Small, dark bumps (ticks)

HOME CARE

■ Relieve swelling by applying ice.

■ Apply calamine lotion to relieve itching.

■ Give a nonprescription antihistamine to relieve itching and swelling.

■ If a tick is still attached to the skin, touch the protruding portion of the insect with the still-hot tip of a blown-out match; the tick will usually fall off the skin.

PRECAUTIONS

■ Protect children with appropriate clothing and insect repellents. Use mosquito netting if necessary.

■ If your child is allergic to certain insect bites or stings, make sure that your doctor tells you what to do if the child is bitten or stung.

■ If your child develops hives or breathing difficulties after being bitten or stung by a scorpion, black widow spider, bee, wasp, or hornet, take the child to the nearest emergency room.

■ If your child has been bitten by a tick and a red rash develops at the site, followed by headache, chills, fever, and body aches and stiffness, see your doctor. These symptoms may indicate Lyme disease.

■ Find out which insects are common in your neighborhood and how to protect your child against them.

Jaundice in children

SYMPTOM

- Yellowing of the skin and the whites of the eyes

HOME CARE

- Home treatment cannot be undertaken until an accurate diagnosis has been made.

PRECAUTIONS

- Jaundice caused by a drug will disappear when the child stops taking that particular medication. However, do not discontinue any medication without your doctor's approval.

- All other types of jaundice in children are potentially serious and require prompt medical attention.

Jaundice in newborns

SYMPTOM

■ Yellow tinge to the skin and the whites of the eyes

HOME CARE

■ Watch your newborn baby closely for signs of jaundice in the first week after the baby goes home from the hospital. Inform the doctor if you suspect jaundice.

PRECAUTIONS

■ If jaundice develops or worsens after the baby comes home from the hospital, consult your doctor immediately.

■ Consult the doctor immediately if your jaundiced baby is nursing poorly, seems excessively drowsy, has a fever, or is irritable.

■ Follow your doctor's instructions exactly if your baby has jaundice.

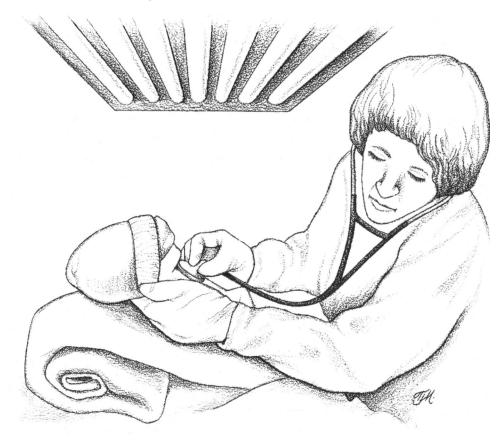

Jaundice in newborns can be treated by exposing the baby to special lights under a doctor's supervision.

Knee pain

SYMPTOMS

- Tenderness or pain

- Swelling

- Difficulty in straightening the leg

HOME CARE

- Home care for knee pain usually involves limiting the child's activity. However, the extent of the limitation depends on what is causing the pain.

PRECAUTIONS

- If the child's knee is swollen, or if the child cannot straighten the leg, a doctor should be consulted. The child should be careful not to put weight on the knee until the doctor has diagnosed the cause of the swelling.

- Treatment for most types of knee pain involves limiting the child's activities.

- Knee pain may indicate a hip problem.

Laryngitis

SYMPTOMS
- Hoarseness
- Dry, hacking cough
- Scratchy throat
- Low-grade fever

HOME CARE
- Use a vaporizer in the child's room.
- Give the child warm drinks.
- Give acetaminophen to reduce fever and relieve pain.
- A nonprescription expectorant cough remedy may relieve a troublesome cough.
- A child with laryngitis should be discouraged from talking.

PRECAUTIONS
- If laryngitis is accompanied by breathing difficulty, the child should see a doctor.
- If laryngitis is accompanied by breathing difficulty and a climbing fever, the child may have an inflammation of the epiglottis. This is a **medical emergency**; take the child to a doctor at once.
- If laryngitis persists, the doctor may recommend that the child see an ear, nose, and throat specialist.

Lazy eye

SYMPTOMS

- Eyes are not parallel.

- Pupils of the eyes are different colors.

- Child has trouble judging distance.

- Child cocks head or moves face in an effort to see clearly.

HOME CARE

- Home care cannot be undertaken until a doctor has diagnosed the condition.

PRECAUTIONS

- A child whose eyes are not parallel all or most of the time should be seen by a doctor.

- If lazy eye is not diagnosed and treated, the condition can become permanent.

- Have your child's eyes checked every year after the age of three or four.

Lead poisoning

SYMPTOMS

- Poor appetite
- Vomiting
- Constipation
- Irritability
- Slow development
- Aggressive behavior
- Seizures
- Personality changes
- Clumsiness
- Paleness
- Fatigue
- Weakness

HOME CARE

- Discourage your child from putting nonfood objects into his or her mouth and swallowing them.
- Have the paint and plaster in your home tested for lead content.
- Watch for changes in your child's behavior.

PRECAUTIONS

- Check your home and yard for possible sources of lead.
- Scraping, sanding, and other tasks involved in remodeling buildings may release lead into the air. Such locations should be avoided by infants, small children, and pregnant women until the work has been completed.

- A person whose work involves exposure to lead should take steps to avoid bringing lead-containing dust into the home on work clothes.
- Sources of lead poisoning can include artist's pigments, exhaust from cars, soil around buildings on which lead-based paint was used, city air, and improperly glazed pottery.

Leukemia

SYMPTOMS

- Paleness, weakness, or fatigue

- Spontaneous bruising

- Red, swollen, or bleeding gums

- Persistent low-grade fever

- Swollen lymph nodes

- Bone pain

- Frequent heavy nosebleeds

- Blood in the urine or stool

- Enlarged spleen or liver

HOME CARE

- Treatment for leukemia must always be regulated by a doctor.

PRECAUTION

- Many common diseases can imitate leukemia. Do not assume that a child has leukemia because he or she has one or more of the symptoms. Have your doctor examine the child to make a diagnosis.

Measles

SYMPTOMS

- Runny nose

- Reddened eyes

- Cough

- Fever

- Rash

HOME CARE

- Give acetaminophen for fever and a cough medication for severe cough.

- Give the child extra liquids.

- Bright light bothers (but does not injure) the eyes; keep the child out of brightly lit areas.

PRECAUTIONS

- A vaccine is available to prevent measles. Be sure that your child receives the vaccination.

- If a child under the age of three years who has not been vaccinated against measles is exposed to the measles virus, call your doctor.

- When a child has measles, the fever and cough should subside as the rash peaks. If they do not, be alert for possible complications, such as pneumonia, encephalitis, and middle ear infection.

Meningitis

SYMPTOMS

- Fever

- Stiff neck

- Headache

- Vomiting

- Exhaustion or collapse

- Convulsions

HOME CARE

- **Meningitis is a medical emergency. Do not attempt home care. Take the child to the doctor immediately.**

PRECAUTIONS

- A child who is very weak and has a stiff neck and fever should be seen by a doctor immediately.

- Laboratory examination of spinal fluid is the only way to diagnose meningitis.

- Meningitis may follow an upper respiratory tract or middle ear infection or a skull fracture.

- The unnecessary use of antibiotics for an upper respiratory tract infection may mask the onset of meningitis.

- Inform your doctor immediately if you discover that your child has been in contact with a person who has meningitis.

Menstrual irregularities

SYMPTOMS

- Severe abdominal pain or backache

- Menstruation before the age of nine years

- Failure to menstruate by the age of 17 years

- Long-term absence of menstruation

- Excessive bleeding

HOME CARE

- Give aspirin, ibuprofen, naproxen, or acetaminophen for pain.

- Encourage the girl to follow her normal schedule of activities during her period.

- Some young women find hot baths or hot soaks placed on the painful area help lessen discomfort.

PRECAUTIONS

- Consult your doctor if there are any symptoms of menstrual irregularities.

- After a girl starts to menstruate, it may take months or even years for her periods to become regular. This does not necessarily indicate a problem.

- Cramps and backaches may be related to tension or anxiety rather than to menstruation itself. However, these symptoms can also be caused by a hormonal imbalance or an abnormal condition of the pelvis. Some women experience pain in the middle of the cycle when they are ovulating. This pain, called Mittelschmerz pain, doesn't mean anything is wrong.

- Make sure that your daughter fully understands the process of menstruation.

Moles

SYMPTOM

■ Flat, dome-shaped, or protruding skin growths that can be up to a half-inch long and vary in color

HOME CARE

■ If a mole requires treatment of any kind, it will be necessary to see a doctor.

PRECAUTIONS

■ A doctor should see any mole that is bleeding, crusting, changing color, or growing rapidly. A doctor should also be consulted if a mole has been partly removed by accident or if the color is extending into the surrounding skin.

■ Most moles are noncancerous. However, a type of mole known as a pigmented nevus can become cancerous; this mole (unlike other types) is present at birth and is dark in color and very large.

■ Moles cannot be safely removed with electrocautery, acids, dry ice, or liquid nitrogen. If removal is necessary, it must be performed, with a scalpel, by a doctor.

■ No child is completely free of moles. Some children have hundreds of them.

Molluscum contagiosum

SYMPTOM

■ Skin eruptions that are at first small, firm, plump, and waxy in appearance. Later they become flatter, with a small central depression.

HOME CARE

■ Call the doctor for instructions about home care.

PRECAUTION

■ Molluscum contagiosum spreads rapidly. Keep the child's clothing and linens separate from those of other family members. Launder the child's belongings frequently to kill the virus.

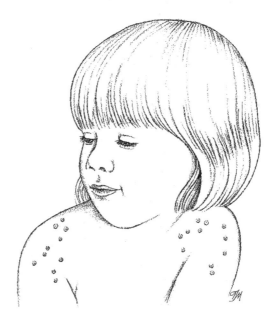

Molluscum contagiosum is a skin infection characterized by plump, round eruptions with indentations in the centers.

Motion sickness

SYMPTOMS

- Nausea

- Paleness or greenish tinge to the skin

- Excessive perspiration

- Vomiting

- Anxiety

HOME CARE

- Give the child an antinausea remedy recommended by the doctor. Give this medication as directed before and during the journey.

- Keep the child cool.

- Restrict the child to a light diet before and during the trip.

- Use a child-restraint seat that raises the child high enough to allow for easy viewing out the front window.

PRECAUTIONS

- Some children are more susceptible than others to motion sickness.

- Motion sickness is not brought on by the child, and the child cannot control it.

- If prolonged motion sickness causes severe vomiting, it may lead to dehydration, which is an emergency situation that requires medical care.

- A child who is susceptible to motion sickness may have attacks every time he or she travels.

Mumps

SYMPTOMS

- Fever
- Loss of appetite
- Headache
- Swelling of the salivary glands

HOME CARE

- The child with mumps needs rest. Give acetaminophen for pain and fever.
- Do not give the child spicy foods.
- Isolate the child from other family members.

PRECAUTIONS

- Make sure that your child is vaccinated against mumps.

- One attack of mumps almost always provides lifelong immunity. Consult your doctor if a child who has already had mumps seems to have it again. The problem is most likely some other disease of the salivary glands.

- If mumps involves the ovaries or pancreas, the child will have abdominal pain. If the testes are involved, they will be swollen and tender.

- If a child who has not been vaccinated against mumps is exposed to the disease, vaccination shortly after exposure can prevent development of mumps.

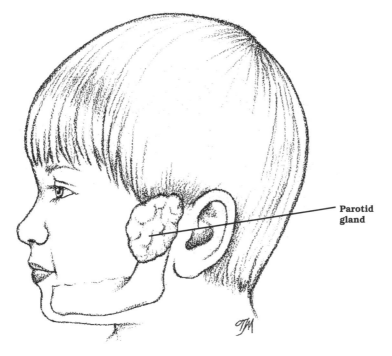

Parotid gland

Mumps is caused by a virus that infects the salivary glands, particularly the parotid glands, which results in swelling.

Nephritis

SYMPTOMS

■ Discoloration of the urine

■ Puffy eyes

■ Headache

■ High blood pressure

HOME CARE

■ Most cases of nephritis are mild and pass unnoticed. If the symptoms are marked enough to be recognized, the child requires medical attention.

PRECAUTIONS

■ If the child's eyes are puffy or the urine is scanty and dark, the child may have nephritis.

■ If symptoms of nephritis are pronounced enough to be noticed, take the child to the doctor.

■ Nephritis usually follows a strep infection. Watch for the condition to follow a strep throat or impetigo, even if the infection has been treated with antibiotics.

Nightmares

SYMPTOMS

- Child awakens screaming

- Confusion on awakening

- Frantic activity on awakening

- Sleepwalking

HOME CARE

- Rouse the child slowly and gently.

- Hold the child and speak soothingly and reassuringly.

- If the child is sleepwalking, make sure he or she cannot fall or get hurt.

PRECAUTIONS

- Frequent nightmares indicate that the child is under excessive stress. Try to identify and relieve the problem. If necessary, enlist the doctor and school personnel to help pinpoint the source of the child's distress.

- Be alert to the school, social, and family pressures that can cause a child to have nightmares.

- Be sure you know how much television your child is watching and that the program content is suitable.

- A child who sleepwalks must be protected from falls and other injuries.

Nosebleeds

SYMPTOMS

■ Bleeding from one or both nostrils or from the mouth

■ Vomiting blood

HOME CARE

■ To stop a nosebleed, compress the entire soft portion of the nose—not just the nostrils—between the thumb and fingers for ten minutes by the clock.

■ Teach your child at an early age how to stop a nosebleed.

■ To prevent nosebleeds, apply petroleum jelly or an antibiotic cream to the insides of the nostrils morning and evening for up to 14 days.

■ Use a vaporizer or humidifier in the child's room.

PRECAUTIONS

■ A child with a nosebleed should not lie down.

■ Stay calm, and do not let the child panic.

■ Do not use cold compresses, nose drops, or other household remedies; they are not necessary.

■ Do not pack the child's nose with cotton or gauze.

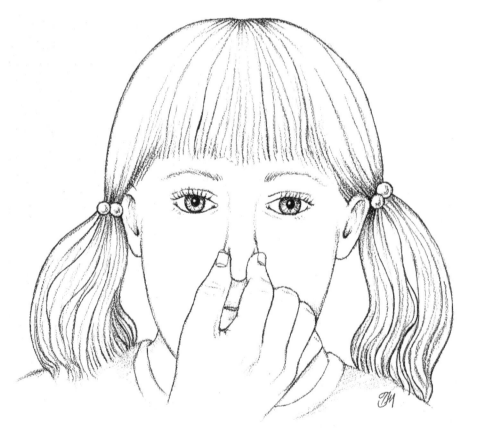

Teach your child to control a nosebleed by pinching the entire soft portion of the nose between thumb and forefinger for ten minutes.

Pigeon toes

SYMPTOM

■ Toeing in (turning inward of the front part of the foot)

HOME CARE

■ None.

PRECAUTIONS

■ Most cases of pigeon toes correct themselves; however, if the child is toeing in after the age of one year, consult a doctor.

■ Never allow a shoe salesperson to recommend orthopedic or corrective shoes for your child. The prescription must always be made by a qualified medical professional.

■ If your child sits on the floor a lot, encourage him or her to sit cross-legged, not on the haunches.

Pinworms

SYMPTOMS

- Itching or burning in the anal or genital area

- Bed-wetting

- Abdominal cramps

HOME CARE

- There is a nonprescription drug available that kills pinworms; consult your pharmacist. Your doctor can also prescribe a medication to get rid of the pinworms.

- Keep the fingernails of the infected child cut and scrubbed to avoid spreading the pinworms.

- Launder the child's clothing and linens to kill the worm eggs.

PRECAUTIONS

- If one member of the family has pinworms, other family members may also be affected.

- Do not blame a child's case of pinworms on the family dog or cat. Pinworms do not live in these animals.

- Be aware that pinworms may be the cause of recurrent inflammation of the vagina or bladder.

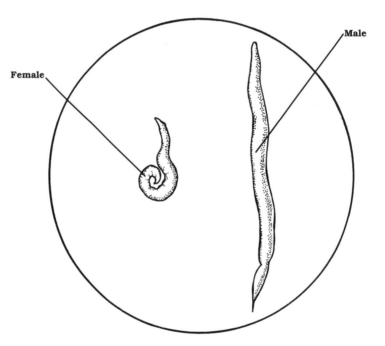

Adult pinworms are one-quarter to one-half inch in length, white, and about as thick as sewing thread.

Pityriasis rosea

SYMPTOMS

- Round or oval scaly patch followed by a rash

- Itching

- Headache

- Lethargy

- Joint pain

- Sore throat

HOME CARE

- No treatment is necessary.

- If the rash causes itching, you may give the child a nonprescription antihistamine.

- Exposure to sunlight and bathing with a mild soap may help clear the rash faster.

PRECAUTIONS

- The first patch may look like ringworm, eczema, or impetigo. The subsequent rash may be confused with ringworm.

- The condition may last for up to eight weeks but is harmless.

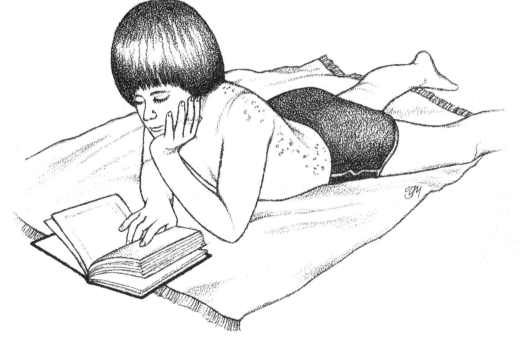

Exposure to sunlight seems to shorten the duration of the rash of pityriasis rosea.

Pneumonia

SYMPTOMS
Bacterial pneumonia:

- Mild upper respiratory tract infection

- High fever

- Chills

- Cough

- Rapid breathing

- Chest pain

Viral pneumonia:

- Headache

- Fatigue

- Fever

- Sore throat

- Severe, dry cough

HOME CARE

- Bacterial pneumonia requires medical attention.

- Viral pneumonia usually clears up on its own.

PRECAUTIONS

- Watch for signs of pneumonia in a child whose resistance has been lowered by a cold or infection.

- If a cold suddenly gets worse and is accompanied by high fever, cough, chills, chest pain, or rapid breathing, call your doctor.

- Flaring of the nostrils, grunting when breathing out, and pulling in of the chest by an infant are signs that call for **immediate medical attention**.

- If a child coughs up a discharge tinged with blood, consult a doctor.

Poisoning

POSSIBLE SYMPTOMS

- Rapid breathing
- Ringing in the ears
- Nausea
- Overexcitement
- Unconsciousness
- Burns on lips, mouth, and tongue
- Abdominal pain
- Vomiting
- Blood in vomit

EMERGENCY TREATMENT

1. Get the poison away from the child, and make sure that there is none left in his mouth. Try to find out what the child took, how much, and when.

2. Call your local poison control center for instructions. Do not wait for symptoms to appear, and do not call your doctor, the hospital, or anyone else first.

3. Be prepared to answer questions about your child's age and weight; what your child ate or drank, how much, and when; whether he has vomited or lost consciousness; and whether you have syrup of ipecac. Have the poison container at hand, if possible; you may be asked to read the label over the phone.

4. Exactly follow the instructions of the poison control center.

PRECAUTIONS

- Keep the phone numbers of the local poison control center, your doctor, and emergency services (fire, police, ambulance) next to your telephone. Don't wait for an emergency to look them up.

- Always keep syrup of ipecac in your medicine cabinet. Check the expiration date periodically.

- Never induce vomiting in a child who is not fully conscious.

- Be aware that in the case of some poisons, vomiting should not be induced. See page 170 for examples.

- Keep all poisonous substances (see page 170 for a list of common poisons) out of the reach of children, preferably in a locked cupboard to which only you have the key.

- Never store a dangerous substance in anything but its original container.

- Do not keep medications in unlabeled containers.

- Make sure all medications have child-resistant caps.

- Many drugs and vitamin and mineral supplements look and taste like candy. Teach your child that medicine isn't candy, and don't present medicine or vitamins as a treat.

- Be aware that more children are fatally poisoned by adult aspirin than by children's aspirin.

- Iron tablets taste sweet but can be deadly.

- Keep your child away from dangerous substances in other people's homes and be alert to the possibility that visitors to your home may bring such substances with them.

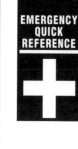

Poisoning

COMMON POISONS

Adhesives (such as glue and paste)
Aftershave
Alcoholic beverages
Ammonia
Antifreeze
Art materials
Aspirin and acetaminophen
Auto wax
Baby powder
Batteries
Benzene
Bleach
Boric acid
Carbon tetrachloride
Cleaning products
Correction fluid
Cosmetics
Deodorants
Dishwasher detergent
Disinfectants
Drain cleaners
Fertilizers
Floor wax
Fungicides
Furniture polish
Gasoline
Grease remover
Hair-care products
Houseplants (some)
Ink
Insecticides and pest strips
Insect repellent
Iodine
Kerosene
Laundry products
Laxatives
Lighter fluid
Lye
Medications of any kind
Moth repellents
Motor oil
Mouse and rat poison
Mouthwash
Nail polish and remover
Naphtha
Oil of wintergreen

Oven cleaner
Paint and paint thinner
Perfume
Pet medications
Petroleum distillates
Plant sprays
Room deodorizers
Rubbing alcohol
Rust remover
Scabicides
Shampoo
Shoe polish
Soaps
Solvents
Swimming pool and aquarium
    chemicals
Tobacco
Toilet bowl cleaner
Turpentine
Vitamin and mineral supplements
Weed killer
Windshield washer solution

DO NOT INDUCE VOMITING OF:

Acids
Ammonia
Benzene
Bleach
Carbon tetrachloride
Cleaning fluid
Correction fluid
Dishwasher detergent
Drain cleaner
Gasoline
Glue
Insect spray
Kerosene
Lye
Oven cleaner
Paint thinner
Petroleum distillates
Polishes
Solvents
Tobacco products
Turpentine

Poison ivy

SYMPTOMS
- Blistered rash
- Itching

HOME CARE
- To remove the irritant from the skin, bathe the child immediately with soap and water and scrub the fingernails.
- Contaminated clothing and shoes should be laundered.
- Applying calamine lotion to the rash and giving nonprescription antihistamines by mouth may help relieve itching.

PRECAUTIONS
- If the child scratches the rash, the skin may become susceptible to impetigo. Watch for signs of infection.
- Teach your child to recognize and avoid poison ivy.
- Dress your child in long pants and socks when he or she is in the woods or other areas where poison ivy grows.
- If the rash continues to spread after several days, it means that the child is still coming in contact with the plant. Try to locate the source of the contact.

Polio

SYMPTOMS

- General bodily discomfort
- Fever
- Sore throat
- Nausea
- Sore, stiff muscles
- Stiff neck or spine

HOME CARE

- Be sure that your child is adequately protected against polio by immunization.

PRECAUTIONS

- If you suspect that your child has polio, take the child to the doctor.
- A child needs the full series of immunizations (including boosters) to receive long-lasting immunity.
- If the child originally received the Salk polio vaccine, he or she must have boosters or receive a full series of the Sabin vaccine in order to be fully protected.
- Polio is caused by one of three different viruses, and recovery from infection by any one of the three confers immunity against that virus only. It is, therefore, possible to have three separate attacks of polio.

Puncture wounds

SYMPTOM
- A wound that is deeper than it is long or wide

HOME CARE
- Wash the wound carefully and apply a nonirritating antiseptic.

- If no foreign body remains in the wound, cover the area with a sterile bandage and inspect it regularly for signs of infection.

- If a foreign body remains in the wound, take the child to the doctor.

PRECAUTIONS
- A puncture wound in the head, neck, abdomen, or chest or in a joint requires **immediate medical attention**.

- Never try to remove a foreign body (for example, a needle or a knife blade) from a puncture wound yourself.

- A puncture wound that is still tender after a day or two should be seen by a doctor.

- Redness, swelling, or stiffness of the joint at the site of a puncture wound is a **medical emergency**. Take the child to the doctor immediately.

- Make sure that your child's tetanus immunization status is always current.

Rashes

SYMPTOM

■ Red patches, blisters, or spots on the skin

HOME CARE

■ If the rash causes itching, have the child take warm baths, or apply a soothing lotion, such as calamine.

PRECAUTIONS

■ Do not be concerned about a rash that disappears within a few days and does not recur.

■ Certain distinctive rashes are symptoms of specific diseases. A rash caused by a disease will be accompanied by other symptoms.

Reye's syndrome

SYMPTOMS
- Severe vomiting

- Unusual drowsiness

- Overactivity or confusion in a child recovering from a viral infection

HOME CARE
- **Do not attempt home treatment.** Consult a doctor immediately.

PRECAUTIONS
- Reye's syndrome usually attacks children and teenagers who are recovering from a viral infection. Children between the ages of 5 and 11 years are at the highest risk.

- **Do not** give aspirin to a child who has chicken pox or influenza. Reye's syndrome has been associated with the use of aspirin in treating viral infections. Acetaminophen, an aspirin substitute that has not been linked to Reye's syndrome, can be used instead. Sponge baths may also help to bring down a fever.

- Reye's syndrome is fatal in 25 percent of cases. Early diagnosis and treatment are vital.

Ringworm

SYMPTOM

■ Scaly, red rash

HOME CARE

■ Ask your doctor to suggest a nonprescription antifungal ointment, and apply it to the infected area until the skin is clear.

PRECAUTIONS

■ If a rash does not improve after several days of home treatment, see your doctor. The rash may not be ringworm.

■ If home treatment seems to make the rash worse, discontinue treatment and see your doctor. The child's skin may be sensitive to the medication you are using.

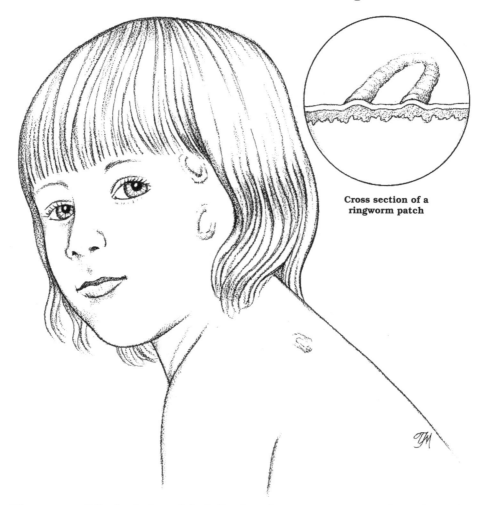

Cross section of a ringworm patch

Ringworm of the body is a skin infection that appears as oval, scaly, red patches that enlarge while healing proceeds from the center.

Rocky Mountain spotted fever

SYMPTOMS

- Headache

- Fever

- Loss of appetite

- Rash

HOME CARE

- This condition requires medical attention.

- Watch carefully for symptoms in a child who has been bitten by ticks. If you suspect that the disease is present, take the child to the doctor at once.

PRECAUTIONS

- Never remove ticks from a dog with your fingers. Use tweezers.

- Use a tick repellent to keep your dog free of ticks.

- Do not allow your child to touch wild rabbits.

- If your child is bitten by a tick, observe the child closely for a week afterward.

- Note that Rocky Mountain spotted fever **always needs medical attention**. It can be fatal if left untreated.

Roseola

SYMPTOMS

- High fever

- Runny nose

- Slight redness of the throat

- Slight enlargement of the lymph nodes in the neck

- Rash

HOME CARE

- To help control fever, give acetaminophen and have the child take lukewarm baths.

PRECAUTIONS

- Roseola does *not* cause coughing, vomiting, diarrhea, eye or ear discharge, or extreme fatigue or collapse. Any of these symptoms should be brought to your doctor's attention.

- Fever caused by roseola typically cannot be kept down consistently with acetaminophen.

- Another common illness that may produce a high fever but few other symptoms is infection of the urinary tract. This is more common in girls.

Rubella

SYMPTOMS
- Swollen lymph nodes
- Rash on face, spreading to body
- Low-grade fever
- Slight loss of appetite
- Slight redness of throat and whites of eyes

HOME CARE
- Give acetaminophen to relieve fever.
- Keep your child isolated from pregnant women.

PRECAUTIONS
- Rubella contracted during the first three months of pregnancy presents a 50-50 chance of damage to the fetus. Before trying to become pregnant, a woman should be tested to find out if she is immune to rubella. If she is not immune, she should be vaccinated at least three months before trying to become pregnant.
- A pregnant woman who has been exposed to rubella should consult an obstetrician immediately.
- All children should be immunized against rubella.

Scabies

SYMPTOMS

■ Severe itching

■ Small red dots or black or gray lines on the skin

HOME CARE

■ Give nonprescription antihistamines to relieve itching.

■ Carefully follow the doctor's instructions for treating scabies.

■ Carefully launder the infected child's undergarments, bedding, and towels to destroy the mites.

PRECAUTIONS

■ If mites attack the skin around a nursing mother's nipples, scabies can occur on her baby's face.

■ Secondary infection can occur if the child scratches the infested skin.

■ Consult a doctor before using any medications for scabies.

■ Consult a doctor before applying any medication to the face of a baby with scabies.

■ Lindane ointment and lotion, which are sometimes prescribed to treat scabies, are poisonous and should be kept out of the reach of children.

■ If treatment does not clear up scabies, the person may be reinfested. Consult your doctor.

■ Scabies is easily transferred from one person to another.

Scoliosis

SYMPTOMS

■ Visibly curved spine

■ Standing position with one hip thrust forward

HOME CARE

■ Check the child's posture periodically.

PRECAUTION

■ Scoliosis can worsen rapidly. See your doctor if you suspect scoliosis.

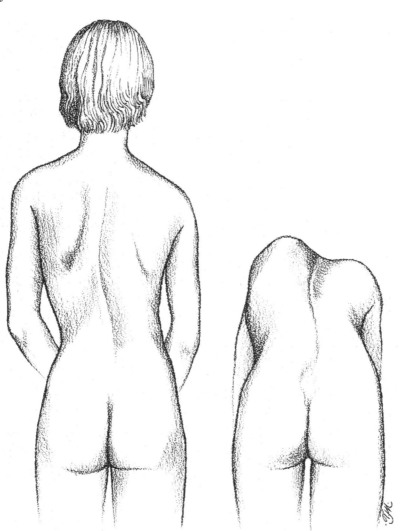

Severe scoliosis can be seen from the back when the child stands up, and even mild scoliosis is evident when the child bends forward at the waist. Bending forward causes the chest to rotate, making one side of the back prominent.

Scrapes

SYMPTOM

- A skin wound that is longer and wider than it is deep

HOME CARE

- Wash the wound with soap and water and look carefully for embedded dirt or any other foreign matter.

- Stop bleeding by covering the wound with gauze and applying gentle pressure.

- If there is no dirt embedded in the wound, apply a nonstinging antiseptic, cover the scrape, and keep it covered until it has completely healed.

- If necessary, scrub the wound gently to remove embedded dirt. Liberally apply antibiotic ointment twice a day during healing. Keep the area covered with a sterile bandage.

- If a scrape is on an area that is subject to constant movement (such as a joint), ointment should be applied periodically to prevent cracking.

PRECAUTIONS

- Do not treat at home any wound that involves the full thickness of the skin (bleeds evenly) or has deeply embedded dirt. Take the child to the doctor.

- If dirt is left in a scrape, it may cause infection or become sealed under the skin.

- A scrape that bleeds evenly over its entire surface requires medical attention.

- Tetanus may develop after a scrape, so keep your child's tetanus immunization status up to date.

- Impetigo may begin at the site of an abrasion.

Shingles

SYMPTOMS

- Listlessness

- Fever

- Pain and tenderness along a nerve

- Blistery rash

- Enlarged lymph nodes

HOME CARE

- Give acetaminophen—not aspirin—to relieve pain.

PRECAUTIONS

- People who have shingles may transmit chicken pox. Consult your doctor if a child who has not had chicken pox or is at high risk from the complications of chicken pox is exposed to someone with shingles.

- A child who is taking steroid medications is at high risk of contracting chicken pox from someone with shingles.

- If shingles involves the eye, consult an ophthalmologist (eye specialist).

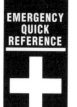

Shock

SYMPTOMS

- Weakness

- Faintness

- Rapid, weak pulse

- Paleness

- Cold, clammy skin

- Cold sweat

- Chills

- Dry mouth

- Nausea

- Rapid, shallow breathing

- Restlessness

- Confusion

EMERGENCY TREATMENT

1. Stop any bleeding and make sure that the child's airway is open.

2. Get professional help immediately. Call the police or the paramedic squad.

3. If there is possible neck or back injury, do not move the child. If there is a head injury, have the child lie flat without elevating the feet. Otherwise, keep the child lying flat with the legs raised.

4. Keep the child warm.

5. Do not offer food or water.

PRECAUTION

- **Shock can be fatal** if the victim does not get immediate professional emergency care.

Shortness of breath

SYMPTOM

■ Breathing rate higher than normal

HOME CARE

■ None, unless shortness of breath is caused by anxiety. Ask your doctor for advice.

PRECAUTIONS

■ Do not be concerned if your child breathes more rapidly during a fever. Fever increases the breathing rate.

■ High doses of aspirin increase the breathing rate.

■ Contact your doctor if your healthy child breathes rapidly while at rest.

Sickle cell anemia

SYMPTOMS
- Weakness
- Fatigue
- Swelling of the joints
- Pain

HOME CARE
- See your doctor for instructions about home care.

PRECAUTIONS
- Sickle cell trait and sickle cell disease occur most often in persons of African descent and are found in many black Americans. Children of black parents and children with a family history of sickle cell disease should be tested before the age of one year.

- A child with sickle cell disease may get frequent infections and illnesses. Treat all infections immediately.

- If a child with sickle cell disease runs a high fever, call the doctor.

- A child with sickle cell disease should have frequent checkups.

- A child with the disease may need special treatment before surgery or dental work.

- No special treatment is needed if the child has sickle cell trait.

Sinusitis

SYMPTOMS

■ Yellow or milky discharge from the nose

■ Fever

■ Pain

■ Stuffy nose

■ Cough

■ Red, swollen eyelids

■ Headache

HOME CARE

■ Protect the child against sinusitis by giving decongestant cold remedies for a cold and having the child use saline nose drops or by treating an allergy with antihistamines. Consult your doctor about the type and duration of such treatment.

■ Give acetaminophen for pain. Warmth applied to the face also helps relieve pain.

PRECAUTIONS

■ A child with symptoms of sinusitis accompanied by a high fever should be seen by a doctor.

■ See a doctor if the child has a puslike discharge or other symptoms of sinusitis on one side of the nose only.

Sore heels

SYMPTOM
- Pain and tenderness

HOME CARE
- Pad the heels of the child's shoes and temporarily restrict activities that involve running and jumping.

PRECAUTIONS
- Inability to move the foot up and down may indicate a torn Achilles tendon. This condition needs medical attention.

- Have the child seen by a doctor if home treatment does not promptly relieve sore heels.

- Pain may recur following a new injury. Repeat the treatment.

Sore throat

SYMPTOMS

- Pain

- Swollen lymph nodes in the neck

- Difficulty in swallowing

HOME CARE

- Have the child gargle with salt water and drink extra fluids.

- Give acetaminophen to relieve pain.

- Keep the child isolated until the cause of the sore throat has been diagnosed.

PRECAUTIONS

- A doctor should examine any child with a sore throat accompanied by any of the following symptoms: swollen or tender lymph nodes in the neck, persistent difficulty in swallowing, puslike discharge from the eyes or nose, earache, sinus pain, breathing difficulty, chest pain, rash, stiff neck, weakness or exhaustion, confusion, repeated vomiting.

- Any child with a sore throat and fever that are still getting worse after 24 to 36 hours should be seen by a doctor.

- A child with a sore throat should be kept away from other children, particularly infants, until a diagnosis has been made.

Speech problems and stuttering

SYMPTOMS

■ Marked delay in achieving speech

■ Continued stuttering or stammering

HOME CARE

■ Speak to and listen to your baby in order to encourage speech.

■ Correct a child's speech gently. Do not finish your child's sentences or respond before he or she finishes a sentence. Never punish or ignore the child for incorrect speech or try to make the child practice speaking.

■ Do not get angry or anxious if the child stutters, and don't let other children tease or ridicule the child.

■ Do not use "baby talk" when speaking to your baby.

PRECAUTIONS

■ Consult your doctor if your child's speech patterns do not appear to be developing according to the normally accepted timetable.

■ Children learn to speak by imitation. Speak, sing, and read to your child.

■ A child who is not speaking clearly should not be forced to practice speaking, be deliberately misunderstood or teased, or have attention drawn to his or her speech.

■ Consult a doctor if your child speaks only in a monotone, has a marked nasal quality to his or her speech, or seems to be regressing rather than improving in vocabulary or pronunciation.

■ Stuttering between the ages of two and five years old is not a problem unless it persists for several months.

■ Severe, constant, or prolonged stuttering requires professional attention.

Sprains and dislocations

POSSIBLE SYMPTOMS

- Pain
- Swelling
- Tenderness
- Stiffness
- Internal bleeding
- Visible malformation
- Inability to use the joint

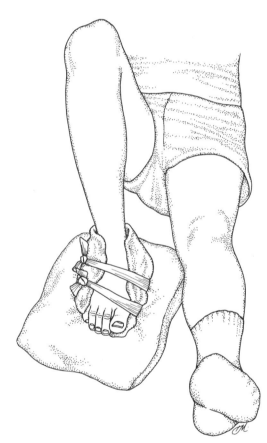

A sprain can be treated by immobilizing, elevating, and resting the affected area and by applying cold compresses soon after the injury. A dislocation should not be treated at home.

HOME CARE

- A dislocation should not be treated at home.(A possible exception is elbow dislocation in a child who has had previous elbow dislocations; see *Dislocated elbow* for the specific instances in which home treatment may be acceptable.)

- A sprain can be treated by immobilizing and then resting the affected area.

- Cold compresses applied to the area help relieve swelling.

- Aspirin or acetaminophen can be given for pain.

PRECAUTIONS

- A sprain that does not improve rapidly may indicate a bone fracture and should be examined by a doctor.

- After a dislocation has been corrected, the joint may remain unstable for some time.

- A severe sprain that is improperly treated can result in a permanently weak joint.

- A sprain that is still swollen or painful to move is not healed.

- Elastic bandages do not adequately support or protect a sprained ankle.

Stomachache, acute

SYMPTOMS

- Sudden abdominal pain
- Crampy pain
- Diarrhea
- Vomiting

HOME CARE

- Apply mild heat to the abdomen.
- Treat constipation by changing the child's diet (including more roughage, such as is found in most fruits, vegetables, and unrefined grains) or by using a glycerin suppository.
- If the child seems to develop a stomachache at mealtime, the problem may be the need to have a bowel movement.

PRECAUTIONS

- Do not try to relieve stomach pain by giving a laxative or placing ice on the stomach.
- If the child's pain does not seem to be due to constipation, digestive tract upset, or emotional stress, take the child to the doctor.
- If the stomach pain is accompanied by fever and painful urination, the child should be seen by a doctor.
- If pain is accompanied by a fever and a cough, see a doctor.
- If any stomach pain persists or gets worse, consult a doctor.
- Severe, crampy stomach pain accompanied by blood or mucus in the stool requires a doctor's attention.

- Be concerned if the stomach pain causes the child to bend forward while walking.
- Severe pain that follows injury to the abdomen or lower chest may indicate internal injury and requires a doctor's attention.

Stomachache, chronic

SYMPTOM

■ Recurrent abdominal pain not accompanied by any other symptoms

HOME CARE

■ If constipation is most likely causing the stomachaches, give the child a high-fiber diet including plenty of fruits and juices. For immediate relief, use a glycerin suppository.

■ If you have any reason to believe that milk intolerance may be causing the stomachaches, ask your doctor if you should temporarily remove milk and milk products from the diet.

■ Try to remove any source of stress that may be causing the stomachache.

■ Record the pattern of the pains so that you can explain the condition to the doctor if necessary.

PRECAUTIONS

■ Stomach pain due to emotional stress is not a product of the child's imagination; it is as real as a pain produced by a physical condition and should be treated accordingly.

■ Do not try to relieve stomach pain by giving laxatives or by placing ice on the stomach.

Strep infections

SYMPTOMS

- Headache

- Fever

- Sore, red throat

- Swollen lymph nodes in the neck

- Vomiting

- Abdominal pain

- Rash (sometimes)

HOME CARE

- Give aspirin, ibuprofen, or acetaminophen to relieve pain and fever, and take the child to the doctor.

PRECAUTIONS

- Keep infants away from groups of children, who may be carriers (persons who harbor a disease-causing organism and can pass it on to others without getting the disease themselves) of the strep bacteria.

- Even if your child appears to be better, do not discontinue treatment until he or she has taken all the medication prescribed by the doctor.

- A strep infection imparts immunity only to the particular type of bacteria that caused it. (There are over 60 types of streptococcus organisms.)

- If a child who is being treated with antibiotics for a strep throat does not respond to the medication within 24 to 48 hours, inform the doctor; the child may have infectious mononucleosis as well.

Styes

SYMPTOMS

- Swelling, pain, and redness of the eyelid

- Formation of pus and a "head"

HOME CARE

- Bathe a stye with warm water several times a day.

- You may give aspirin or acetaminophen to help reduce pain.

- Apply antibiotic ointment to prevent reinfection.

PRECAUTIONS

- Styes do not cause redness of the white of the eye. Consult your doctor if redness appears.

- See a doctor if a stye recurs or if it is accompanied by fever, headache, loss of appetite, or lethargy.

- Washcloths and towels used by the infected child should be kept separate from those used by other family members.

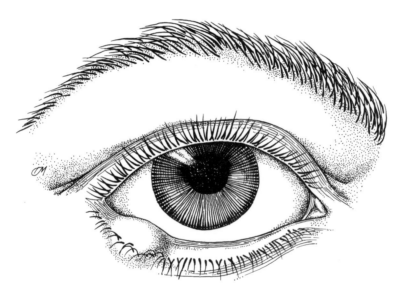

A stye is a boil that occurs in the oil or sweat glands in the upper or lower eyelid.

Sudden infant death syndrome

SYMPTOMS

■ None

HOME CARE

■ If an infant is considered to be in a high-risk category, the doctor will make recommendations for home care to guard against sudden infant death syndrome (SIDS).

PRECAUTIONS

■ Every parent should know how to revive an infant who has stopped breathing. The best way to learn the proper technique is to take one of the courses in cardiopulmonary resuscitation (CPR) that are offered by local hospitals and community organizations. If, for some reason, taking such a course is not possible, ask your doctor to demonstrate the technique.

■ Certain factors, including premature birth, low birth weight, and lack of medical care for the mother during pregnancy, make some babies more at risk than others.

■ SIDS is more common in families in which it has occurred before.

■ No one knows what causes SIDS. There are many different theories, some contradicting others.

Sunburn

SYMPTOM

- Red, blistering, painful skin

HOME CARE

- Prevent sunburn by regulating the child's exposure to the sun and using an appropriate sunscreen.

- If the child does get burned, apply cold water compresses to the burned area, followed by cocoa butter, burn ointment, or a paste of baking soda and water.

- Give aspirin or acetaminophen for pain and nonprescription antihistamines for itching.

- Avoid breaking the blisters of sunburn.

PRECAUTIONS

- The sunscreen used on a child should contain para-aminobenzoic acid (PABA), titanium dioxide, or sulisobenzone.

- Sunscreens come off in water. Follow the instructions for reapplying the product after the child has been swimming.

- Remember that children and babies can be burned by sunlight coming through an open window.

- Use sunburn medication sparingly; it can be absorbed through the skin and cause side effects.

- Skin damage from overuse of sunlamps is often seen in teenagers.

- Some medications increase sensitivity to the sun. Ask the doctor if a medication your child is taking has this effect.

- A child who has a sunburn accompanied by fever or extreme fatigue or weakness needs a doctor's care.

- Fair-skinned babies and children can burn even on cloudy days or in the shade.

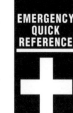

Swallowed objects

EMERGENCY SYMPTOMS

■ Choking

■ Inability to breathe or cry

EMERGENCY TREATMENT

■ Call the police or paramedic squad.

■ See the section on *Choking* (page 71).

OTHER SYMPTOMS

■ Gagging

■ Pain in the throat or chest

■ Difficulty in swallowing

■ Abdominal pain

■ Vomiting

HOME CARE

■ Ask your doctor whether immediate medical attention is necessary.

■ Examine the stools until the swallowed object has passed. If it does not appear within one week, notify the doctor.

PRECAUTIONS

■ An object lodged in the esophagus (the tube through which food passes on its way to the stomach) must be removed promptly (within hours) by a doctor.

■ Do not give the child a laxative in an effort to speed passage of a swallowed object.

■ No medication or other agent is available to speed up or make safer the passage of a swallowed object through the digestive tract.

■ Any object that has not left the body within one week should be reported to the doctor.

■ Keep small objects out of the reach of babies and toddlers. Examine toys for parts that might be swallowed.

Swimmer's ear

SYMPTOMS

■ Itching or clogging of the ear canal

■ Discharge from the ear canal

■ Pain

■ Fever

■ Swollen, tender lymph nodes in the area of the ear

HOME CARE

■ To relieve pain, give aspirin or acetaminophen and apply warm compresses to the outside of the ear.

■ Try to prevent swimmer's ear in a susceptible child by drying the ear canals after each swimming session. To do this, place a few drops of rubbing alcohol or glycerin in each ear.

■ After administering any eardrops, keep the child's head tilted for a little while so that the drops can penetrate deeply into the ear canal.

PRECAUTIONS

■ Severe pain, fever, or swollen lymph nodes near the ear or failure to respond to home treatment within a few days indicates that the child should be seen by a doctor.

■ Never attempt to clean inside a child's ear canal.

Teething

SYMPTOMS

- Drooling
- Fretfulness
- Sleeplessness
- Loss of appetite
- Pain or discomfort
- Chewing on fingers or objects

HOME CARE

- Give the baby zwieback toast, teething biscuits, or a teething ring to bite on. This will help the teeth erupt.
- To ease pain, give aspirin or acetaminophen, rub the gums with a cold object, or have the child bite on a cold object.
- Distract the baby with activities.

PRECAUTIONS

- Do not be too quick to assume a baby's symptoms are caused by teething; look for other causes. A baby may be fretful, wakeful at night, or unwilling to eat for many reasons other than teething.
- Teething does not cause fever, cough, or discharge from the nose.
- Diarrhea and constipation are not related to teething unless there has also been a significant change in the child's diet.
- Do not try to force-feed a child whose eating and drinking habits change during teething.
- Drooling from teething may cause the face to become chapped, but rashes are due to other causes.
- Overuse of teething ointments and solutions that contain local anesthetics can be harmful.
- **Never** apply aspirin directly to the gums.

Testis, torsion of

SYMPTOMS

■ Increasing pain and swelling of the testis

■ Discoloration of the skin of the scrotum

■ Nausea

■ Vomiting

■ Lower abdominal pain

■ Fever

HOME CARE

■ None. Torsion of the testis is an **emergency** and requires immediate professional care.

PRECAUTIONS

■ Do not attempt to treat this condition at home. The child must see a doctor **immediately**.

■ If pain near a testis increases and the testis is swollen, tender, or discolored, take the child to a doctor at once.

■ Lower abdominal pain or pain in the groin may indicate torsion in a boy who has an undescended testis that has not been corrected.

■ If pain increases following an injury or bruise to the testis, suspect torsion.

■ **Never delay treatment** of torsion of the testis. Hours count.

Testis, undescended

SYMPTOM

■ Failure of one or both testes to rest in the scrotum at birth

HOME CARE

■ Check periodically to see if the testis has descended. If it has not descended by the age of one year, consult your doctor.

PRECAUTIONS

■ An undescended testis that is not treated may become twisted, injured, or cancerous.

■ An undescended testis should be treated before the child is four years old. If an undescended testis is not corrected before the age of four years, body heat may cause it to become damaged and unable to produce sperm.

■ Do not worry the child by discussing the condition.

Tetanus

SYMPTOMS

- Muscle stiffness, especially of the jaw and neck

- Difficulty in swallowing

- Pain in the extremities

- Muscle spasms

- Convulsions

HOME CARE

- Treat all wounds, even minor ones, promptly.

PRECAUTIONS

- Tetanus can be fatal. Be sure your child is properly protected by immunization.

- Tetanus can enter the body through a cut or puncture wound, as well as a scratch, burn, insect bite, or other minor wound. All wounds should be treated at once.

- All family members should be vaccinated against tetanus.

- If a mother has not been immunized against tetanus, her newborn baby is susceptible to tetanus.

- Tetanus can infect a newborn baby through the stump of the umbilical cord. If a baby is delivered at home, be certain that strict antiseptic techniques are employed during and immediately after the birth.

Thrush

SYMPTOM

■ White, flaky plaques (patches) on the tongue and the inside of the mouth

HOME CARE

■ Follow the doctor's instructions for treating thrush.

■ Sterilize objects that are placed in the baby's mouth.

PRECAUTIONS

■ Thrush often follows antibiotic treatment and may also accompany nutritional deficiencies or long-term illness.

■ A nursing mother may have to use medication on her breasts to avoid reinfecting the child.

■ A nursing mother should be treated for diseases that could reinfect her child.

■ White plaques that occur only on the tongue are probably not due to thrush.

■ If thrush recurs frequently, it may be because objects that are placed in the baby's mouth are not being adequately sterilized. Consult your doctor.

■ Treat thrush only with products recommended by your doctor. Overuse of nonprescription products can burn the membranes of the mouth.

Thyroid disorders

SYMPTOMS
Underactive thyroid:

■ Excessive sleepiness

■ Choking while nursing

■ Severe constipation

■ Noisy breathing

■ Retarded growth

■ Protruding tongue

■ Hoarse cry

■ Thick, dry skin

■ Goiter (in some cases)

Overactive thyroid:

■ Irritability

■ Restlessness

■ Behavior problems

■ Hand tremors

■ Increased appetite without weight gain

■ Excessive sweating

■ Protruding eyeballs

■ Goiter (in some cases)

HOME CARE

■ Take your child for regular checkups.

■ Be aware of signs that might indicate thyroid malfunction.

PRECAUTIONS

■ Some symptoms of underactive thyroid may appear in older children whose thyroid is normal. Only a doctor can diagnose thyroid malfunction.

■ A cyst on the neck should be seen by a doctor. It could be an abnormally positioned thyroid gland.

Tics

SYMPTOM

■ Jerky, spasmodic muscle movements

HOME CARE

■ Try to find out if any type of stress may be causing the problem.

■ Do not nag or punish the child or call attention to the tics.

PRECAUTION

■ Everyone in the child's environment must cooperate in ignoring the tics.

■ Tics that persist for more than a few weeks or accompany other symptoms or unusual types of behavior may indicate a potentially serious problem and require professional attention.

■ Tics can be caused by physical conditions. The diagnosis should be made by a doctor.

Tonsillitis

SYMPTOMS

■ Sore, red throat

■ Inflamed tonsils, often with white or yellow spots

■ Fever

HOME CARE

■ Treat as you would treat a cold or sore throat.

■ Give acetaminophen for fever and pain.

■ Give the child plenty of fluids.

PRECAUTIONS

■ Drooling accompanying a sore throat should be brought to the attention of your doctor **immediately**.

■ Between the ages of three and nine years, children often have enlarged tonsils and adenoids. This enlargement is normal and should not be confused with infection.

■ White, cheesy material on the tonsils is normal and does not indicate infection.

■ If a child is eating poorly, the cause is usually something other than enlarged tonsils.

Toothache

SYMPTOMS

■ Pain

■ Redness and swelling of the gums

HOME CARE

■ Give aspirin or acetaminophen for pain.

■ Apply an ice pack to the jaw.

PRECAUTIONS

■ Do not apply heat to the site of a toothache.

■ A careful program of dental hygiene is the first defense against toothache. Your child should brush his or her teeth at least once daily and use dental floss if possible.

■ Have your child see the dentist regularly beginning at age two or three years.

■ **Never** apply aspirin directly to the site of a toothache.

■ Provide extra fluoride if the water in your area is not fluoridated. Ask your doctor or dentist about this.

Toxic shock syndrome

SYMPTOMS

- High fever

- Vomiting

- Diarrhea

- Sunburnlike rash

- Peeling of the skin on the palms of the hands and the soles of the feet

- Blurred vision

- Confusion

HOME CARE

- Toxic shock syndrome requires **immediate** medical attention. Do not attempt home care.

PRECAUTIONS

- Although rare, toxic shock syndrome can be fatal.

- This disease develops very suddenly and progresses rapidly.

- Toxic shock syndrome is not limited to menstruating women and girls. It has also occurred in children, men, and nonmenstruating women.

- Tampon use may promote an environment favorable to the growth of the causative bacteria. If tampons are used, they should be used alternately with sanitary napkins whenever possible, changed frequently, and not used at night.

- Toxic shock syndrome can affect patients recovering from burns or surgery and persons with boils or abscesses.

Toxoplasmosis

SYMPTOMS

- Minor illness produces few symptoms

- Severe illness causes high fever

HOME CARE

- Prevention is the best home care.

PRECAUTIONS

- Toxoplasmosis in a pregnant woman can harm the fetus.

- A pregnant woman should avoid eating raw or undercooked meat.

- A pregnant woman should not handle or clean a cat's litter box during the pregnancy.

- It is not necessary to get rid of the family cat if someone in the household is pregnant. However, do not introduce a new pet, especially a cat, during the first three months of a pregnancy.

Ulcers

SYMPTOMS
- Abdominal pain
- Vomiting of blood
- Blood in stools

HOME CARE
- The only home care recommended in the case of a suspected ulcer is to give the child an antacid by mouth. The child should be under a doctor's care.

PRECAUTIONS
- Ulcers do not usually cause ordinary stomachaches in children.
- Intense, highly motivated children, particularly those with family problems, may be susceptible to ulcers.
- If a child is under stress, his or her abdominal pain is more likely to be caused by the stress than by an ulcer.
- When more than one member of a family has ulcers, the cause is more likely to be shared stress than a hereditary factor.
- Black, tarry stools can be caused not only by the presence of blood but also by the ingestion of iron supplements and some foods.

Urinary tract infections

SYMPTOMS

- Frequent, urgent, or painful urination
- Dribbling of urine
- Bed-wetting
- Inability to control urination
- Abnormal urine
- Fever
- Abdominal or back pain
- Chronic diarrhea
- Vomiting
- Redness of external genitals

HOME CARE

- Do not attempt home treatment. If symptoms are present, the child should be seen by a doctor.

PRECAUTIONS

- Attempted home treatment can cause a low-grade, chronic infection.
- In many cases, there will be a fever but no other symptoms, and the infection will not be evident in the course of a physical examination.
- A urine sample should be collected at the midpoint of urination.
- An infant in whom such an infection is suspected should be examined as soon as possible to find the underlying cause.

Vaginal bleeding

SYMPTOM

- Bleeding that is not due to normal menstruation

HOME CARE

- If there is a burning sensation on urination, have the child urinate while in a bathtub of water (to dilute the urine) and then bathe in fresh water.

- Bleeding due to minor bruises or lacerations can be treated at home. All other abnormal vaginal bleeding requires medical attention.

PRECAUTIONS

- If a girl is less than nine or ten years old and has vaginal bleeding with or without breast development, she should be seen by a doctor.

- If there is any suspicion of sexual molestation, contact your doctor immediately.

- Any girl whose mother took diethylstilbestrol (DES) during pregnancy should be seen by a gynecologist at the beginning of puberty whether or not bleeding is present.

- A baby girl may have a bloody discharge from the vagina during the first two weeks of life. This is usually a normal response to the withdrawal of the mother's hormones, but mention it to your doctor.

Vaginal discharge

SYMPTOM

■ Discharge that is irritating, pus-like, bloody, or foul smelling

HOME CARE

■ Have the child take sitz baths to which a cup of vinegar has been added.

■ Check for signs of pinworms or urinary tract infection.

■ Teach your daughter simple preventive measures, such as wearing cotton underpants, avoiding the use of chemical products in the genital area, and practicing proper techniques for cleaning herself after using the toilet.

PRECAUTIONS

■ Any girl whose mother took diethylstilbestrol (DES) while pregnant should be examined by a gynecologist (a specialist in disorders of the female reproductive system) at the beginning of puberty, whether or not vaginal discharge is present.

■ The use of chemicals in the bathwater (such as bubble bath) or vaginal sprays can cause vaginal discharge.

■ Discharge from the vagina is normal during the first two weeks of a baby girl's life and for one to two years before a girl starts menstruating. This discharge does not irritate or have a foul odor.

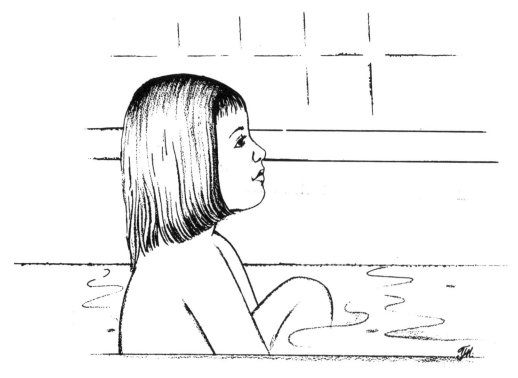

Have your child take sitz baths to which a cup of vinegar has been added.

Viral infections

SYMPTOMS

■ Vary according to the virus

HOME CARE

■ In the case of illness caused by an intestinal virus, give acetaminophen to relieve pain and fever. (Refer to the appropriate section for treatment of diseases caused by a specific virus.)

PRECAUTIONS

■ Call the doctor immediately if your child has any of the following symptoms: stiff neck or back, severe headache and vomiting, extreme weakness or collapse, confusion.

■ Consult your doctor if any of the following symptoms appears: rash resembling red sandpaper or red goose bumps; puslike discharge from eyes, nose, or ears; reddish-purple spots; tender, red, enlarged lymph nodes; severe earache; blood in the stools; severe cough; breathing difficulty.

■ Because there are so many different types of viruses, diagnosis can be very difficult.

■ Immunity against any one virus is short-lived, so a child can have one viral infection right after another.

Vision problems

SYMPTOMS

- Tilting or cocking of the head

- Looking out of the corner of the eye

- Squinting

- Crossed eyes

- Sensitivity to light

- Headaches

- Dislike of reading

- School problems

HOME CARE

- Have your child's eyes examined regularly, and be aware of the symptoms that might suggest that the child has a vision problem.

PRECAUTIONS

- A child's vision should be checked annually from the age of four years or younger.

- If your child holds books very close to the eyes when reading or cannot see the television screen from a distance, have the child's eyes checked.

Vomiting

SYMPTOM

- Forceful ejection of the contents of the stomach

HOME CARE

- Vomiting after coughing is normal, particularly in infants and young children.

- Solid foods, milk, and aspirin tablets aggravate vomiting and should not be given.

- Have the child sip ice water, carbonated beverages, tea with sugar, flavored gelatin water, apple juice, or commercial electrolyte solutions (available from your pharmacist).

PRECAUTIONS

- Prolonged or severe vomiting can cause dehydration (loss of body fluids). The younger the child, the more serious dehydration can be. Call your doctor if an infant has been vomiting for more than 12 to 24 hours or if an older child has been vomiting for more than two to three days.

- Consult your doctor if vomiting is accompanied by abdominal pain, fever, or headache.

- Abdominal pain accompanied by vomiting may indicate appendicitis.

- If vomiting and diarrhea occur at the same time, control the vomiting first.

- Some phenothiazine drugs that are given to control vomiting in adults can have serious side effects in children and should not be given.

- If the child is taking a medication, vomiting may hinder its action.

Warts

SYMPTOM

- Rough, raised growths anywhere on the skin

HOME CARE

- As a rule, leave warts alone.

- With the approval of your doctor, you can use an appropriate commercial product to safely remove most warts other than those on the eyelids or face.

PRECAUTIONS

- No treatment is successful in all cases, and warts may spread during treatment or recur afterward.

- At home, do not treat warts on the eyelids or face or warts that involve the cuticles or extend under the nails.

- If the surrounding skin becomes red or painful, discontinue home treatment.

- Most warts are harmless unless they are annoying, bleed often, or become infected.

Whooping cough

SYMPTOMS

- Runny nose

- Low-grade fever

- Severe, strangling ("whooping") cough followed by vomiting of mucus

HOME CARE

- Isolate the child from other young children.

- If the vomiting is severe, feed the child several small meals a day, rather than three large ones.

PRECAUTIONS

- Make sure that your child is adequately immunized against whooping cough. It is especially important that all infants be immunized because whooping cough in infants is often fatal.

- Whooping cough is more common than many parents and doctors believe, and 90 percent of cases are never diagnosed.

- A child who has been exposed to whooping cough should be seen by a doctor.

- A mild cough may indicate mild whooping cough, which the child can spread to others.

- Any cough that is getting progressively worse after two weeks should be brought to the attention of your doctor.

- Whooping cough is highly contagious. The infected child should be kept away from other people.

- Whooping cough can be caused by three types of bacteria, and recovery from one type does not confer immunity against the other two.

Understanding Your Child's Condition

As a concerned parent, you want to know more than what to do immediately to help your child. You want to know what's wrong with your child and why; what signs to look for; what precautions to take; what you can do at home; and what the doctor is likely to do.

You'll find those answers and more here. You'll find a clear description of each condition, what causes it, and, in some cases, when and in whom it is most likely to occur. Under "Signs and Symptoms," you'll find clues that should alert you that your child may have the condition, along with brief details on how the doctor will reach a firm diagnosis. Under "Home Care," you'll find measures you can take to make the child more comfortable. You'll also learn when home treatment should not be attempted. Under "Precautions" are listed measures to prevent your child from getting the disease and practical suggestions about how to take care of the child if he or she does get sick. This section also alerts you to possible complications that require medical attention and points out developments that are normal and don't need a doctor's care. Under "Medical Treatment," you'll learn how a doctor generally treats the condition. You'll also learn if any follow-up care or testing will be necessary.

In short, you'll get the information you need to play an active role in your child's health care.

Acne

Acne is a condition of the skin that occurs most commonly during adolescence. Acne usually appears on the face, but it may also appear on the chest and back. In its mildest form, acne appears as large blackheads and whiteheads (blind blackheads). The formation of pimples occurs in a more severe case. In the worst cases, cysts and scars form.

For generations it was mistakenly thought that acne was caused by a lack of cleanliness and a diet of junk foods. Now it is believed that acne is caused by the action of hormones during the adolescent years. Pimples are caused by normal skin germs breaking down the oil in the blackheads and forming irritating substances. The pus that results is not a sign of infection.

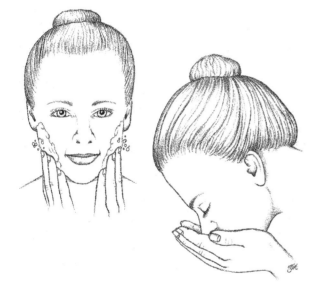

Wash the affected area twice a day with a mild soap to control acne.

SIGNS AND SYMPTOMS

The skin breaks out in red bumps, which may or may not be open. Lumps under the skin indicate that the acne has formed cysts.

HOME CARE

Wash the affected area with mild soap twice a day. After washing, apply acne preparations containing sulfur, resorcinol, salicylic acid, or mild benzoyl peroxide. Changes in the teenager's diet are unnecessary. Your doctor may suggest the use of a blackhead spoon (available at most pharmacies) for removal of large, unsightly blackheads.

Acne in young infants should not be treated with any medication. Simply wash with clear water. Notify your doctor if the condition gets worse.

PRECAUTIONS

■ To avoid making a case of acne worse, adolescents should stay away from products that can irritate the skin, such as motor oil, gasoline, and oil-containing cosmetics.
■ Do not squeeze or pick pimples—scarring may result.
■ Acne in young infants should not be treated with any medication.
■ If acne does not improve, or if cysts develop, see your doctor.
■ Never allow X-ray treatment of acne.

MEDICAL TREATMENT

Acne treatment has vastly improved in the past few years. Doctors now have a number of drugs that they can use to treat acne. Applying vitamin A ointment or liquid or prescription-strength benzoyl peroxide is often the first line of treatment. Long-term treatment using antibiotics taken by mouth is safe and effective. Applying antibiotics on the skin is another common treatment for acne; the medicine is applied once or twice a day. Disfiguring scars can be removed by a dermatologist or plastic surgeon without hospitalization once the acne has been brought under control.

RELATED TOPIC: Boils

Anemia

Anemia occurs when there is too little hemoglobin in the blood. Hemoglobin is the substance that carries oxygen in the blood and gives the blood its red color. Normally, hemoglobin is contained within the red blood cells (RBCs). A child can be anemic because there are too few RBCs, because each RBC contains too little hemoglobin, or as a result of both conditions.

There are more than 30 types of anemia, each with its own cause and treatment. The most common is iron deficiency anemia. Anemia can occur at any age. Some forms run in families; others are acquired.

Among the most common causes of anemia are a poor diet that does not include enough of the nutrients needed to manufacture hemoglobin (iron, protein, folic acid, vitamin B_{12}, and copper); the loss of blood by internal or external bleeding; failure to absorb nutrients, even though they are ingested; the formation of abnormal (short-lived) RBCs; inability of the bone marrow to produce RBCs fast enough; and the too-rapid destruction of normal RBCs within the body. In addition to the many diseases that are forms of anemia, many other illnesses can produce anemia.

SIGNS AND SYMPTOMS

Most cases of anemia produce no symptoms. However, tiredness, shortness of breath, rapid pulse, and jaundice (yellowing of the skin and the whites of the eyes) may be clues. If a child looks pale, check the nail beds, the insides of the eyelids, and the membranes inside the mouth for additional colorlessness. Also watch for these possible causes of anemia: vomiting of blood, blood in the stools (red or tarry, black bowel movements), excessive menstruation, a grossly inadequate diet, chronic diarrhea, and exposure to poisonous substances.

If you think your child might have anemia, see your doctor. The presence and type of anemia can be determined only by laboratory tests. Periodic examinations and a medical history taken by a doctor can help detect anemia early, an important factor in treatment. If one family member has anemia, watch for symptoms in other family members.

HOME CARE

Never attempt to treat anemia yourself. The wrong treatment can be harmful and will make a proper medical diagnosis difficult. All children should receive a balanced diet to prevent anemia caused by lack of proper nutrition; your doctor can give you advice on this.

PRECAUTION

■ Iron overdosing is a common cause of poisoning among children in this country. If iron supplements are prescribed by your doctor, keep them out of the reach of children. Some iron medicines are sweet, and children might mistake them for candy.

MEDICAL TREATMENT

To evaluate your child for anemia, the doctor will conduct a physical examination, take a medical history, and perform a complete blood cell count. Your doctor may also need to take a reticulocyte (young RBC) count, a platelet (a blood element that aids in clotting) count, and measurements of iron and of the iron-binding capacity in the blood. More extensive testing, if necessary, may include hemoglobin electrophoresis, sickle cell test, urinalysis, test of stools for hidden blood, examination of bone marrow, test for poisons, examination of both parents' blood, X ray of the intestinal tract, and tests of the chemical content of the blood. These tests will determine the type of anemia that is present.

The treatment prescribed may include adding supplemental iron and vitamins to the diet and changing the diet. Iron or vitamin injections are usually not necessary. In rare cases, a blood transfusion may be prescribed.

As treatment proceeds, be sure additional tests are scheduled to check on the effectiveness of the treatment. The proof of proper treatment is in the cure.

RELATED TOPICS: G6PD deficiency; Sickle cell anemia

Animal bites

Animal bites that break the skin may result in serious complications. Animal bites often become infected by bacteria from the animal's mouth and may cause tetanus (lockjaw) and rabies.

Tetanus is a serious disease caused by a type of bacterium that lives in soil, dust, and the intestines and wastes of animals and humans. The bacterium can easily enter the body through puncture wounds or scratches caused by animal bites and claw wounds. A vaccine to prevent tetanus is available.

Rabies is a fatal disease of the central nervous system that may affect any mammal. It is caused by a virus that can be identified in the brain of an affected animal. Rabies is transmitted through the saliva of the sick animal. It is most commonly found in the United States among skunks, foxes, cattle, dogs, bats, cats, and raccoons.

SIGNS AND SYMPTOMS

Even in younger children, an animal bite is usually obvious from its appearance. It is

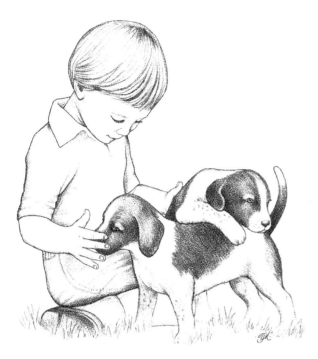

Make sure that your child's tetanus immunization is current and that your pets have been vaccinated against rabies.

sometimes difficult to tell a bite from a claw wound; however, claw wounds should be treated in the same way as bites because a claw wound can also contain bacteria from the animal's saliva. If the bite has caused a bruise but there is no break in the skin, you do not need to worry about rabies or tetanus.

HOME CARE

Scrub the wound with soap and water for five to ten minutes and flush with water. Apply antiseptic to minor wounds. Consult your doctor immediately for advice concerning rabies, tetanus, and repair of the wound. Your doctor will need to know when your child was most recently vaccinated against tetanus.

The likelihood that an animal bite will become infected is very high. If redness begins spreading out from the wound or if the wound becomes more tender, call your doctor.

If at all possible, the animal that bit the child should be inspected for rabies. Because catching an animal can be extremely dangerous, call the local police, health authorities, or animal control agency, and allow them to deal with the animal. If the animal is a pet, find out if it has been vaccinated against rabies. In some states, all animal bites must be reported to the police.

PRECAUTIONS

■ Make sure that your child's tetanus immunization status is up to date.
■ Always contact your doctor about treatment in the case of animal bites.
■ Be sure that your own pets (dogs and cats) receive regular rabies shots.

MEDICAL TREATMENT

Because of the high possibility of infection, your doctor may decide not to stitch the wound. However, if the wound is located where scarring is not desirable (such as on the face), the doctor may choose to stitch the wound. Treatment begins with removal of injured tissue and thorough cleansing. Antibiotics taken by mouth may be prescribed. If necessary, your doctor may give the child a tetanus booster or antitoxin (a substance that counteracts the poisonous effects of the tetanus bacterium).

The decision to give antirabies vaccine, with or without antiserum, is difficult to make. There is a possibility of serious reactions. However, with new antirabies vaccines now being tested, the likelihood of serious reactions may be lessened. Your doctor will arrange for examination of the animal for rabies. If the animal is not caught, the decision depends on the likelihood of rabies in your area, the circumstances of the bite (provoked or unprovoked), and the species of the animal. Local and state health departments can provide information to help you make this decision.

RELATED TOPICS: Bruises; Cat scratch fever; Cuts; Puncture wounds; Scrapes; Tetanus

Anorexia nervosa

Anorexia nervosa means literally "nervous loss of appetite." Actually, however, persons with this condition—almost always female and from middle-class homes—do not lose their appetites. Rather, they willfully suppress the urge to eat in an unhealthy desire to lose more and more weight. In short, they starve themselves because they mistakenly believe that they are fat and need to diet.

After a certain point, anorexia nervosa leads to the cessation of menstruation. It also causes the destruction of healthy muscle and organ tissue that the body must use as an energy source in the absence of food. Ultimately, anorexic patients may starve themselves to death.

Anorexia nervosa is considered to be principally caused by serious psychological problems. Anorexic youngsters are usually obedient, successful children who try to do everything expected of them by parents, teachers, and friends. The anorexic's strenuous dieting and exercising may represent a desire to gain absolute control over at least one part of her life.

Anorexic girls may also try to deny the onset of adulthood by dieting away all the signs of mature femininity: breasts, curved hips, and rounded thighs. The lack of menstrual periods, too, is a reminder of childhood.

In addition, the current preoccupation of our culture with thinness as the ideal of attractiveness fuels the anorexic's desire to starve herself to the "perfect" weight. Frequently, the condition arises after a casual remark that the girl is slightly overweight.

The anorexic's fear of becoming fat is accompanied by a distorted body image that makes it impossible for her to realize how unattractively thin she has become. Often when an anorexic looks in the mirror, she perceives herself as fat when in reality she is exceedingly thin.

SIGNS AND SYMPTOMS

The anorexic develops an aversion to eating, which cannot be overcome by threats or appeals to reason. The dieting is accompanied by overly vigorous exercise to burn off the few calories that she does consume. Although she refuses to eat more than tiny amounts of certain foods, she is often obsessed with the subject of food and may prepare elaborate meals for others.

The anorexic may go on eating binges, after which she forces herself to vomit. Excessive use of laxatives is also common.

After a certain percentage of body fat has been lost, menstruation will automatically cease. Fine, downy hair may begin to grow all over the patient's body.

HOME CARE

An anorexic child should be under a doctor's care. The doctor will tell you how to take care of the child at home.

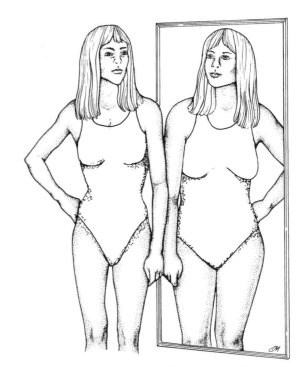

Because of an anorexic's distorted body image, she may perceive herself as fat when in reality she is exceedingly thin.

PRECAUTION

■ If the condition is not controlled, the anorexic may starve to death.

MEDICAL TREATMENT

The doctor will first attempt to rule out a physical cause of the child's extreme weight loss, such as cancer, infectious disease, disorders in the digestive organs, or problems in absorbing the nutrients from food. If the patient has lost more than 25 percent of her original body weight, if she displays the classic behavior, and if the onset of symptoms occurs before the age of 25, a diagnosis of anorexia is usually warranted.

Hospitalization and forced feeding may be necessary if the disease has led to severe malnutrition. However, most anorexics can be treated on an outpatient basis by a family physician, a psychiatrist, or a specialist in eating disorders.

The psychological problems that underlie anorexic behavior should be exposed and resolved. In the meantime, however, the youngster must be persuaded to gain weight and reassured that her doctor and parents will not allow her to become overweight. Healthy attitudes toward body weight and normal eating patterns must be restored.

Appendicitis

Appendicitis is an inflammation of the appendix, caused by infection. The appendix is a blind pouch about the size of your little finger that is located where the small intestine joins the large intestine. In 99 percent of all children, the appendix lies in the lower right quarter of the abdomen.

Appendicitis can occur at any age. If the inflamed appendix is not surgically removed, the infection worsens until the appendix bursts. Then the infection spreads throughout the abdomen. An infected appendix may perforate (rupture) within hours of the initial pain or may not rupture for a day or two. A ruptured appendix can lead to death.

SIGNS AND SYMPTOMS

Persistent abdominal pain in your child should be considered a symptom of appendicitis until proved otherwise. Typically, the pain of appendicitis is constant; it does not come and go like the pain from cramps. Once it starts, it grows continuously worse. The pain may start in the pit of the stomach, but more often begins in the area of the belly button. Usually it soon moves to the lower right quarter of the abdomen. The pain is made worse by jumping, walking, or just moving about. Bumps in the road encountered during the drive to the doctor's office cause more pain. The abdomen is tender to gentle pressure in the lower right quarter, more tender than in other areas. There may be nausea and vomiting, but these symptoms usually appear only after the pain has started.

Generally, there is a low-grade fever (100°F oral, 101°F rectal), but the temperature may range anywhere from normal to 104°F. Bowel movements are usually normal, but there may be diarrhea. Diagnosis may be difficult because not all of these signs are present in all cases. Because diagnosis is so difficult and the condition is so serious, call your doctor if you have any reason to suspect appendicitis.

HOME CARE

Try applying gentle heat, as with a heating pad turned to "low." If the pain gets worse, it is probably appendicitis. **Never apply cold;** this can mask the symptoms of appendicitis.

Do not give painkillers. Aspirin can affect the blood's ability to clot, so it should not be given in case the child needs surgery. Acetaminophen is safe but useless in this situation.

Allow only clear liquids by mouth. However, once you suspect that there is a strong possibility of appendicitis, do not give your child any food or drink until you consult your physician.

Never give a laxative or an enema.

PRECAUTION

■ If pain persists in the lower right quarter of the abdomen despite home treatment measures, call your doctor.

MEDICAL TREATMENT

The only acceptable treatment for appendicitis is an appendectomy (surgical removal of the appendix). Therefore, your doctor must be reasonably sure of the diagnosis. In addition to the abdomen, your child's chest and throat will be examined because a throat infection and pneumonia can cause symptoms of appendicitis. A rectal examination will also be performed, and a white blood cell count and urinalysis will be done. An X-ray examination may be ordered.

If the test results strongly suggest appendicitis, the doctor may operate immediately. If not, he or she may admit your child to a hospital for observation for a few hours until the diagnosis becomes more certain. Unnecessary surgery is to be avoided, but the rule of safety is to operate on a child who may have appendicitis rather than postpone surgery until the appendix ruptures.

RELATED TOPICS: Stomachache, acute; Stomachache, chronic

Arthritis

Arthritis is an inflammation of any joint or joints. Arthritis most often affects joints in the fingers, toes, wrists, ankles, elbows, knees, shoulders, hips, jaw, and spine. Six types of arthritis occur in childhood: rheumatoid arthritis, arthritis associated with acute rheumatic fever, infectious arthritis, allergic arthritis, postviral arthritis, and arthritis of rubella.

Rheumatoid arthritis can occur at any time past the age of one year. The cause is as yet unknown. It may affect one or several joints. The joints become swollen, warm, stiff, and mildly to moderately painful, but not usually red. The neck is affected in 50 percent of the cases. Arthritis may appear months before or after other signs of illness, such as fever, irritability, loss of appetite, and a fine pink rash.

Arthritis associated with *acute rheumatic fever* usually affects many joints, which become red, swollen, and extremely tender. Other symptoms of general illness (including fever) are also present.

Infectious (purulent) *arthritis* is an inflammation within a joint caused by one of various bacterial diseases (including staphylococcal, streptococcal, pneumococcal, and salmonella infections). This type of arthritis most often occurs in infants less than one year old. In older children and adults, it can be caused by puncture wounds near the joints. In this type of arthritis, the joint is tender, swollen, and red. The child usually has a fever.

In *allergic arthritis* the joints are stiff, swollen, and red, but pain is slight. The disease is caused by an allergic reaction to insect stings, medications, foods, or small particles inhaled from the air. It is generally accompanied by hives.

Postviral arthritis occurs after an illness caused by a virus. The symptoms are similar to those from other causes of arthritis, especially rheumatoid arthritis. Postviral arthritis corrects itself without treatment.

Arthritis of rubella occurs as a complication of rubella (German measles) or as a reaction to rubella vaccine, especially in older children. Arthritis of rubella usually corrects itself without treatment and usually causes no permanent damage.

SIGNS AND SYMPTOMS

Arthritis should be considered whenever there is pain and a limited ability to move any joint, unless there has been a physical injury to the joint. Deciding if a child has arthritis is best left to the doctor.

HOME CARE

No home treatment is safe until a doctor's diagnosis has been made. Trying to treat the condition at home may only delay proper treatment. Also, home treatment may make diagnosis more difficult for the doctor. If your doctor is not immediately available, pain relievers containing aspirin or acetaminophen will tem-

porarily reduce the discomfort. Rest or immobilize the affected joints.

PRECAUTIONS

■ Infectious arthritis is an acute emergency, and delay of treatment for 24 hours may result in permanent damage to a joint.
■ Rheumatoid arthritis and rheumatic fever require prompt treatment to minimize damage but are not considered emergencies.
■ Rheumatoid arthritis can begin with only a prolonged unexplained fever and no outward signs of arthritis (redness, tenderness, swelling).

MEDICAL TREATMENT

For the evaluation of arthritis, several tests are necessary. These tests may include X-ray studies, a wide variety of blood tests, blood culture, analysis of a sample of fluid drawn from the joint, electrocardiogram, and stool culture. Treatment may include antibiotics, drainage of the joints, large doses of aspirin (aspirin substitutes do not have the same effect), or oral steroids. If large doses of aspirin are prescribed and taken over a period of time, aspirin blood levels should be tested regularly.

If the condition is diagnosed as allergic arthritis, the doctor may suggest using oral antihistamines to relieve the symptoms. If it is diagnosed as arthritis of rubella, no treatment is necessary.

RELATED TOPICS: Growing pains; Hip problems; Knee pains; Puncture wounds; Sprains and dislocations

Asthma

Asthma is often an allergic reaction of the bronchial tree (the system of air passages leading into the lungs). It is a major and potentially dangerous form of allergy because it causes breathing difficulty. During an asthma attack, there are spasms in the smooth muscles of the bronchial tubes, and thick mucus collects in these tubes.

Asthma is often caused by an allergy to small particles breathed in from the air (animal dander, pollens, dust, feathers, molds). Less commonly, asthma is caused by an allergy to certain foods, medicines, and insect stings. Attacks may also be brought on by physical exertion, upper respiratory tract infections, emotional stress, or exposure to irritants, such as smoke and chlorine. The tendency to have allergies runs in families.

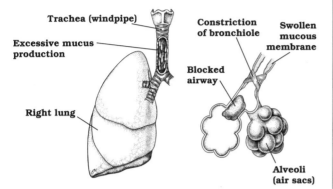

The difficult breathing characteristic of asthma occurs when the bronchioles (small respiratory tubes) constrict or become clogged with mucus or when the membranes lining the tubes become swollen. Stale air is trapped in the tiny air sacs, called alveoli, and less fresh air can be inhaled.

SIGNS AND SYMPTOMS

The major symptoms of asthma are shortness of breath, cough, a sensation of "air hunger," difficulty in breathing out, and wheezing. Wheezing is a high-pitched whistling sound heard more when the child is breathing out than when breathing in. The child usually does not have a fever.

Carefully noting when asthma attacks occur may help you and your doctor find an allergic cause of asthma. Do attacks begin after the child has been around a cat, dog, horse, or other animal with fur? Do attacks come in certain seasons (such as during tree, grass, or ragweed pollination)? Be alert to these and other possible causes of allergies.

Some children have exercise-induced asthma. They have symptoms only when they exert themselves, such as when playing sports. A third of Olympic athletes have this type.

HOME CARE

The first time your child has an attack that might be asthma, do not try to care for the child at home. Contact your doctor immediately. The doctor will determine if the child has asthma and will select a specific treatment.

After a doctor has diagnosed asthma, home care is important. Prescribed medications should be given as soon as an attack begins. Medicines are less effective if an attack is under

way. Rid your home of any identified causes of asthma allergy—pets, feather pillows and comforters, house dust, and sources of mold. Avoid exposing your child to airborne irritants such as insecticides, smoke, and paint fumes.

You and your child can monitor your child's asthma by regularly using a peak-flow meter. This simple device measures a child's lung capacity and how quickly the child can force the air out of the lungs. If there is a decline in peak flow, the asthma is getting worse.

PRECAUTIONS

■ Do not use over-the-counter aerosol medications on children. They can be dangerous and make other medications less effective.
■ Do not use aminophylline or theophylline given in the form of rectal suppositories. Rectal medications are not reliably absorbed, and the child may receive an improper dose.
■ Do not let an asthma attack go untreated. Frequent attacks of asthma that are untreated or improperly treated can cause permanent damage to the lungs and bronchial tubes.
■ Not all wheezing is caused by asthma. Have your doctor check your child if you suspect asthma.

MEDICAL TREATMENT

The treatment for asthma should produce good results. Your doctor will begin treatment by taking a detailed medical history and performing a general physical examination. An X ray of the child's chest may be ordered. The diagnosis can be confirmed if asthma medicines relieve the symptoms.

There are many different medicines used to treat asthma. Theophylline is the old standby, used for many years. It is a bronchodilator, a drug that opens up the bronchioles, or air passages in the lungs, and increases the flow of air through them. Currently, more children are started on other bronchodilators, some as pills, some as inhalers. Steroids are used to treat severe attacks as well as to prevent attacks.

The doctor may also order a series of skin tests of materials to which the child may be allergic. The substances identified as causes of allergic asthma must be removed from the child's surroundings wherever possible. Children also may be desensitized to substances that cause allergic reactions. Desensitization involves giving weekly to monthly injections of increasing amounts of the irritating substances over a period of one to ten years.

Severe attacks may require hospitalization for administration of oxygen and of intravenous medications and fluids.

Children with asthma should always take their medicines with them when they travel.

RELATED TOPICS: Bronchiolitis; Bronchitis; Croup; Hay fever and other nasal allergies; Hives; Hyperventilation

Athlete's foot

Athlete's foot is an infection of the skin of the feet. It is caused by one of several fungi that grow best in moisture. The mildest cases cause itching, scaling, and cracking between the toes, particularly between the fourth and fifth toes. Athlete's foot may spread to the soles of the feet as small blisters and scaling. In severe cases, it may spread to the ankles and legs. It may invade and deform the toenails. Scratching may cause additional (secondary) infections. The condition is most common during adolescence, but it may occur at any age—even in infants.

SIGNS AND SYMPTOMS

The scaling and cracked appearance of the skin and the itching that accompanies it are symptoms that may indicate athlete's foot.

HOME CARE

Apply over-the-counter fungicidal ointment, such as Whitfield's ointment, once or twice a day (half strength for delicate skin). Or you may use ointments containing undecylenic acid or tolnaftate (available without a prescription).

To decrease sweating of the feet, avoid rubber-soled or plastic-soled shoes. Use cotton socks to absorb moisture. Socks that have not been dyed may be best since some dyes can irritate the skin.

Many "incurable" cases of athlete's foot are not athlete's foot at all but contact dermatitis caused by the treatment. Contact dermatitis is a skin rash or inflammation caused by some irritating substance. In some people, the ointments used to treat athlete's foot may cause such irritation; the athlete's foot fungus has actually been cleared up, but the skin remains irritated. If treatment for athlete's foot does not relieve the symptoms, check with your doctor

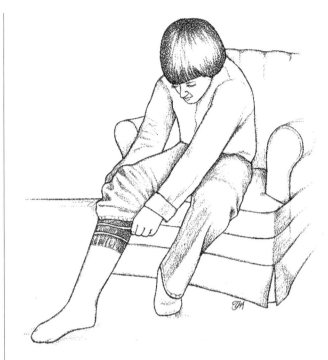

To control and prevent athlete's foot, have your child wear only cotton socks, preferably undyed.

to determine if the skin irritation is contact dermatitis.

PRECAUTIONS

■ Continue treatment until the skin is completely clear; fungal infections that are not completely treated flare up again.
■ If improvement is not prompt and lasting, see your doctor. The condition may not be athlete's foot but contact dermatitis.

MEDICAL TREATMENT

The diagnosis is confirmed by scraping the skin to obtain a sample for culturing and then identifying the fungus under a microscope. The doctor may prescribe other fungicidal ointments or lotions or a fungicide taken by mouth. If a secondary infection has developed, the doctor may prescribe oral antibiotics and may recommend soaking the area in a solution of potassium permanganate or aluminum sulfate and calcium acetate.

RELATED TOPICS: Eczema; Rashes

Backaches

Backache is pain, soreness, or stiffness occurring anywhere in the back. Backache is almost as common in children as in adults. Almost as soon as children are old enough to complain of pain and to explain where the pain is, they complain of occasional backaches. Backache may occur more frequently during adolescence.

Most back pains are the result of strenuous activities that cause stress to the muscles and ligaments of the back. These back problems are usually minor and often correct themselves without treatment.

More serious causes of back pain are arthritis, infections and abnormalities of the kidneys, malformations and abnormal curvatures of the spine, compression fractures (usually caused by injuries), and a defect of the growth plates of the vertebrae (the bones of the spine), called Scheuermann's disease.

SIGNS AND SYMPTOMS

Backache caused by stress causes pain and slight tenderness in the muscles that run along the spine. The pain is aggravated by bending and twisting, but it is less noticeable when resting. If physical activities are limited, the condition improves slowly day by day.

Backache caused by kidney problems often occurs on only one side. There may be other symptoms of urinary problems, such as burning during urination, frequent urination, or discoloration of the urine.

Backache caused by a sprain is limited to one spot near the spine or to a longer area along the spine.

Backache caused by a disease of the vertebrae or by scoliosis (abnormal curvature of the spine) may also be limited to one spot near the spine or to a longer area along the spine. Some abnormal curves in the spine can be seen. Minor curves to one side or the other can best be seen with the child undressed and bending forward to touch the floor with both hands. Even a slight curve causes the back to appear lopsided in this position.

HOME CARE

If there is no visible deformity, no fever, and no sharp pain in one location, home care is safe. The pain can be relieved with aspirin or acetaminophen, mild heat from an electric heating pad or a lukewarm bath, and bed rest. If the mattress is not extra-firm, a bed board under the mattress (a piece of plywood will do) may help relieve the discomfort. Have your child avoid any strenuous physical activity until the pain has been gone for at least a week.

PRECAUTIONS

■ If the child has a fever, urinary symptoms, severe pain, or a sharp pain in one area, see your doctor.
■ Do not use muscle-relaxant medications on children unless your doctor has prescribed them.

MEDICAL TREATMENT

In addition to a careful medical history and physical examination, your doctor may order a urinalysis, an X-ray examination of the spine, a CT scan or MRI, and blood studies. Specific treatment depends upon the cause of the back pain. In some cases, the doctor's treatment may be the same as home care. Treatment might also include antibiotics, orthopedic exercises, a back brace, or even hospitalization and traction.

RELATED TOPICS: Arthritis; Scoliosis; Urinary tract infections

Baldness

Baldness is a loss of hair either in one spot or over the entire scalp. Some infants are born bald or nearly so and develop a full head of hair during their first two years. Rarely do babies born bald remain bald for life. Other babies are born with a full head of hair. They may remain that way, or their original hair may be replaced by a second and permanent growth. Rarely is hair lost during infancy and never replaced.

Infants commonly rub off a band of hair at the back of the head against the crib or playpen mat. Hair that is rubbed off in this way will grow back. Drawing the hair tightly into pigtails, braids, or ponytails also may result in temporary bald spots. Children with the habit of twisting and playing with strands of hair may also lose hair. Emotionally disturbed children may pull out their hair by the handfuls; this condition, called trichotillomania, requires treatment of the child's emotional problems.

Alopecia areata is a condition that results in the sudden appearance of round or oval areas that are totally bald. The scalp may be completely normal in appearance or slightly pink. Although temporary, the condition may last for months or years. Rarely is the entire head involved. The cause is unknown.

Ringworm of the scalp produces scattered bald spots. The scalp is scaly, and the bald spots are studded with broken-off stubbles of hair.

Hereditary baldness occurs primarily in males. It causes baldness at the temples or the top of the scalp. Occasionally this type of baldness starts during adolescence.

Hyperparathyroidism (malfunction of the parathyroid glands) may result in scattered baldness. The disease is accompanied by other signs of illness.

Impetigo and other infections of the scalp produce temporary bald spots.

Teenagers often fear that they are going bald when they see loose hair after combing. Usually this condition is merely a normal thinning of the hair that does not worsen.

SIGNS AND SYMPTOMS

Inspect the scalp closely for signs of ringworm or infection. Look for broken or regrowing hairs. Watch to see if the child is rubbing his or her head against the playpen or crib, or if the child has a habit of twisting or pulling the hair.

HOME CARE

Alopecia areata is treated with patience and time. Hereditary and congenital baldness (baldness present at birth) can be treated only with understanding and love; a hairpiece may help.

PRECAUTIONS

■ Do not treat baldness with over-the-counter preparations that promise growth of hair.
■ Do not consult cosmetologists. See a qualified dermatologist.

MEDICAL TREATMENT

Alopecia areata is sometimes successfully treated with steroids either applied to the skin or locally injected. Hyperparathyroidism must be diagnosed by blood tests; it is treated with prescribed doses of vitamin D and a special diet.

RELATED TOPICS: Impetigo; Ringworm

Bed-wetting

Many children cannot remain dry through the night before they are four or five years old. About ten percent of all children over the age of five are bed wetters. Children of any age may have occasional accidents at night, especially if they are ill or in exhausted sleep; this is not true bed-wetting.

In five to ten percent of cases, children who are bed wetters have a physical disease, such as an infection or abnormality of the urinary tract, diabetes, or a neurologic (nervous system) disorder. If a toilet-trained child suddenly begins bed-wetting, the cause may be physical. If bed-wetting develops a year or more after night training has been established, or if a child wets himself or herself both day and night, a physical disease is likely.

However, most cases of bed-wetting are not caused by an identified physical disorder. Some cases seem to be hereditary, with brothers, sisters, and parents also having been bed wetters. Some are caused by overemphasis by the family on toilet training. Others are caused by taking children out of their night diapers too soon or by waking children to urinate in an effort to train at night. Some children have emotional problems that cause bed-wetting. Still, the cause of many cases of bed-wetting remains unknown.

SIGNS AND SYMPTOMS

A child who frequently and consistently wets the bed after the age of five years has a bed-wetting problem.

HOME CARE

Before beginning any home treatment of bed-wetting, see your doctor. The doctor can perform tests to determine whether bed-wetting is being caused by a physical disease, such as a urinary tract infection or diabetes.

If the doctor finds no physical cause, the best home treatment is to ignore bed-wetting as much as possible. Do not take a child out of night diapers until the child consistently remains dry. Do not make a big fuss about daytime training. Do not try to shame a child into remaining dry at night.

Many parents have found that wetness alarms, which awaken the child as soon as urination begins, are effective.

Withholding liquids during late afternoon and evening hours is not usually successful and may seem like punishment to the child. Behavior modification techniques (rewarding success and reacting neutrally toward failure) rarely work. Rubber sheets and plastic pants are helpful until the child stops bed-wetting.

Until then, patience, calmness, and understanding may be the best treatment.

PRECAUTIONS

■ Do not let a minor problem like bed-wetting become a major destructive factor in your relationship with your child. Anger and frustration between parent and child are more costly than extra laundry.

■ Do not allow other children to taunt a bed wetter.

MEDICAL TREATMENT

Before planning treatment, your doctor will conduct a physical examination and order a urinalysis. If the doctor suspects a serious medical cause, which is quite rare, X-ray studies of the urinary tract or consultation with a urologist may be suggested. Behavior modification is usually the first treatment tried. If this isn't successful and the family and child do not want to wait for the bed wetter to outgrow the bed-wetting, drug therapy may be started. Imipramine (an antidepressant) may be given by mouth at bedtime for a trial period. Drugs that lessen bladder spasms may be used. There is a nasal spray (DDVP) that often controls bed-wetting.

RELATED TOPICS: Diabetes mellitus; Urinary tract infections

Birthmarks

Birthmarks are any unusual marks or blemishes present on an infant's skin at birth. Almost 50 percent of all infants are born with red or salmon-colored marks on the mid-forehead, upper eyelids, upper lip, or back of the scalp and neck. These marks, which are sometimes quite extensive, fade and disappear during the first years of life.

Many black and Oriental babies and Caucasian babies who are destined to become brunettes have smooth, blue-black marks on their backs and buttocks. These birthmarks are called Mongolian spots. They are often mistaken for large bruises. They gradually disappear and are almost always gone by adolescence.

One in ten babies develops one or more strawberry marks during the first month of life. These are usually not visible at birth, or they may look like slightly pale spots on the skin. As the child grows, the marks become brilliant red. They are often raised, and vary in size from a quarter inch to two inches across. They may appear on any part of the body and increase in size for weeks or months. The strawberry marks then gradually fade and shrink. In almost all instances, they are gone by age five or six years.

Two uncommon but permanent birthmarks are port wine marks and pigmented moles. Both may be tiny or large and may appear anywhere on the skin. They grow in proportion to the growth of the child's body. Port wine marks are smooth, flat, and purplish. Pigmented moles are brown to black, are often slightly raised, and may have dark hairs.

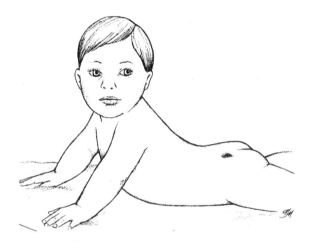

Many babies have smooth, blue-black marks, called Mongolian spots, on the backs and buttocks. These marks are almost always gone by adolescence.

SIGNS AND SYMPTOMS

Each type of birthmark is recognized by its typical appearance and behavior. Mongolian spots are often mistaken for bruises, until it becomes obvious that the spots are not fading.

HOME CARE

In most cases, no treatment is necessary. Strawberry marks are made up of countless, closely packed capillaries (tiny blood vessels). They should be protected from scratching or rubbing, which can cause bleeding. If bleeding occurs, it can be controlled by pressing lightly with gauze directly on the bleeding point. If desired, port wine marks can be hidden by cosmetics when the child is older.

PRECAUTIONS

■ Strawberry marks occasionally become infected if the overlying skin is broken. If there is any discharge, odor, or redness of the skin surrounding a strawberry mark, call your doctor.

■ Strawberry marks rarely require treatment; in almost all instances, it is best to allow them to disappear by themselves. In rare situations, they may cause anemia or bleeding that requires correction.

MEDICAL TREATMENT

The doctor may decide to surgically remove some pigmented moles. Strawberry marks rarely require surgical removal, because they usually become smaller with time. Port wine marks are now treated with laser therapy, often with excellent results.

RELATED TOPICS: Anemia; Moles

Blisters

Blisters occur when there is a buildup of clear or almost clear fluid between layers of the skin. They may be caused by heat burns; chemical burns; friction (rubbing); bacterial or fungal infection; hand, foot, and mouth disease; allergy to insect bites; or allergy to certain plants. Blisters range from the size of a pinhead to several inches across.

SIGNS AND SYMPTOMS

Blisters are obvious from their typical appearance—a raised bubble of skin containing clear fluid. The cause of blisters is sometimes determined by their location. When blisters appear on the palms or heels, they are usually due to rubbing; most blisters on the feet are caused by ill-fitting shoes or by not wearing socks. Blisters on the soles and toes may be caused by a fungus. Blisters on the cuticles or backs of fingers almost always mean an infection.

HOME CARE

Do not break open blisters caused by rubbing or by burns. Protect them with gauze and bandages. If a blister is accidentally opened, trim away the major portion of loose skin, cleanse with soap and water, and cover with a bandage. If the blister becomes infected (redness and increasing tenderness are signs of infection), it should be soaked in an Epsom-salts solution or

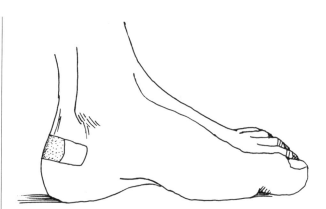

A blister should be protected with a bandage while it heals.

Burow's solution (which is available without a prescription). An infected blister should be checked by a doctor.

PRECAUTIONS

■ Red streaks extending from a blister indicate spreading infection. If red streaks appear, see your doctor.

■ Soaking unbroken blisters in an Epsom-salts solution that is too weak causes marked enlargement of the blisters. Use at least one-half cup of Epsom salts to a quart of water.

MEDICAL TREATMENT

Your doctor will determine the cause of the blister and look for signs of infection. Infected blisters are opened, and the fluid is cultured to determine the type of infection. Soaks or oral antibiotics may be prescribed individually or in combination.

RELATED TOPICS: Athlete's foot; Blood poisoning; Burns; Chicken pox; Hand, foot, and mouth disease; Herpes simplex; Impetigo; Poison ivy

Blood poisoning

Blood poisoning is the spread of a bacterial infection into the bloodstream. In popular usage, blood poisoning refers to the development of red streaks from an infected wound or blister. These red streaks resemble broad, wobbly, red pencil marks. The streaks quickly (within hours) extend in the direction of the heart. They are signs of the infection traveling along the lymph vessels of the affected part of the body. If ignored, the spreading germs can—within hours or days—reach the bloodstream.

As the bacteria travel along the lymph channels and enter the lymph nodes, the nodes swell, become tender, and sometimes redden as their cells fight and kill the germs. If the lymph nodes succeed in fighting off the poisonous bacteria, the infection is halted. A fever below 100°F or the absence of a fever indicates that the germs have not reached the bloodstream. A sudden, quickly rising high fever (over 101°F) generally means that they have entered the bloodstream.

SIGNS AND SYMPTOMS

In a good light, the pink or red, slightly wavy lines are easily seen just under the skin. These lines may be one inch to several feet long. The lymph nodes toward which these red streaks lead are often swollen and tender.

Blood poisoning can occur during early infancy, when natural resistance to infection is low; symptoms include irritability, fever, and poor feeding. Beyond infancy, blood poisoning results in high fever, chills, and prostration (extreme exhaustion or collapse).

HOME CARE

If blood poisoning occurs, call your doctor. Elevate the affected part of the body. Apply warm soaks of Epsom-salts solution (one-half cup in a quart of water) to the entire area. If there is an unopened infected blister at the source, soak the blister, too. Give aspirin or acetaminophen for pain and fever.

PRECAUTIONS

■ Always contact your doctor. Blood poisoning is best treated with antibiotics.
■ If a child with blood poisoning has a high fever or is prostrate (in a state of collapse), **contact a medical facility promptly.**

MEDICAL TREATMENT

Your doctor will give your child antibiotics by mouth or by injection. The doctor may open and drain the point of infection. Culture of the blood or of material from the site of the original infection may be necessary. Laboratory tests, including blood studies and a urinalysis, may be necessary. Hospitalization may be necessary if the blood poisoning is severe.

RELATED TOPICS: Blisters; Cuts; Fever; Glands, swollen; Puncture wounds

Boils

Boils are local infections that occur beneath the skin. They are almost always caused by a bacterium called hemolytic *Staphylococcus aureus*—"staph" for short. Boils are identified by redness, pain, and the formation of pus in the center, which tends to "point" (come to a head) and drain through the skin. Pus is a mixture of live and dead white blood cells, liquefied dead tissue, and live and dead staph germs. Pus is therefore infectious; it can spread boils to other areas and to other persons.

A small superficial boil is a pimple or pustule. (An acne pimple is not a true boil.) A large boil with several heads is a carbuncle. A boil on the edge of the eyelid is a stye. When many boils are present at one time, the condition is called furunculosis. Abscesses are collections of pus in parts of the body other than the skin, as in muscles, brain, bone, and internal organs. Abscesses are like boils, but often they are caused by organisms other than staph germs.

Staph germs are often harmlessly present in the nose and throat or on the skin of healthy persons. Staph germs on the skin cause no problems unless there is a cut or break in the skin. If the germs enter the body through a break in the skin, they cause infections.

SIGNS AND SYMPTOMS

Boils are easily recognized by their redness and pain and by the formation of pus in the center.

HOME CARE

Boils are treated with frequent or constant soaks with warm Epsom-salts solution (one-half cup per quart of water). When a boil comes to a head and drains, the drainage must be caught on a clean cloth or gauze pad. The surrounding skin should be cleansed frequently with soap and water to avoid more boils.

PRECAUTIONS

■ See your doctor if boils develop on the face. The lymph and blood vessel drainage from this area is such that spread of infection to the central nervous system is a possibility. Be especially careful that drainage from a boil does not come in contact with the eyes.
■ Never squeeze a boil. Squeezing breaks down the wall surrounding the boil. When this wall is

broken down, the infection rapidly spreads outward.

■ Treat all minor wounds and insect bites properly to lessen the likelihood of infections and the formation of boils.

MEDICAL TREATMENT

Your doctor may open and drain the boil, culture pus, and order sensitivity studies on the organisms found. These studies will help your doctor identify the antibiotic that will most effectively fight the infection. The doctor may prescribe antibiotics to be taken by mouth. Many staph germs have become resistant to penicillin. Other antibiotics that may be used include erythromycin, oxacillin, cloxacillin, methicillin, and cephalosporin.

For repeated attacks of boils, your doctor may recommend nose and throat cultures of the patient and the entire family to identify carriers of the staph germs. Antibiotic ointments and antiseptic baths may be prescribed.

RELATED TOPICS: Acne; Cuts; Insect bites and stings; Puncture wounds; Scrapes; Styes

Botulism

Botulism is a specific type of food poisoning. Botulism is caused by the toxin (poison) produced by *Clostridium botulinum*, a bacterium that is related to the tetanus germ and that is prevalent everywhere. The botulism germ grows in anaerobic (without oxygen) environments (such as tightly closed jars that have not been properly sterilized). Botulism is primarily caused by eating improperly prepared canned or preserved foods that have not been adequately reheated. The foods most likely to cause poisoning are seafood, mushrooms, meat, and vegetables. The toxin and germs are undetectable outside the laboratory. Foods contaminated with botulism may look, smell, and taste normal.

With improvements in commercial food preparation and the decline in home canning in the first half of the 20th century, botulism had become a rare illness in the United States. With the current increased interest in home canning and "natural" foods (those without preservatives), botulism is threatening a comeback.

Adults and children past infancy can be poisoned by botulism only if they eat food in which the botulism germ has already formed the toxin. Recent cases of fatal botulism among infants, however, suggest that the botulism germ can grow in an infant's immature intestines to form the dangerous toxin within the infant's body. The only natural food so far identified as a source of botulism germs for infants is honey. Therefore, you should not give honey to an infant. Other raw or improperly cooked foods may eventually be identified as potential sources of the germ.

SIGNS AND SYMPTOMS

Symptoms of botulism are nausea, vomiting, diarrhea, and abdominal pain followed in 12 to 48 hours by double vision, dilated pupils, and difficulty in speaking, swallowing, and breathing. There is no fever and no loss of awareness or alertness. **Death may result.**

Suspect botulism if your infant develops symptoms within a week of eating raw or home-prepared foods. Suspect the disease if more than one member of your family develops similar symptoms after eating the same food. If symptoms of stomach or intestinal upset are followed by paralysis that starts at the eyes and moves downward, botulism may be the cause. Home diagnosis, however, is totally unreliable. Consult your doctor immediately if symptoms of botulism occur.

HOME CARE

None. Call your doctor immediately if you suspect botulism.

PRECAUTIONS

■ Do not give babies unwashed, unpeeled raw foods or improperly cooked foods.
■ Do not give honey to infants.
■ Do not use foods that come in damaged or dented store-bought cans. Damaged cans may have leaks through which the botulism germ can enter the food.
■ Certain home-preserved foods (for example, vegetables and meats) should be reheated for ten minutes at a temperature of at least 180°F before eating because of the danger of botulism.
■ When canning or preserving foods at home, follow preparation and sterilization directions carefully.

MEDICAL TREATMENT

Diagnosis is made by identifying the toxin in samples of the food eaten and in the patient's stomach contents, stools, and blood. Treatment includes injection of the antitoxin (a substance that counteracts the effects of the poison). Stomach washing, laxatives and enemas, antibiotic therapy, and hospitalization may be necessary. Immunization to prevent botulism is available, but only for persons at high risk.

RELATED TOPICS: Dehydration; Diarrhea in older children; Diarrhea in young children; Dysentery; Food poisoning; Vomiting

Bowlegs and knock-knees

Bowlegs and knock-knees are two conditions in which the legs are not as straight as they are in most persons. In bowlegs, the legs bend outward so that the knees are farther apart than usual. In knock-knees, the legs bend inward so that the knees are closer together.

Theoretically, when a child stands straight, the ankle bones should touch or almost touch each other, and the knee bones should touch or almost touch each other. With an infant lying on the stomach or back, the legs can be pulled straight with the toes and knees pointed straight ahead to determine whether the bones of the knees and ankles come together. If the

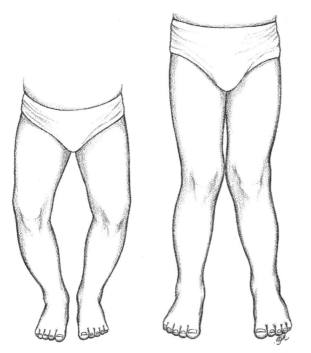

Very young children often appear bowlegged (as shown on the left). Preschoolers may stand knock-kneed (as shown on the right). Both conditions may correct themselves as the child grows older.

ankles touch but the knees do not, the child is bowlegged. If the knees touch but the ankles do not, the child is knock-kneed.

By these standards, however, all infants, children, and adults are bowlegged or knock-kneed to some degree, so you should not become alarmed. Most infants appear bow-legged, and when they start to walk, they walk "cowboy" style. This condition usually corrects itself by age two. Most preschoolers stand knock-kneed, especially if they are plump. This condition also corrects itself.

True bowlegs and knock-knees either are due to rickets (vitamin D deficiency) or are inherited. Although common 50 years ago, rickets is now rare in the United States. An unusual form of bowlegs, often occurring on only one side, is Blount's disease, in which the top of the tibia (shin bone) becomes deformed.

SIGNS AND SYMPTOMS

Have the child stand with the legs straight and the toes pointed forward. Then observe if there is any distance between the knees or between the ankles. Remember that the distance between the ankles or the knees varies from person to person and that these differences are usually normal. If you think that there might be a problem, ask your doctor.

HOME CARE

In most cases, no home care is needed. To prevent rickets, children should receive about 400 international units of vitamin D daily. This amount is found in many commercial infant formulas and in most commercial milk. Some vitamin D is present in breast milk, but the amount varies. If your child is being breast-fed, ask your doctor whether the child is receiving enough vitamin D.

PRECAUTIONS

■ If you think your infant or child is bowlegged or knock-kneed, watch to see if the condition worsens after several months. If it does, consult your doctor.
■ Do not use orthopedic shoes without your doctor's prescription.
■ Do not give your child vitamin D supplements unless your doctor has prescribed them. Overdoses of vitamin D can be harmful.

MEDICAL TREATMENT

In most instances, the doctor will examine your child and then prescribe no treatment—except to wait and watch. X-ray studies of the knees may be necessary, as well as blood tests for rickets. Use of orthopedic shoes or night splints is rarely necessary. For Blount's disease, braces or corrective operations on bones may be required.

Bronchiolitis

Bronchiolitis is an inflammation of the lungs, which is caused by a viral infection. Bronchiolitis occurs during the first two years of life, most often at about age six months. It is almost always caused by a respiratory virus.

The early symptoms are similar to those of bronchitis. Bronchiolitis may develop in an infant who has been exposed to an older child or adult with a cold. The illness may last for several days. Infants who are subject to bronchiolitis may develop asthma in later years.

SIGNS AND SYMPTOMS

The first symptoms of bronchiolitis are nasal congestion, fever, loss of appetite, and a mild cough. These symptoms may then progress to frequent, severe coughing; rapid, difficult breathing; wheezing (a whistling sound heard when the child breathes out); irritability; and cyanosis (a bluish discoloration of the skin). The child's extra efforts to breathe may cause flaring of the nostrils, as well as drawing in of the flesh in the spaces between the ribs and of the abdomen just below the ribs.

HOME CARE

Do not attempt to treat bronchiolitis on your own. Diagnosis and treatment should be handled by your doctor. See your doctor if your infant has a frequent cough, even if only for short periods. See your doctor if your child has difficulty in breathing other than that caused by nasal congestion.

PRECAUTIONS

■ Bronchiolitis can be a serious illness. See your doctor.
■ Do not give cough medicine to a child with bronchiolitis. Cough medicines may be dangerous to a child who is already having difficulty in breathing.
■ An infant with rapid breathing can suffer dehydration (a serious loss of body fluids) because of loss of vapor from the breath.

Dehydration in infants can be dangerous. Give the child extra fluids by mouth.

MEDICAL TREATMENT

In some areas, bronchiolitis is the most common reason for hospitalizing infants. An infant with bronchiolitis may require oxygen or intravenous fluids. A chest X-ray examination, nose and throat cultures, and blood studies may be ordered. Antibiotics are of no use because they are not effective in treating viruses. If a child has repeated attacks of bronchiolitis, one injection of epinephrine may be given to determine if the child has an allergy; if the epinephrine relieves the symptoms, it is likely that the attacks are caused by an allergy.

RELATED TOPICS: Asthma; Bronchitis; Common cold; Coughs; Dehydration; Frequent illness; Pneumonia; Shortness of breath; Viral infections

Bronchitis

Bronchitis may be thought of as a cold that spreads to the trachea (windpipe) and to the bronchi (the air passages leading into the lungs). It may start with the signs of a common cold—nasal congestion and discharge, sneezing, watery eyes, and scratchy throat—but it may also develop without the appearance of any cold symptoms.

Most cases of bronchitis are caused by viruses. These germs cannot be combated by antibiotics. Bronchitis is contagious and is passed on in the same manner as a cold. If the disease occurs frequently, the child may have an underlying allergy. (Sometimes children with asthma tend to have repeated attacks of bronchitis.)

SIGNS AND SYMPTOMS

The major symptoms of bronchitis are a dry, hacking cough; a low-grade fever (100°F oral, 101°F rectal) or no fever; and tightness and pain in the center of the chest. Often the child experiences a loss of appetite and feels generally weak and uncomfortable. After a few days, the cough loosens. Occasionally, a rattling sound can be heard in the chest when the child takes a breath, but there is never any real difficulty in breathing (except from nasal congestion). The entire illness may last about a week.

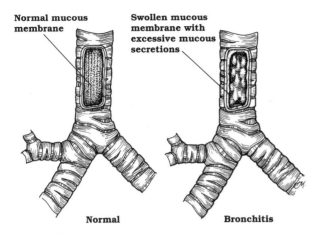

In bronchitis, the mucous membranes that line the bronchial tubes (the air passages leading into the lungs) swell and secrete more mucus, resulting in clogging of the bronchial tubes and reduced airflow into the lungs.

There is rarely high fever or prostration (extreme exhaustion or collapse). There is never pain on the side of the chest. No blood appears in the sputum (discharge coughed up out of the lungs).

HOME CARE

Treatment for bronchitis is similar to that for the common cold. Limited activity is recommended during the fever stage and the time when the cough is the worst. Encourage your child to drink liquids to avoid dehydration (serious loss of body fluids).

Give acetaminophen for fever and body aches. Phenylephrine or oxymetazoline nose drops may be used. If the cough is exhausting or keeps the child from sleeping, cough medicine might help.

A humidifier or vaporizer may make breathing easier. (Be sure to keep it meticulously clean, however. Otherwise, it can actually become a source of infection if microorganisms are allowed to grow in it.)

PRECAUTIONS

■ See your doctor if any unusual symptoms occur, such as pain on the side of the chest or blood in the sputum.
■ See your doctor if bronchitis occurs more than once a year.
■ See your doctor if the condition worsens after three to four days.
■ Do not use oral decongestants, which may aggravate a dry cough.

MEDICAL TREATMENT

Your doctor will perform a physical examination, with special attention to the chest. Throat or sputum cultures, a chest X-ray examination, and blood studies may be necessary. If bronchitis occurs frequently, the doctor will investigate the possibility of an allergy, a foreign body in the bronchial tubes, or a lowered resistance to infection.

The usefulness of antibiotics and some types of cough medicines is debatable. Antibiotics usually are not helpful for most types of bronchitis (those caused by viruses), and some cough medicines can aggravate the condition.

If a child has repeated attacks of bronchitis, your doctor may give epinephrine by injection to determine if the child has an allergy; if epinephrine relieves the symptoms, it is likely that the attacks are caused by an allergy.

RELATED TOPICS: Bronchiolitis; Chest pain; Common cold; Coughs; Cystic fibrosis; Frequent illness; Viral infections

Bruises

Bruises are made up of blood that has escaped from capillaries (tiny blood vessels) or larger blood vessels and can be seen through the skin. They vary from pinhead-size to several inches across. Bruises usually are black and blue in color. If they are near the skin's surface, they appear maroon or purple. Bruises of the whites of the eyeballs are always blood-red. As blood in a bruise moves back into the bloodstream, a bruise often becomes yellow or green.

If the escape of blood has been deep in the tissues—as with torn ligaments or broken bones—it may take days to reach the surface of the skin as a visible bruise. Escaped blood often travels to other parts of the body (for example, the blood from a bruise on the forehead may produce a black eye).

Most bruises are caused by physical injuries. Normally active children always seem to have one or more bruises. Children with fair complexions bruise more easily than children with darker complexions. The areas most likely to bruise are the shins, knees, arms, and thighs. Bruises may take days or weeks to disappear, depending on their size.

A different type of bruise, called a spontaneous bruise, may be a cause for concern. Spontaneous bruises suddenly appear even though no injury or blow to the skin has occurred. Spontaneous bruises may appear because the capillaries are abnormally fragile (sometimes due to vitamin C deficiency), because the capillaries have been injured by infections or by allergic reactions, or because of a lack of proper clotting of the blood. Bruises often are caused by injuries that were simply not noticed at the time; however, if bruises appear in areas not likely to be injured, or if a great many bruises appear, it is less likely that they were caused by unnoticed injuries—these may be spontaneous bruises.

There is another type of bruise known as a petechia. Petechiae are pinhead to one-eighth inch in size. They are dark red or maroon in color and often appear by the hundreds. Forceful vomiting or coughing can sometimes cause many petechiae to appear on the head and neck. Petechiae may also appear in one smaller area when caused by a blow to the skin.

SIGNS AND SYMPTOMS

Bruises are easily recognized when an area of the skin is discolored (black, blue, purple, red, green, or yellow). Bruises can be distinguished from other skin marks or rashes by a simple test. A bruise of any size does not blanch (turn white or pale) when pressed; all other red or purple marks or skin rashes will blanch when pressed.

HOME CARE

Applying cold compresses soon after an injury will help decrease bleeding and lessen bruising. Ice should not be placed directly on the skin. Wrap the ice cubes or cold packs in a thin cloth. A bag of frozen peas is a convenient and moldable ice pack.

Applications of heat 24 hours or more after the injury can help the body absorb the blood in the bruise. Do not be concerned about the color of the bruise or the different colors the bruise turns in the process of healing.

PRECAUTIONS

■ Spontaneous bruising should always be examined by a doctor. Spontaneous bruising may be a sign of illness.

■ Petechiae scattered over the body can indicate an urgent situation. If there is also fever or prostration (extreme exhaustion or collapse), a true emergency exists. Don't waste any time— **see your doctor at once.**

MEDICAL TREATMENT

For bruises caused by injuries, a doctor's treatment is the same as home care. If there are spontaneous bruises, including petechiae that are scattered over the body, your doctor will perform a complete physical examination. The examination may include a complete blood cell count; platelet count; blood coagulation studies; nose, throat, and blood cultures; spinal tap; and bone marrow studies. The patient may be hospitalized to be given intravenous fluids and antibiotics.

Burns

Burns are injuries of the skin caused by excessive heat, by chemicals (acids and alkalis), or by electricity. The seriousness of a burn depends on the size, the location, and the depth of the skin burned. Burns are classified as first degree (the least serious), second degree, and third degree (the most serious). *First-degree burns* cause reddening of the skin and pain; they may blister after one or two days. (Sunburn is a good example of a first-degree burn.) *Second-degree burns* redden and blister immediately. *Third-degree burns* are the deepest and cause the death of a full depth of skin; the skin blisters or appears scorched (blackened) or dead white.

If more than ten percent of the skin surface has suffered second-degree or third-degree burns, a serious emergency exists. Any second-degree or third-degree burn should be treated immediately by a doctor. A person with severe burns may go into shock, which is life-threatening and requires immediate medical treatment. Burns of the fingers, joints, and face may be serious because burns in these locations may cause scarring and deformity.

SIGNS AND SYMPTOMS

Redness, blistering, or scorching of the skin are the obvious signs of a burn.

HOME CARE

Do not try to treat second-degree or third-degree burns at home; they must be treated by a doctor. If a burn is blistered, charred, or scorched, cover it with a clean, wet cloth. Keep the child warm, and see your doctor at once. Do not apply ointments or other treatments to burns that will need a doctor's care.

First-degree burns (reddened skin only) can usually be cared for at home. Immediately apply cold compresses to the burn or place the burned area under cold running water. Continue applying cold until the pain lessens (up to one-half hour).

First-degree burns treated at home must be covered to prevent infection. The covering should not stick to the burn, but it should keep out air and germs until the burn has healed. (If air is kept from the burn, there should be no further pain.) Apply a light layer of antibiotic cream or a cream containing silver sulfadiazine to the burn. (Silver sulfadiazine requires a prescription, but your doctor may prescribe it over the telephone.) Then cover the area with several thicknesses of sterile gauze. Change the dressing every 24 to 48 hours until the burn has completely healed. For simple sunburn, apply over-the-counter sunburn products, if needed, and leave uncovered.

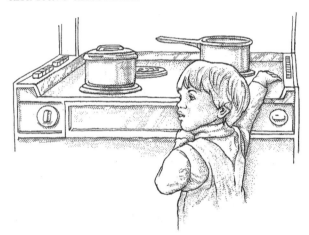

Watch children closely when they are around the stove. Turn pot handles toward the back of the stove so that children cannot grab them.

PRECAUTIONS

■ If a severely burned child becomes weak, pale, cold and clammy, or shows any other signs of shock, keep the child warm and get medical help immediately.
■ Do not break open blisters that are caused by burns.
■ Electrical burns often occur when young children chew on live electrical wires and extension cords. A physician should examine any electrical burn.

■ Water over 115°F can scald. If there are young children in the home, turn down the thermostat on the water heater.
■ Watch young children when they are in the kitchen, especially when near the stove or near hot foods or beverages.
■ Keep matches and cigarette lighters out of your child's reach.
■ Do not keep gasoline or other flammables in the house. Keep them locked away outside.
■ Avoid flammable garments.
■ Keep childproof plugs in electrical outlets.
■ Keep your child's tetanus immunization status up to date. (This is particularly important in the event of second- or third-degree burns.)
■ Do not leave young children home alone—not even for a moment.

MEDICAL TREATMENT

A child will usually be hospitalized for any third-degree burn, for second-degree burns that cover more than ten percent of the skin, and for second-degree burns of the face, fingers, or joints. In the hospital, the proper dressings can be applied; antibiotics and intravenous fluids can be administered, if necessary; and the child's condition can be monitored for complications. Plastic surgery may be necessary.

RELATED TOPICS: Blisters; Shock; Sunburn; Tetanus

Cat scratch fever

Cat scratch fever is caused most often by a germ—probably a virus—transmitted by a minor scratch or bite from a kitten or young cat, which is not itself ill. The puncture wound or scratch does not heal in the time expected. One to two weeks later, the wound is still red, sometimes with a small amount of pus. One to six weeks after the incident, the lymph nodes near the wound become swollen, tender, and red. The child has a low-grade fever (100°F oral, 101°F rectal). Eventually the lymph nodes may break down and discharge pus through the skin.

SIGNS AND SYMPTOMS

The signs of cat scratch fever are a minor cat scratch or bite that has not healed; large, tender lymph nodes; and a low-grade fever. There may be pus in the wound. If you do not know that your child has been scratched by a cat, it may be difficult to tell cat scratch fever from any other infected wound.

HOME CARE
Scrub all cat scratches and bites immediately with soap and water for ten minutes. Then apply an antiseptic. If the wound becomes infected, see your doctor.

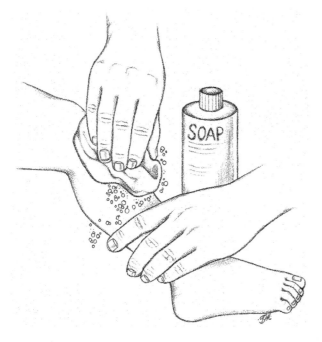

Scrub all cat scratches and bites immediately with soap and water for ten minutes.

PRECAUTIONS
■ Unsupervised play between cats and young children is dangerous to both the child and the animal.
■ Do not allow children to tease or torment cats or any other animals.

MEDICAL TREATMENT
Your doctor will rule out other illnesses by blood tests and cultures. Treatment with broad-spectrum antibiotics is occasionally helpful. Cat scratch fever may require surgical incision and drainage or complete removal of a lymph node.

RELATED TOPICS: Animal bites; Glands, swollen; Puncture wounds

Chest pain

Chest pain is common during childhood. Although chest pain in adults can be serious, it is rarely a symptom of serious disease in children.

A very common form of chest pain in children is the so-called stitch in the side—a stabbing pain in the lower chest, more often on the left side than the right. This pain occurs with exercise and will stop after a minute or two of rest. This type of pain may be caused by gas pains in the large intestine, contraction of the spleen, or spasm of the diaphragm (the muscular partition between the chest and abdominal cavities). Regardless of the cause, it is harmless.

Pain in the area of the sternum (breastbone) is common when a child has bronchitis or a head cold combined with a cough. A frequent, hard cough often makes the diaphragm sore, causing a pain just below the ribs. Pain on one side of the chest may be caused by pleurodynia (pain from inflammation of the muscles between the ribs) or by shingles.

Injuries to the chest area may cause pain that is worsened by deep breathing and movements of the chest. While the discomfort may be the result of a muscle strain or bruise, a physician should rule out other possibilities, such as a fractured rib.

There are a few causes of chest pain in children that are more serious, but these are also uncommon. Pleurisy (inflammation of the lining of the chest cavity) that develops as a complication of pneumonia may cause chest pain, accompanied by fever, difficulty in breathing, and coughing.

Another more serious cause of chest pain is spontaneous pneumothorax, which occurs when a small bubble on the surface of the lung bursts and air escapes into the chest cavity, causing gradual collapse of the lung. This condition comes on suddenly, often with sharp pain, and causes increasing shortness of breath.

A hernia of the diaphragm causes chest pain that is usually worse when the child is lying down and that lessens or is absent when the child is sitting or standing.

Heart pain in children, even those with serious heart conditions, is so rare that it is practically unknown.

SIGNS AND SYMPTOMS

Chest pain may occur alone or with other symptoms. The exact location of the pain and the circumstances that bring on or worsen the pain are clues to the type and cause of chest pain. Other symptoms (cough, fever, rash at the site of the pain, and shortness of breath) are also clues to the cause.

HOME CARE

Most cases of minor chest pain can be treated at home with aspirin or acetaminophen, mild heat, and reassurance. If chest pain is caused by a hard cough, cough medicines may help. Pleurisy, spontaneous pneumothorax, and hernia of the diaphragm should be treated by a doctor.

PRECAUTIONS

■ If chest pain is accompanied by shortness of breath, high fever, a cough producing blood flecks, or prostration (collapse), **get medical help immediately.**

■ If there is persistent pain beneath either armpit that is made worse by breathing, see your doctor.

■ Do not give cough medicines if the child is having difficulty in breathing.

MEDICAL TREATMENT

Your doctor may recommend X-ray examination of the chest and blood studies. Pneumothorax is treated by hospitalization, close observation, and possibly puncture of the chest wall to remove trapped air.

RELATED TOPICS: Bronchitis; Pneumonia; Shingles; Viral infections

Chicken pox

Chicken pox is caused by a highly contagious virus. The chicken pox virus is transmitted by contact with a person who has the disease or via droplets or airborne particles from such a person. Symptoms may appear within 12 to 21 days after being exposed to a person with chicken pox. One attack of chicken pox makes a person immune for life, unless the attack is extremely mild. A vaccine to prevent chicken pox is likely to be available soon.

SIGNS AND SYMPTOMS

Chicken pox may start with the symptoms of a mild cold, but often a rash is the first sign. The rash worsens for three to four days and then heals in three to four days. The child is contagious from 24 hours before the rash appears until all blisters of the rash have dried. Fever can be low or as high as 105°F; fever is the worst on the third or fourth day after the appearance of the rash.

The key symptom of chicken pox is the rash. Each new spot, or pock, resembles an insect bite. Within hours the pock develops a small clear blister in the center, which may be hard to see without good light. Most blisters break and are replaced by a brown scab. The rash usually begins on the trunk and moves outward to the limbs and face. However, the rash may appear anywhere on the skin, including the scalp and the mucous membranes of the mouth, genitals, anus, and eyelids. It becomes quite itchy. The pocks never appear in bunches or groups. New pocks continue to appear for three to four days.

HOME CARE

Bed rest is not necessary, but your child should be isolated from other people. Cut the child's fingernails to lessen scratching. To reduce the itching, bathe your child in lukewarm water with cornstarch added, or apply calamine lotion (without phenol) to the skin. Give acetaminophen—**not aspirin**—for fever or pain.

PRECAUTIONS

■ **Do not** give aspirin to a child with chicken pox. Aspirin use during chicken pox *may* be a factor causing Reye's syndrome, which is a life-threatening illness.

■ Encephalitis (inflammation of the brain) is a rare complication of chicken pox. If high fever, collapse, headache, vomiting, or convulsions occur, **see your doctor immediately**.

■ Chicken pox can be dangerous to newborns. If a young infant is exposed to chicken pox or develops chicken pox, call your doctor.

■ Chicken pox is also dangerous to children taking steroids or other immunosuppressant drugs and to children with immune mechanism deficiencies, which hinder the child's ability to fight infectious diseases. If such a child develops chicken pox or is exposed to it, call your doctor.

■ Even if a child has already been exposed to someone with chicken pox, prevent any further exposure.

■ If the pocks become infected (characterized by increasing redness, soreness, and formation of pus), call your doctor.

■ The lymph nodes of the neck, armpits, groin, and back of the skull ordinarily swell with chicken pox; however, if they become red and tender, report this to your doctor.

■ **Do not** apply calamine lotion with phenol.

■ When your child is bathed, pat the skin dry without breaking the blisters or disturbing the scabs to avoid scarring.

■ If spontaneous bruises (bruises not caused by injuries) appear, or if ruptured blood vessels appear under the skin, see your doctor.

MEDICAL TREATMENT

If pocks have become infected, your doctor will usually culture material from the infected pocks and will treat your child with oral antibiotics for five to ten days. (Antibiotics do not influence the course of chicken pox, however; they work only against the secondary infection.) If there are signs of encephalitis, your child will probably be hospitalized for tests and treatment. Spontaneous bleeding under the skin may be treated with oral medications, or your doctor may order hospitalization.

If a child at high risk is exposed to chicken pox, your doctor will probably give him or her an injection of zoster immune globulin.

RELATED TOPICS: Bruises; Encephalitis; Rashes; Reye's syndrome

Child abuse and neglect

More than two million children are abused or seriously neglected every year. More than 50 percent of reported cases are of child neglect, 30 percent are of physical abuse, and 15 percent are of sexual abuse.

Most abused children are abused by someone they know: a parent, relative, sibling, or friend. Most adult abusers were abused themselves as children. Young parents, parents with chemical-dependency problems, single parents, and parents living in poverty are more likely to abuse their children. But abuse occurs in families of every socioeconomic, ethnic, educational, and religious background.

Child neglect may be physical (withholding clothing, food, shelter, or other physical necessities), emotional (withholding love, attention, comfort, affection), or medical (withholding necessary medical care).

SIGNS AND SYMPTOMS

In some cases, the signs and symptoms of neglect or abuse are obvious; in others, they are very subtle and difficult to detect. Abused or neglected children may believe what they are experiencing is normal and may see no need to mention it. In addition, they may be afraid to tell anyone what's happening because they fear more abuse, fear that no one will believe them, or feel that they've done something to provoke the abuse and that they deserve it. Most abused children will not initiate discussion about their abuse or neglect.

There are the obvious signs of unexplained or excessive bruises and burns. The subtle signs are more common, but they are also more difficult to detect. A child's behavior may change; he or she may become more fearful and withdrawn. The child's self-esteem may decrease, and academic performance may suffer. The child may be frequently absent from school. A sexually abused child may exhibit sexual behavior that is inappropriate for his or her age, may describe sexual acts, or may use age-inappropriate words related to sexual acts.

An abused child may have a number of physical complaints such as unexplained or inappropriately explained bruises, burns, or broken bones. The child may frequently complain of abdominal pain, headaches, or genital discomfort. The child may have urinary tract infections, sexually transmitted diseases, or unexplained weight loss. A child previously capable of using the toilet may have trouble controlling urination or bowel movements.

HOME CARE

If the child is acutely injured, use appropriate first aid or, if the injuries are severe, contact a doctor or emergency room for further instructions. In most cases, the abuse has been going on for a while and there are no serious acute medical problems.

Any time there is a suspicion of abuse or neglect, the child needs to be seen by a doctor. In many states, any person suspecting abuse is obligated to report it to the proper authorities.

Many parents, particularly if they were abused in childhood, fear they will lose control and abuse their own children. The best treatment in such a situation is prevention. There are support groups for parents and there are emergency numbers a parent can call when they fear they are losing control and may abuse a child. Individual counseling with a qualified professional may also be helpful.

PRECAUTION

■ Disbelieving or doubting a child who tells you of an abusive situation may lead to perpetuation of the abuse.

MEDICAL TREATMENT

Much of what the doctor does depends on when the abuse occurred. If there are concerns about serious injuries, the doctor will examine the child immediately. On the other hand, if the abuse occurred in the past, the doctor may decide not to examine the child. Instead, he or she may refer the child to a doctor who specializes in handling this type of case. An abused child may be very resistant to any examination, even when suffering from pain or other abuse-related injuries.

Any health-care worker is required to report any case of abuse, even if only suspected, to the state child-protection agency. If this is done, keep in mind that the health-care worker has no choice and is doing it for the child's well-being.

Choking

Choking is one of the few true emergencies of childhood—minutes may determine life or death. Choking is caused when the airway becomes obstructed, resulting in inability to breathe. A swallowed object is the most common cause of choking.

Choking is easily identified by two key signs: the child frantically tries to breathe, and the child is not able to cry out or to speak. If choking continues, the child quickly becomes blue, convulsive, limp, and unconscious. If an object completely blocks the air passage, you have only a few minutes to reestablish an airway before brain damage or death can occur.

Objects that present a particular danger of choking if a child puts them in his or her mouth are peanuts, tablets, glass eyes of toy animals, hard or hard-coated candies, beads, popcorn, and tiny toys or small parts from toys.

Solid particles of food from the stomach may choke a child who breathes in while vomiting. A baby who has been vomiting is safest from choking when lying on his or her stomach.

Choking may also occur in a child who has croup. However, it is easy to tell choking that is the result of croup from other choking by one important distinction—a child choking on a foreign object cannot speak or cry out, while a child with croup can do both. Choking caused by croup is treated differently from other choking (see the article on *Croup* for treatment of that form of choking).

SIGNS AND SYMPTOMS

Choking on an object is easily identified by two major signs: frantic, unsuccessful efforts to breathe and inability to talk or cry out.

HOME CARE

Seconds count! Scream for help. A second adult on the scene should phone the police or paramedic squad for help. (Police are usually more quickly available in most communities than an ambulance, the fire department, or a doctor.)

Give the child **one minute** to cough up the object. If the child's efforts are unsuccessful, perform the following maneuvers.

If the child is an infant: Lay the baby face down on your forearm, with your hand supporting her head. The baby's head should be lower than her chest. Using the heel of your hand, give four quick blows to the baby's back between the shoulder blades. Then place your free hand on the back of the baby's head and, holding her between your forearms, turn her faceup, with her head still lower than her body. Put two fingertips on the baby's chest between the nipples. Press quickly and fairly hard four times. (You are trying to squeeze the upper abdomen and lower chest, which will force up the diaphragm so that air is pushed out of the lungs. The rush of air out of the lungs may pop the object out of the airway.) Repeat the cycle of four blows and four presses for as long as the baby is still choking. **Don't give up.**

If the child is a toddler or an older child: Stand behind the child. Reach around the child, lock your hands together, and place them just below his breastbone. Use a quick upward motion while pulling his stomach in. (You are trying to squeeze the upper abdomen and lower chest, which will force up the diaphragm so that air is pushed out of the lungs. The rush of air out of the lungs may pop the object out of the airway.) Repeat if necessary.

Only if these efforts are unsuccessful should you attempt to get the object out with your fingers or tweezers (there is a danger of pushing the object farther into the airway).

If breathing stops, begin resuscitation once the airway is clear. Continue until trained help arrives.

PRECAUTIONS

■ When an object completely blocks the air passage, the child seldom reaches a doctor in time. However, the object may be only partially blocking the airway, even though you may not think so. Do not abandon your efforts to help a choking child until medical help arrives.
■ Never give mouth-to-mouth resuscitation until the obstructing object has been removed. To do so may force the object farther down the throat.
■ A baby who has been vomiting should be placed on his or her stomach to lessen the chance of choking on the vomit.
■ Prevention of choking is most important. Examine all toys for loose eyes or other small parts. Keep tablets under lock and key. Do not give peanuts, popcorn, or hard candies to toddlers, and be sure to clean up after adult gatherings before children can wander unattended into a room and find such hazardous treats.

MEDICAL TREATMENT

The doctor may need to perform a tracheotomy (make an opening through the neck into the windpipe) on the spot. Then oxygen, artificial respiration, and intravenous fluids will be administered.

RELATED TOPICS: Convulsions with fever; Convulsions without fever; Croup; Swallowed objects

Circumcision

Circumcision is the removal of the cuff of skin (the foreskin) that covers the glans (the head of the penis) in most boy babies. The natural opening in the foreskin is usually large enough to allow urine through (rarely is there no opening at all). It is also important to be able to pull back the foreskin so that the smegma (the waxy material that normally forms under the fore-

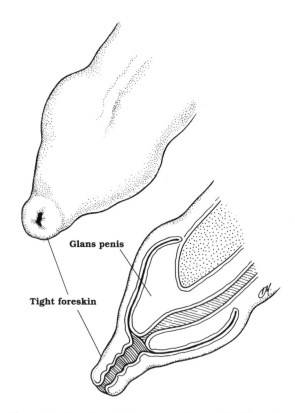

Glans penis

Tight foreskin

In phimosis, the foreskin cannot be pulled back.

skin) can be removed during bathing. In a condition called phimosis, the opening is not large enough to allow the foreskin to be pulled back to uncover the glans. The foreskin can sometimes be stretched by a doctor when the opening is too small to allow the foreskin to be pulled back; however, sometimes circumcision is necessary.

If the penis is uncircumcised, it sometimes happens that the pulled-back foreskin cannot be drawn forward again and may act as a tourniquet, cutting off the blood supply to the glans; this condition, called paraphimosis, is treated by circumcision.

Circumcision has been practiced throughout the world for centuries, both for religious and social reasons. It has been commonly performed on newborn boys in the United States since World War II. Its advantages are easier cleansing and lessened possibility of paraphimosis. However, contrary to what many people believe, circumcision does not protect against cancer of the penis. The disadvantages of circumcision are a slight chance of infection or bleeding after the operation (less than one percent), the brief pain of the operation, and the chance of accidental injury to the glans during the operation (a rare occurrence).

In recent years many doctors have declared that circumcision is unnecessary surgery. However, many other doctors feel that the advantages outweigh the disadvantages. The decision to circumcise male infants remains with the parents. Parents should ask questions and gather as much information as possible to help them make the decision.

MEDICAL INDICATIONS FOR PERFORMING CIRCUMCISION

Circumcision is required only when boys are born with no opening in the foreskin, when the opening is too small to allow passage of urine, or when paraphimosis has developed and must be immediately corrected.

HOME CARE

A circumcision should be covered until healed (two to five days) with a nonstick bandage and gauze coated with petroleum jelly. The area should not be submerged in bathwater until the wound has healed.

PRECAUTIONS

■ Any bleeding of the circumcised penis beyond a few drops should be reported to your doctor.
■ If there are any signs of infection (pus, spreading redness, swelling of the shaft of the penis), see your doctor.
■ During bathing, any part of the foreskin remaining after healing of the circumcision should be pulled back to expose the base of the glans for cleansing.
■ Boy babies born with malformations of the penis should not be circumcised because the foreskin may be used later during surgery to correct the malformation.

MEDICAL TREATMENT

Your doctor or religious leader will perform the circumcision, using one of a variety of approved techniques. Ask for specific directions for care of the circumcision. In a rare instance of post-operative infection, the doctor will perform cultures of blood and material from the circumcision site and begin antibiotic therapy.

Colic

Colic is a relatively common condition characterized by fussiness and long spells of crying that affects many infants (10 to 20 percent of babies in the United States). Often, babies with colic appear to be suffering from cramplike abdominal pains. However, other babies with colic don't act like they are experiencing any such abdominal discomfort—instead, their crying seems related only to general irritability. (In some babies, both factors may be at work.) Colic usually starts during the first few weeks of life and lasts one to six months (an average of three months).

SIGNS AND SYMPTOMS

The signs of colic are seen in the typical behavior of colicky infants. A baby with colic cries for hours a day, particularly in the late afternoon and evening. The child often pulls the legs up, clenches the fists, screams, and turns red. The child may feed briefly but often stops feeding and returns to crying. Rocking and cuddling also stop the cries only briefly. In other respects, the infant is normal—the baby gains weight well, has normal bowel movements, and doesn't spit up any more than most infants do.

A variation of this typical form of colic occurs in the infant who wakes frequently (every two hours or so), cries fretfully, takes one to two ounces of formula or a few minutes at the mother's breast, falls into a fitful sleep, and wakens later to repeat this pattern.

HOME CARE

First check for obvious causes of crying and discomfort. Consider diarrhea or constipation, loose diaper pins, severe diaper rash, a trapped arm or leg, and signs of illness—fever, nasal discharge, cough, reddened eyes, vomiting, hernia (a lump in the groin), or sores. The baby may also be either too hot or too cold.

See whether your baby responds promptly to talking and cuddling and remains comfortable. (A baby in pain can be distracted, but only temporarily.) Giving the child a pacifier may help.

Offer your baby a feeding. If your baby takes an ample feeding and falls asleep comfortably for several hours, the child was hungry, not colicky. Keep the baby partially upright in an infant carrier between feedings to avoid regurgitation of food into the esophagus.

If the baby is being breast-fed, check that the mother's nipples are not bleeding—swallowed blood causes cramps. It has also been suggested that if a breast-feeding mother drinks too much cow's milk, this may cause cramps in the infant.

If your baby seems to be having abdominal discomfort, applying warmth to the abdomen may temporarily relieve the problem. Place a cloth diaper over the infant's abdomen, and then place a hot-water bottle filled with warm (not hot) water on top of the diaper. On occasion, you may want to try inserting a glycerine suppository or lubricated thermometer to induce a bowel movement.

PRECAUTIONS

■ Make sure that formula is properly prepared.
■ When bottle-feeding your baby, make sure that the nipple is kept full; this will keep your baby from swallowing too much air.
■ Make sure that the bottle's nipple hole is large enough so that the baby can finish feeding in a reasonable time (20 to 25 minutes).
■ Carefully burp the baby in different positions after each feeding.

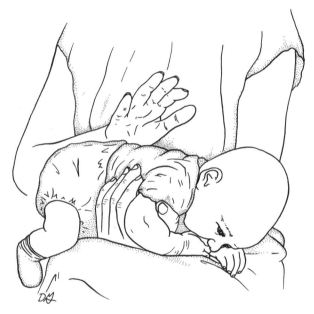

After each feeding, carefully burp the baby in different positions.

MEDICAL TREATMENT

Your doctor will check for signs of illness, such as sores in the mouth or urinary tract problems. A urinalysis may be ordered. Your doctor may also recommend a change in formula to investigate the possibility that the child is allergic to the formula. It is sometimes suggested that a breast-feeding mother try eliminating all milk products from her diet. The doctor may also temporarily stop any solids already started to determine if the child is allergic to certain foods. Unfortunately, only rarely is a cause for colic found.

RELATED TOPICS: Constipation; Coughs; Diaper rashes; Diarrhea in young children; Fever; Food allergies; Hernia; Vomiting

Common cold

A cold is a viral infection of the upper respiratory tract. The infection causes discomfort in the throat, nose, and sinuses. A cold sometimes also affects the eyes (connected to the nose by the tear ducts), the ears (connected to the nose by the eustachian tubes), and the lymph nodes of the neck (connected to the nose by lymph channels). A cold is transmitted from person to person through the air or by droplets on the hands or on objects (for example, toys, drinking glasses, and handkerchiefs). Symptoms may develop within two to seven days after exposure to a cold virus. People of all ages are subject to catching colds, but younger children and infants are particularly at risk from colds.

Many years were spent trying to develop a vaccine against the cold germ. Then it was discovered that there is not just one cold germ. Colds are caused by many different viruses, and all respiratory viruses can cause common colds. An attack by one type of virus makes a person immune to only that virus. Often this immunity lasts only for a short time.

Many cold viruses can cause complications such as croup, laryngitis, bronchitis, bronchiolitis, viral pneumonia, and encephalitis. All cold viruses can make a child more susceptible to bacterial infections, such as ear infections, sinus infections, lymph infections, and bacterial pneumonia. No child's cold should be taken lightly.

SIGNS AND SYMPTOMS

The symptoms of a cold are nasal congestion, sneezing, clear nasal discharge, scratchy sore throat, and fever up to 103°F. In general, the younger the child, the higher the fever. Symptoms may also include reddened, watery eyes; dry cough; mild swelling and tenderness of the lymph nodes in the neck; and mild pain in the ears.

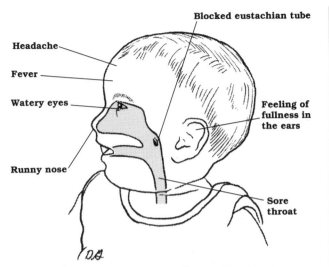

A common cold may cause discomfort in the nose, sinuses, eyes, ears, and throat.

It is often difficult to tell a cold from other illnesses that have similar symptoms. Usually it is assumed to be a cold if the familiar cold symptoms occur but symptoms of other illnesses do not. Another clue is that a cold lasts only three to ten days.

HOME CARE

Your child should drink a lot of liquids but should eat only if he or she wants to eat. Give acetaminophen for fever or pain. Bed rest is not necessary, but the child should avoid strenuous physical activities while fever is present.

Nose drops or oral decongestants and a nasal aspirator may be used to relieve nasal stuffiness and discharge. (Unless instructed to do so by your doctor, do not use nose drops for more than two or three days. Also, because of the risk of contamination, never use the same bottle of nose drops for more than one person or for more than one week at a time.) Cough medicines may ease a severe cough. Remember, however, that overuse of any of these medications can cause more harm than good. Chest rubs and vitamin C treatments have *not* been proved helpful.

A humidifier or vaporizer may make breathing easier. (Be sure to keep it meticulously clean, however. Otherwise, it can actually be a source of infection if microorganisms are allowed to grow in it.)

Isolate the child from others, particularly from infants and the elderly.

PRECAUTIONS

■ The following symptoms do *not* usually occur with a common cold and may be signs of another illness: fever lasting more than two to three days; puslike discharge from the eyes, nose, or ears; large, red, tender lymph nodes in the neck; breathing difficulties; chest pain; severe headache; stiff neck; vomiting; chills accompanied by shaking; prostration (collapse). If any of these symptoms occurs, call your doctor.
■ Some viruses that cause common colds stay in the body for one to two weeks, so the child remains contagious for the entire time of the cold.
■ Infants should not be exposed to anyone with a cold, even a mild cold. Infants are not protected against the common cold by the mother's antibodies; young infants can become seriously ill from these viruses.

MEDICAL TREATMENT

Your doctor will perform a physical examination to check for signs of other illnesses and for signs of complications. The doctor sometimes will order blood tests and a throat culture.

RELATED TOPICS: Bronchiolitis; Bronchitis; Chest pain; Coughs; Croup; Earaches; Encephalitis; Fever; Glands, swollen; Headaches; Laryngitis; Pneumonia; Shortness of breath; Sinusitis; Viral infections; Vomiting

Concussion

A concussion is an injury to the brain. It is caused by a fall or by a blow to the head from a blunt object. In many ways, a concussion is like a bruise of the brain. There is swelling in the brain, and sometimes blood escapes into the brain tissue. Since a concussion is an injury to the brain matter itself, it may occur even if the skull is not fractured. Concussions range from mild to serious.

Most children suffer one or more blows to the head at some time during childhood. Typical reactions to head injuries are immediate crying, headache, paleness, vomiting once or twice, a lump or cut at the site of injury, and sleepiness for one or two hours. These are **not** the signs of a concussion—they are usual reactions to a blow on the head.

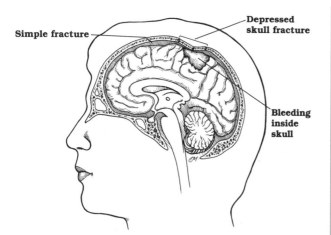

Simple fracture

Depressed
skull fracture

Bleeding
inside
skull

Every child who suffers a concussion should be examined by a doctor in case there has been a skull fracture, which may cause bleeding inside the skull.

SIGNS AND SYMPTOMS

Any of the following are signs of a possible concussion: unconsciousness at the instant of the injury, no memory of the accident or of events that occurred before the accident, confusion (the child doesn't recognize his or her parents or know his or her own name), persistent vomiting, inability to walk, eyes not parallel, pupils of different sizes (however, some children normally have unequal pupils), pupils that do not become smaller when a bright light is shined into the eyes, blood coming from the ear canal, bloody fluid that does not clot coming from the nose, headache that continues to become more severe, stiff neck (the chin cannot be touched to the chest with the mouth closed), increasing drowsiness, slow pulse (less than 50 to 60 beats per minute), and abnormal breathing.

There are two rare forms of concussion in which symptoms do not develop until hours (called epidural bleeding) or weeks (called subdural bleeding) after the injury.

HOME CARE

If the child shows any signs of a concussion, see your doctor. If there are no signs of a concussion, or if you are waiting to see the doctor, have the child rest in bed. Bed rest is the most essential treatment for a head injury that does not penetrate the skull. Keep the child lying quietly, with the head on a pillow. Check the child frequently. The child may sleep but **must** be awakened every hour so you can check on his or her condition until the child feels well. Keep the child in bed until at least one day

after he or she seems fully recovered. Give only aspirin or acetaminophen for headache.

PRECAUTIONS

■ **Do not** attempt home treatment if there are any signs of a concussion.

■ **Do not** treat a head injury at home if the scalp is depressed (pushed in) at the site of the injury or if gentle tapping of the skull produces the dull sound of a broken melon. (These symptoms rarely, if ever, occur without other signs of concussion.)

■ **Do not** give painkillers, sedatives, or any medication stronger than aspirin or acetaminophen to a child with a head injury.

MEDICAL TREATMENT

Your child may be hospitalized for observation. A computed tomographic (CT) study may be ordered. (X rays of the skull are less commonly ordered now that CT scans are generally available.) An echoencephalogram (which uses sound waves to visualize structures in the brain), an electroencephalogram, and a spinal tap may sometimes be helpful. If the concussion is serious, your doctor may consult a neurosurgeon (a surgeon who specializes in disorders of the nervous system).

Conjunctivitis

Conjunctivitis, or pinkeye, is an infection of the transparent membrane (conjunctiva) that covers the white of the eye and lines the inside of the eyelids.

Conjunctivitis is highly contagious. It is spread by contact with discharge from the eye or by contact with hands or objects (washcloths, toys, handkerchiefs) that have touched the infected eye. Symptoms of conjunctivitis may develop within one to three days after contact with the infection. Conjunctivitis usually spreads quickly to the other eye.

Conjunctivitis may exist alone. It may also develop as a complication of sore throat, tonsillitis, earache, or sinusitis.

SIGNS AND SYMPTOMS

Conjunctivitis causes redness of the entire white of the eye. There is a buildup of yellow pus. The eyelids may swell and redden. There is a burning sensation in the eye. Vision is always normal, and light rarely bothers the eye.

Conjunctivitis is different from other conditions that also cause reddened eyes. *Eye allergies* cause itching and tearing but never pain or pus. *Viral infections* cause pain and tearing but no pus. *Foreign bodies* in the eye cause pain, sensitivity to light, and tearing, but no pus; furthermore, redness caused by a foreign body usually appears in only one part of the white of the eye. *Glaucoma* causes pain, enlargement of the pupil, tearing, and sensitivity to light, but no pus. If your child has reddened eyes, consider these other possible causes.

HOME CARE

If you suspect conjunctivitis, call your doctor. Your doctor may wish to see the child; however, if your description of the symptoms is detailed, the doctor may prescribe antibiotic eyedrops or ointment over the telephone.

Always place the antibiotic in the eyes as frequently as directed. Treat both eyes even if only one seems affected. Continue treatment for 24 hours after the eyes appear normal.

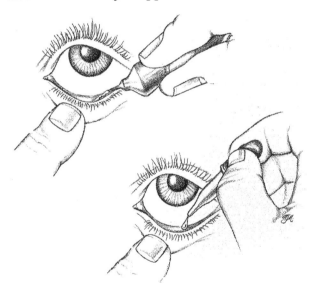

To place eyedrops or ointment into the eye, gently pull down the lower lid to form a pouch. Place the prescribed amount of medication into the pouch. Do not touch the eyedropper or ointment tube to the eye. Direct the child to close the eyes but not to rub them.

Since conjunctivitis is so contagious, isolate your child from other people. Watch other members of the family for possible symptoms.

PRECAUTIONS

■ With medication, the condition should improve quickly—usually within 24 hours. If the eyes don't begin clearing in that time, call your doctor.

■ If eye ointments are used, vision will be blurred for a few minutes after each application. Any other vision problems should be reported promptly to your doctor.

■ Be certain to notify your doctor of any other signs of illness, such as a head cold; nasal discharge; sore throat; earache; fever; or swollen, tender lymph nodes. Conjunctivitis may be a complication of another disease.

MEDICAL TREATMENT

The doctor will carefully examine the outside and inside of the eyeball, including looking under the eyelids for hidden foreign bodies. Your doctor may stain the eyeball with special drops to look for injuries or ulcers (scratches on the surface of the eye). The doctor may also culture any discharge from the eye, nose, or throat. Antibiotics taken by mouth might be prescribed. If necessary, your doctor may consult an ophthalmologist (a specialist in eye diseases).

RELATED TOPICS: Common cold; Earaches; Eye allergies; Eye, blocked tear duct; Fever; Glands, swollen; Sinusitis; Sore throat; Tonsillitis

Constipation

Constipation is a condition in which the stools (bowel movements) are too hard. The function of the colon (large intestine) is to store unabsorbed food waste and to absorb and hold water from the liquid material received from the small intestine. If the colon absorbs too much water, the stools become hard.

The frequency of bowel movements is not a factor in constipation. Passage of six too-firm stools a day is considered constipation. Passage of one normal or soft stool every third or fourth day is not constipation. Many normal, healthy children have a bowel movement only every few days and are not constipated. The hardness of a stool is judged by appearance and by diameter. A stool greater than twice the usual diameter is probably too hard.

In more than 95 percent of cases, constipation is not caused by any physical abnormality. In such cases, constipation can usually be cured by changes in the diet or by using medications that soften the stools.

In children, there are two common causes of constipation. The first is a diet low in roughage, which holds water in the stools. Foods that prevent constipation are all fruit juices and all fruits (particularly those eaten with the skin on) except bananas; all vegetables, especially if eaten raw, except peeled potatoes; and unrefined grains (whole-grain cereals and breads).

The second common cause of constipation in children is that the child is resisting the normal impulse to move the bowels. (This often occurs when parents put too much pressure on the child during toilet training.) As a result, the colon continues to absorb water from the retained stools, which then become too hard. As the stools become harder, bowel movements become painful. Fear of such pain makes the child even more determined to postpone bowel movements. Constipation enlarges the colon, causing a loss of muscle tone, and the physical impulse to empty the bowel becomes weaker. This cycle can lead to chronic constipation.

SIGNS AND SYMPTOMS

The major sign of constipation is stool that is too hard, too dry, and larger in diameter than usual. Constipation can cause pain in the anus during bowel movements. Red blood may appear on and around the stools. Other symptoms are cramps in the abdomen and an eventual loss of appetite.

If constipation continues for days or weeks, *paradoxical diarrhea* may develop. In this condition, loose, watery stools seep around the hard stool in the colon and are passed as diarrhea. When this happens, it can be difficult to tell whether the child has constipation or diarrhea.

HOME CARE

For immediate temporary relief, use a glycerine suppository or disposable commercial enema. For a long-term cure, increase the amount of roughage and decrease the amount of constipating foods in your child's diet. (Check with your doctor to find out which foods tend to cause constipation and how you can ensure that your child's diet is nutritionally adequate.) If constipation occurs during toilet training, stop training efforts.

PRECAUTIONS

■ Check with your doctor before giving laxatives to a child. Laxatives may force passage of a hard stool and cause pain that leads to further holding back by the child.
■ Enemas, suppositories, and laxatives are habit-forming. They should never be used on a regular basis.
■ Do not assume that a child is constipated simply because bowel movements do not occur every day.

MEDICAL TREATMENT

Your doctor will perform a rectal examination and a careful examination of the child's abdomen. X-ray studies of the bowel may be performed to look for possible physical abnormalities.

RELATED TOPICS: Diarrhea in older children; Diarrhea in young children; Stomachache, acute; Stomachache, chronic

Convulsions with fever

Convulsions are uncontrolled contractions or spasms of the muscles. If a child who has a fever goes into convulsions, there are two possible causes. The convulsions may be caused by the fever itself or by certain diseases involving the brain that also cause fever.

Febrile convulsions (convulsions caused by the fever itself) occur in five to ten percent of all children. How quickly the temperature rises or falls is more important than how high the temperature is. A sudden change of only 2°F or 3°F may cause convulsions, but a gradual rise of 5°F or 6°F may not.

Febrile convulsions may be thought of as chills accompanied by shaking that become extreme. They are most common between the ages of three months and three years. Febrile convulsions occur less and less often from age three to age eight. After the age of eight, febrile convulsions are rare. One episode of febrile convulsions usually means that the child is more likely to have them in the future. However, the tendency to have febrile convulsions does *not* mean that the child will later have epilepsy.

Diseases involving the brain that cause convulsions include meningitis, encephalitis, and abscess of the brain. When convulsions occur with these diseases, the child usually has a fever. However, the disease—not the fever—causes the convulsions.

SIGNS AND SYMPTOMS

During convulsions with fever, a child will fall unconscious, will become rigid, and may stop breathing briefly. The child may turn blue, lose control of the bladder and bowels, and vomit. The limbs, torso, jaws, and/or eyelids will jerk uncontrollably. The child will quickly begin breathing normally again. The seizure activity may last two minutes to 30 minutes or longer. After regaining consciousness, the child will not remember that the convulsions occurred.

Several traits of febrile convulsions can help you distinguish them from convulsions caused by such diseases as encephalitis, meningitis, and brain abscess. A major sign of febrile convulsions is that the child recovers quickly (within minutes). Immediately after a febrile convulsion, the child is alert, can respond, and is not prostrated (in a state of collapse or exhaustion). After a febrile convulsion, the child can bend the neck forward. There is often a family history of febrile convulsions.

After convulsions caused by diseases involving the brain, the child often cannot bend the neck forward and may be in a state of collapse or exhaustion.

HOME CARE

Do not panic! Your child is in no pain and is in more danger from improper treatment than from the convulsion. Protect the child from injury while the convulsion is occurring. Call your doctor immediately.

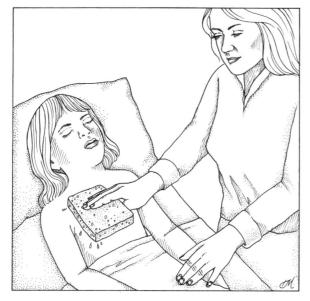

If a child tends to have convulsions with a fever, sponge the child's body with a damp (lukewarm) sponge at the first sign of fever.

PRECAUTIONS

■ **Do not** give aspirin or any other medication by mouth to an unconscious child. An unconscious child cannot swallow and may choke on the medicine.

■ **Do not** give mouth-to-mouth resuscitation to a convulsing child. The breathing muscles are temporarily in spasm during the convulsion, and such forceful artificial respiration may be harmful.

■ **Do not** place a convulsing child in a tub of water to reduce the child's temperature. Accidents such as scalding and injuries against the sides of the tub have occurred; this practice is *not* recommended.

■ If the child cannot bend the neck forward after the convulsions have ended, or if the child has collapsed or is exhausted, report this to your doctor. These may be signs of serious illness.

■ If a child tends to have convulsions when he or she develops a fever, sponge the child's body with a damp (lukewarm) sponge at the first sign of fever.

MEDICAL TREATMENT

Any child who has a febrile seizure needs to be seen by a doctor. If the seizure doesn't stop, call for help and take your child to the nearest emergency room. It is necessary to find the cause of the fever.

Most doctors agree that a child who has experienced a febrile seizure doesn't need to take medicine on a daily basis in an attempt to prevent more febrile seizures.

A child who has had one febrile seizure is more likely to have more when suffering from an illness with fever. Parents should remember that febrile seizures don't lead to epilepsy, nor do they make children more likely to have other neurological problems.

RELATED TOPICS: Choking; Convulsions without fever; Encephalitis; Fever; Meningitis

Convulsions without fever

Convulsions (jerking movements or spasms of the muscles) that occur when a child has no fever may be caused by many conditions. Epilepsy is the best-known cause of such convulsions. Epilepsy is a disorder of the brain that causes repeated attacks, or seizures. There are several forms of epilepsy, which are identified by the type of seizure experienced. (Although some forms of epilepsy cause convulsions, other types do not; therefore the term seizure is more properly used to describe an attack of epilepsy.) The cause of most types of epilepsy is not known.

SIGNS AND SYMPTOMS

Epilepsy must be diagnosed by a doctor. However, epilepsy can be suggested by the typical behavior that occurs in different types of seizures.

In a *generalized convulsive seizure,* the child suddenly loses consciousness and may cry out as the seizure starts. The body stiffens, and the child may fall. Muscle spasms cause jerking or wild thrashing movements. The child may lose control of the bladder and bowels. When the spasms end, the child may fall into a deep sleep and will usually be confused and sleepy on awakening. Sometimes there is a warning sensation (called an aura) before this type of seizure begins, such as sleepiness, headache, yawning, or tingling in the arms and legs.

Generalized nonconvulsive (absence) seizures are so different from major convulsive seizures that they are often not recognized as epilepsy— or may not even be noticed. The child may simply stare into space. There may be rapid blinking or fluttering of the eyelids. The child remains conscious yet may be totally unaware that the seizure is occurring. If it is not recognized as a seizure, it may be mistaken for a learning disability, not paying attention, or simple daydreaming.

In *complex partial seizures* the child remains conscious but may sit motionless or may make repeated or unusual movements.

In *simple partial seizures* the child is conscious and may simply feel tingling in the hands and feet. The child may also perceive bad odors, see flashing lights, or speak unintelligibly.

HOME CARE

Call your doctor any time a child has convulsions.

Of course, you must immediately care for the child during the convulsions. The most important home care is to prevent your child from injury during the thrashing phase of convulsions. Do not put your fingers in the child's mouth in an attempt to grab the tongue to prevent it from being swallowed.

If epilepsy is diagnosed, the doctor will give instructions for caring for the child at home. Until the seizures have been controlled, discourage the child from climbing high ladders or tall trees. Do not allow the child to swim alone. Otherwise, your child can and should live a normal life with only minor changes in activities.

PRECAUTION

■ If you find your child unconscious, do not assume that a fall was the cause. Consider the possibility that epilepsy led to a fall and unconsciousness.

MEDICAL TREATMENT

Your doctor will perform physical and neurologic (nervous system) examinations. The doctor may also order a variety of laboratory and diagnostic tests. A number of prescription medications that control seizures are available. The doctor may order blood tests to determine the amount and type of drug to be used. In difficult cases, your doctor may recommend consultation with a neurologist (a specialist in diseases of the nervous system).

RELATED TOPICS: Choking; Convulsions with fever

Coughs

Coughing is a valuable defense mechanism of the body. It is the body's way of removing any foreign material that enters the respiratory tract (the throat, larynx, trachea, bronchial tubes, and lungs). Coughing is not a disease itself—it is an automatic reflex that is set off by any irritation of the lining of the respiratory tract.

In most cases, coughing helps remove unwanted materials from the body, although sometimes coughing does not succeed. The only harm in a cough is that it may keep a person from sleeping, or it may cause soreness of muscles and exhaustion if the cough is hard and frequent. Coughing may also lead to vomiting in children.

A cough is only as serious as the disease or condition that causes it. As with a fever, a child with a cough is no less ill if you lessen or stop the cough. A child with a mild illness and a cough is still only mildly ill. To correct the cough, cure the disease.

SIGNS AND SYMPTOMS

Coughing is itself a symptom of a disease or an indication that an irritating substance is present in the respiratory tract. Most coughs are caused by viral infections (common colds, croup, bronchitis, bronchiolitis). Some are caused by bacterial infections (sinusitis, epiglottitis, bacterial pneumonia, whooping cough). Other coughs are caused by allergies (asthma) or by inhaling irritating particles.

It is not unusual for young children to vomit after a coughing spell. This is normal and nothing to worry about. It occurs because the child can't bring up and spit out the phlegm that is loosened by the coughing.

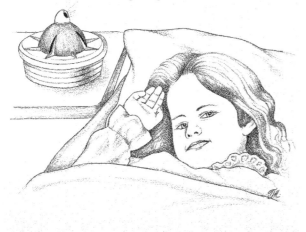

A vaporizer or humidifier will add moisture to the air and help relieve coughs.

HOME CARE

Since coughing is only one symptom of an illness, you must treat the whole illness—not just the cough. When the illness is cured, coughing and other symptoms will be relieved. There are, however, steps you can take to help relieve coughing. Give the child plenty of liquids. Use a vaporizer or humidifier to add moisture to the air. (Be sure to keep it meticulously clean, however. Otherwise, it can actually become a source of infection if microorganisms are allowed to grow in it.)

Cough medicines are sometimes useful. You should be aware, however, that there are various types of cough medicines that differ in their usefulness in the treatment of specific illnesses or kinds of coughs:

Cough suppressants are used to reduce the frequency of the cough by suppressing the cough reflex. They may contain a narcotic (codeine, dihydrocodeinone, or hydromorphone) or a nonnarcotic (dextromethorphan or ben-

zonatate). Consult your doctor before giving your child a narcotic cough suppressant.

Expectorants contain ingredients (such as glyceryl guaiacolate, guaifenesin, ammonium chloride, and antimony potassium tartrate) that may make it easier to cough mucus out of the lungs.

Antihistamines are used if an allergy is causing the cough. They reduce or counteract allergic reactions.

Some cough medicines contain a combination of ingredients and are intended to serve more than one purpose. Many different combinations of drugs are on the market in liquid form or as tablets or capsules. Before purchasing a cough medicine for home use, consult your doctor about the type of cough medicine (if any) that should be used.

Remember also that sometimes it is better not to try to suppress the cough. In some illnesses (especially asthma and pneumonia), coughing helps the child get rid of excess mucus in the lungs or air passages.

Many doctors believe that the cough and cold medications available do little if anything to help suppress a cough.

PRECAUTIONS

■ Do not give cough medicine to a child with croup.

■ Do not give cough medicine to a child with any breathing difficulty unless it has been approved by your physician.

■ Do not give cough medicine to a child who may have inhaled a foreign body.

MEDICAL TREATMENT

Your doctor will concentrate on treating the condition causing the cough, not the cough itself. Narcotic cough medicines and some cough medicines that contain antihistamines must be prescribed by a physician.

RELATED TOPICS: Asthma; Bronchiolitis; Bronchitis; Common cold; Croup; Pneumonia; Sinusitis; Viral infections; Whooping cough

Cradle cap

Cradle cap (seborrheic dermatitis) is a skin condition in which yellowish, scaly, or crusty patches appear on the scalp. The crusty patches are made up largely of oil and dead skin cells. Cradle cap is most common in infants, but it is seen in children through age five. Temporary loss of hair is common.

SIGNS AND SYMPTOMS

The key sign of cradle cap is the yellowish, scaly, crusty appearance of the patches. A greasy scalp film can be scraped off. The patches most often appear on the scalp, but may extend onto the forehead. Patches may also appear in the skin fold behind the ears, on the ears, and in the diaper area. The most typical location in infants is over the soft spot in the scalp called the anterior fontanelle.

HOME CARE

Mild cases of cradle cap on the scalp can usually be cleared up by daily, vigorous shampooing. Use soap on a wet, rough washcloth wrapped around the palm of your hand. If regular soap or shampoos do not clear up the condition, special shampoos that contain coal tar or salicylic acid are useful. If necessary, apply ointments containing sulfur, salicylic acid, or coal tar to the scalp daily.

PRECAUTIONS

■ Be sure that medicated shampoos and ointments do not get into your child's eyes.
■ Stop using medicated shampoos or ointments if the scalp or the skin becomes irritated or red.

MEDICAL TREATMENT

Your doctor will determine whether the condition is cradle cap or some other skin condition, such as a yeast infection or an allergic skin reaction. A topical steroid may be prescribed.

RELATED TOPIC: Eczema

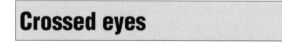

Crossed eyes

Crossed eyes is a condition in which one or both eyes turn inward toward the nose. In many cases, it is caused by improper functioning of the eye muscles.

The eyeballs are turned in all directions by six tiny muscles that lie within the bony socket of the eye. These muscles keep the eyes parallel when the child looks at a distant object (more than 20 feet away) and turn the eyes slightly inward when they are focusing on closer objects.

Infants learn to focus their eyes during the first three to six months of life. The eyes may occasionally turn in (*esotropia*, or internal strabismus) or out (*exotropia*, or external strabismus) in relation to each other during this learning period. These conditions may briefly occur even up to the age of one year and still be considered normal. When an infant's eyes are continuously not parallel, when they are not parallel more and more often at any age, or when they are not parallel past the age of one, the situation is abnormal and requires your doctor's attention.

Although most cases of crossed eyes are caused by improper muscle function, some are caused by a vision problem in one or both eyes. Anything that can cause crossed eyes can also cause the development of a "lazy eye" (*amblyopia ex anopsia*). If lazy eye is not corrected by the age of four to six years, disuse may cause a loss of sight in that eye.

SIGNS AND SYMPTOMS

Watch the relationship of the eyes to each other as the child focuses near and far, looks to either side, and looks up and down. If the eyes seem to turn inward more than usual, consult your doctor.

Be aware, however, that although many young children appear to have crossed eyes, their eyes are actually straight. Many infants and young children have an extra skin fold at

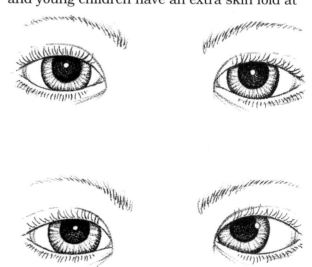

To judge the straightness of a child's eyes, shine a light into the eyes while the child is looking straight ahead. The highlight should be at the same spot in each eye (as shown at the top). If the highlight is at different spots (as shown on the bottom), one eye may be crossed.

the inner corners of their eyes (alongside the nose). This fold of skin appears because of the tininess of the bridge of the nose. This extra fold allows more white of the eye to show toward the temples than toward the nose, creating an illusion of crossed eyes.

Straightness of the eyes is best judged by observing the position of the highlights (the points where light is reflected in the eyes) in both eyes. If the highlights appear in the same position in both eyes, the eyes are parallel.

Some children experience wandering or inward turning of an eye when they are tired. When the children are well rested, their eyes move properly. This shouldn't cause any alarm since it is normal for many children.

HOME CARE

There is no home treatment except under the supervision of your doctor.

PRECAUTIONS

■ If the pupils of your child's eyes are not equally black, smoothly round, and the same size, see your doctor.

■ If your child's eyes are not parallel, see your doctor to avoid the development of a lazy eye.

■ All children should have their vision checked annually beginning at the age of four or five.

MEDICAL TREATMENT

Your doctor will check the eye muscles and vision and inspect the insides of the eyeballs. This examination can be done on any child at any age. If your doctor diagnoses or suspects crossed eyes, you will probably be referred to an ophthalmologist (a physician who specializes in disorders of the eyes). Treatment will depend on the cause. It may include eye surgery, glasses, placing a patch over one eye, daily use of eye drops, or eye muscle exercises guided by a specialist.

RELATED TOPICS: Lazy eye; Vision problems

Croup

Croup is an inflammation and swelling of the larynx (voice box), usually caused by an infection. Croup is common and is passed on in the same way as a cold—by airborne droplets or by direct contact with an infected person.

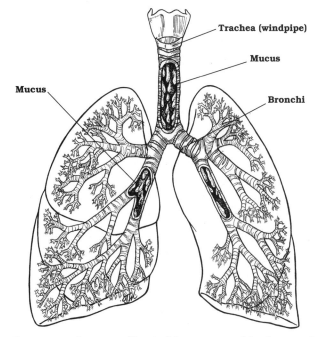

Croup can be complicated by mucous blockage of the windpipe and the bronchi leading into the lungs. This may lead to serious breathing problems and become a medical emergency.

Croup causes a tight, dry, barking cough and hoarseness. Difficulty in breathing develops quickly, with more trouble in inhaling than exhaling. Efforts to inhale cause the crowing sound that is typical with croup. (This is in contrast to asthma, in which there is more difficulty in exhaling, and a wheezing sound is heard when the child breathes out.) Croup can be serious, but milder cases, especially repeated ones, can usually be handled safely at home.

There is a form of croup, *epiglottitis*, that is a life-threatening illness—a true emergency in which minutes count. It is a bacterial infection of the epiglottis (the lidlike structure that covers the entrance to the larynx) and surrounding tissues. It is most common in children between the ages of three and nine years. The fever may rise to 105°F. The difficulty in breathing quickly becomes severe. The child drools, has trouble swallowing, and prefers to sit with the head forward, mouth open, and tongue partially out. The condition rapidly progresses to choking and convulsions—it must be treated immediately.

SIGNS AND SYMPTOMS

The key symptoms of croup are a barking cough, hoarseness, difficulty in breathing, and a crowing sound heard when inhaling. There may be no fever or only a low-grade fever (101°F).

It is important to be always watchful for the signs of epiglottitis: a high fever, difficulty in breathing and swallowing, sore throat, drooling, and preference for the characteristic position of sitting with the head forward, mouth open, and tongue partially out.

Choking on a foreign object may resemble croup, since both share the same symptom of frantic efforts to breathe. However, it is easy to tell choking from croup by one important distinction—a choking child cannot speak or cry out, but a child with croup can do both.

HOME CARE

If a child has serious breathing difficulty, do not try to care for him or her at home. Notify your doctor, and head for the nearest hospital emergency room.

Mild, repeated attacks of croup can often be cared for at home (if there is no serious difficulty in breathing). However, it is best to call your doctor the first time you suspect that your child has croup.

The basic home care for mild attacks is adding moisture to the air to relieve the cough and help the child breathe more easily. A humidifier or vaporizer will be helpful. (Be sure to keep it meticulously clean, however. Otherwise, it can actually become a source of infection if microorganisms are allowed to grow in it.) Steam also may be generated quickly by running a hot shower in a closed bathroom. Sit in the room with your child for a short while. If the symptoms are not relieved, call your doctor.

PRECAUTIONS

■ If your child has a high fever, has difficulty in breathing and swallowing, is drooling, or sits with the head forward, mouth open, and tongue hanging out, **get medical help immediately**.

■ Never give any type of cough medicine to a child with croup or any difficulty in breathing.

■ **Do not** give ipecac as a home treatment for croup. Ipecac may make breathing even more difficult.

MEDICAL TREATMENT

Mild cases of croup can usually be treated at home. In severe cases, the child will be hospitalized, and a croup tent, which provides high humidity, will be used. The doctor may also order an X-ray examination, cultures, and

blood tests. If the condition becomes severe, intubation (insertion of a tube into the airway) may be necessary.

Epiglottitis is always treated as an emergency. The doctor will intubate the child or perform a tracheotomy (in which an opening is made surgically in the windpipe). Intravenous fluids and antibiotics will be given, and the child's condition will be carefully watched.

RELATED TOPICS: Asthma; Choking; Convulsions with fever; Fever

Cuts

Wounds of the skin are classified as abrasions (scrapes), punctures, and lacerations. A laceration is a cut of any size and depth and can be located anywhere on the body.

SIGNS AND SYMPTOMS

A cut is obvious from its appearance and the bleeding that occurs. However, there are signs and symptoms that you should look for to help you decide whether the cut needs a doctor's care or can be treated at home. Major cuts with serious bleeding obviously need a doctor's immediate attention; emergency control of bleeding is the only possible home treatment. For less severe cuts, consider the following characteristics:

First, look at the depth of the cut. If a cut is more than skin deep, it should not be treated at home. Deeper structures (such as muscles, tendons, and nerves) must be repaired with stitches.

Second, look for dirtiness or raggedness in the cut. A cut with ragged edges or with deeply embedded dirt needs professional care to avoid infection and to reduce scarring.

Third, look at the width and location of the cut. A small cut rarely needs stitching to control the bleeding, but stitching may help reduce the amount of scarring. A cut heals leaving a scar the size of the opening of the skin. There is no treatment that will reduce the length of the scar. But the closer the edges of the cut are to each other during the healing process, the narrower the final scar will be. If a homemade bandage can hold the edges together for the seven to ten days required for healing, there may be no advantage to a doctor's treatment. However, if the cut is in an area that moves, such as near a joint or on some parts of the face, it is nearly impossible to keep the edges from gaping unless the wound is stitched.

HOME CARE

First, stop the bleeding. Apply firm pressure directly on the cut for ten minutes (by the clock). Use sterile gauze if it is immediately available. If not, any reasonably clean cloth (for example, a handkerchief, towel, or shirt) will do. Even bleeding from large arteries can be controlled by pressure applied directly on the wound. You rarely need so-called pressure points.

Do not use a tourniquet to stop bleeding from a cut. The only time a tourniquet is necessary is when a limb has been partially or completely amputated. In such a case, the tourniquet may be placed anywhere above the wound. The current thinking is that once the tourniquet has been put on, it should be left on—not released and tightened as was once suggested. Then immediately rush the person to the nearest medical facility.

Second, once the bleeding has stopped, wash the area with soap and water so that the cut is clearly visible. Look at the depth, width, dirtiness, raggedness, and location of the cut to decide if a doctor should treat the wound.

If it seems reasonable to care for the cut at home, apply a nonstinging antiseptic. Draw the edges of the wound together with adhesive butterfly bandages. Then cover the wound with sterile gauze and a bandage to prevent infection. If the cut is near the joint of a finger, splinting the fingers can keep them from moving until the cut has healed. If the cut is between two toes, the area can sometimes be kept from moving by bandaging together those toes. Inspect the wound every day for signs of possible infection. Remove the butterfly bandages after seven to ten days.

PRECAUTIONS

■ If the cut requires stitching, it must be done within eight hours to avoid infection.
■ If a wound becomes infected (characterized by increased tenderness, swelling, discharge of pus, or red streaks spreading out from the wound), see your doctor.
■ Be sure that your child receives tetanus boosters at the ages recommended by your doctor.

MEDICAL TREATMENT

Your doctor has the skill and equipment to handle most cuts that cannot be cared for at home. Your doctor will clean a dirty wound and decide if the wound needs stitching. In some cases, the services of a general surgeon or a plastic surgeon will be required.

RELATED TOPICS: Animal bites; Blood poisoning; Immunizations; Puncture wounds; Scrapes; Tetanus

Cystic fibrosis

Cystic fibrosis is a chronic (lifelong), inherited disease. It affects the lungs, pancreas, sweat glands, and sometimes the liver and other organs. It is the most common serious inherited disease in the United States.

Cystic fibrosis is passed from parents to child through a particular gene. (The genes are the parts of the body's cells that determine such inherited characteristics as hair and eye color and blood type). To inherit cystic fibrosis, a child must receive that particular abnormal gene from both parents. A child who receives the abnormal gene for cystic fibrosis from only one parent will not have the disease. A person who carries the gene but does not have the disease is known as a "healthy carrier." When both parents are healthy carriers, there is a 25 percent risk that any one of their children will receive the gene from both parents and suffer from the disease. Five percent of white persons, two percent of African Americans, and less than one percent of Asian and native African black persons are healthy carriers. One in 2,000 white children in the United States has cystic fibrosis.

SIGNS AND SYMPTOMS

Cystic fibrosis may appear at birth as an obstruction or blocking of the intestines. Symptoms may also appear during infancy or childhood or sometimes as late as adolescence.

Some common symptoms of cystic fibrosis are frequent respiratory infections, including bronchitis and pneumonia; chronic cough; failure to gain adequate weight; constipation or diarrhea with foul-smelling stools; protrusion of the rectum; and clubbing (broadening) of the fingertips and toes. Almost all persons with cystic fibrosis have unusually salty sweat; the first sign of cystic fibrosis is often the very salty taste of the child's skin when kissed.

HOME CARE

If you have any reason to suspect that your child has cystic fibrosis, see your doctor. If cystic fibrosis is diagnosed, home treatment will be directed by your doctor. Treatment at home may include taking antibiotics, following a special diet, taking pancreatic enzymes by mouth, inhaling vapor and medications, and postural drainage (a technique for placing the child in specific positions and tapping over the chest to allow excess fluids to drain from the lungs).

PRECAUTIONS

■ If your child shows any signs of cystic fibrosis, a sweat test should be done. A sweat test is a painless, harmless, inexpensive, and generally reliable test for cystic fibrosis.
■ If there is any history of cystic fibrosis in the family, a sweat test should be considered for all children, even if they appear to be healthy.
■ The sweat test is not reliable before the age of one month and is not as reliable during adolescence.

MEDICAL TREATMENT

The doctor will perform a sweat test and may also order a chest X-ray study. If cystic fibrosis is diagnosed, your doctor will most likely refer you to a medical center where there are specialists in treating cystic fibrosis.

The outlook for a child with cystic fibrosis who is in relatively good health is better now than in the past, but a cure for cystic fibrosis is still being sought. The earlier the diagnosis is made and treatment is started, the better the outcome.

Deafness

Deafness is a partial or complete loss of the sense of hearing. A hearing loss may be slight or severe and may occur in one ear or in both ears. A child may be born with a hearing loss, or it may develop at any age.

Normal hearing involves the following chain of events: Sound waves pass down the ear canal and cause the eardrum to vibrate. Vibrations of the eardrum, in turn, move the three tiny bones in the middle ear. This motion

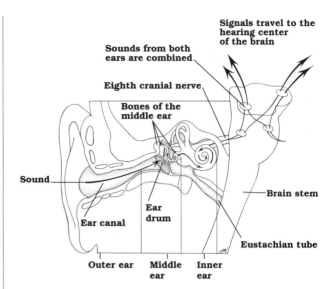

In normal hearing, sound causes vibrations of the eardrum, which are transmitted by the chain of bones in the middle ear to the inner ear, which then sends signals through the auditory nerve to the brain.

of the bones transmits the vibrations across the middle ear to the inner ear. In the inner ear, the vibrations are changed to electrical impulses, which are carried to the brain through the eighth cranial nerve. The brain interprets these electrical impulses as sound.

If any of the structures involved in this process malfunctions or is damaged or diseased, deafness can result. The following problems may lead to hearing difficulties:

Ear-canal problems that may cause hearing loss include a buildup of earwax, a foreign object in the canal, or swimmer's ear (infection of the outer ear).

Eardrum and middle-ear problems may be caused by an inflammation of the middle ear or a blocked eustachian tube (the tube that connects the middle ear and the upper part of the throat).

Inner-ear problems may be caused by injuries or infections.

Eighth cranial nerve problems have several possible causes. A child may be born with a nerve that has not developed properly or that was damaged before birth. (For example, if a pregnant woman contracts rubella, the virus may infect the eighth cranial nerve in the fetus.) After birth, this nerve can be damaged by an injury, a viral infection (such as mumps or measles), or a bacterial infection (such as meningitis). This nerve can also be affected by certain medications.

SIGNS AND SYMPTOMS

Signs of hearing loss usually can be seen in a child's behavior. Suspect hearing loss if any of the following situations occurs: an infant over three months old ignores sounds or does not turn the head toward sound; a baby over one year old does not speak at least a few words; a child over two years old does not speak in at least two-word or three-word sentences; a child over five years old does not speak so that a stranger can understand; a child of any age has learning problems in school; or a child simply does not seem to hear well at home. Any of these symptoms may be caused by hearing loss, but they may also have other causes. Every child should be given a professional hearing test before starting kindergarten.

HOME CARE

Home care for a hearing problem depends on the cause, as well as on the degree of hearing loss. If you think that your child may have a hearing problem, see your doctor. A doctor can more accurately determine if there is a problem and can prescribe the best treatment.

PRECAUTIONS

■ Every woman of childbearing age should consult her doctor about rubella (German measles) immunization.

■ Do not put any object (including cotton swabs) into your child's ear canal for any reason. You may force earwax to become packed into the canal, or you may damage the eardrum or other structures within the ear.

MEDICAL TREATMENT

Your doctor will examine the ear to determine the cause of the hearing loss. Specialists have equipment to test hearing in children of any age past early infancy. If there is any doubt about the cause or treatment of the hearing loss, your doctor may refer you to a center that specializes in speech and hearing disorders. A deaf child should start special education as soon as the condition is discovered, even if the child is as young as one or two years old.

RELATED TOPICS: Common cold; Draining ear; Earaches; Immunizations; Rubella; Speech problems and stuttering; Swimmer's ear

Dehydration

Dehydration is a serious loss of body fluids. It occurs when the body is losing more fluids than it is taking in. When an excessive amount of body fluid is lost, the water, minerals, and salts that are essential to health and to life are lost as well.

Several conditions may cause the body to lose excessive amounts of water, minerals, and salts. Diarrhea, vomiting, and excessive sweating are common causes of dehydration. Illnesses that increase the breathing rate (such as bronchiolitis and asthma) may cause the child to lose water vapor from the lungs. Illnesses that cause excessive urination (such as diabetes) may also cause dehydration.

The smaller the child, the more quickly dehydration can develop. In young infants, the condition can become serious as rapidly as 12 to 24 hours after the start of any cause of dehydration (such as diarrhea or vomiting). A child who is not losing extra fluids will rarely become dehydrated simply by taking in fewer liquids. Except in young infants and in children with diabetes, the kidneys can compensate for a smaller intake of liquids. However, a small intake of liquids in a child who is also losing fluids causes dehydration to occur even more rapidly.

SIGNS AND SYMPTOMS

Except in a child with diabetes, one sign of dehydration is a smaller output of urine. A young child who does not urinate for six to eight hours, or an older child who does not urinate for 10 to 12 hours, may be dehydrated. The child's urine may be dark colored and have a strong odor. Other signs of dehydration include sunken eyes, drowsiness, rapid or slow breathing, tearless crying, and depression (sinking in) of the soft spot at the top of an infant's head. The membranes inside the mouth may feel dry when touched. The skin may feel less resilient than usual (for example, it does not easily return to its original shape when pinched gently between the thumb and the forefinger).

HOME CARE

If a child shows any symptoms of dehydration, call your doctor. If the child is vomiting, stop the vomiting first. With any condition that causes fluid loss (including prolonged high fever), you should encourage your child to drink extra fluids. Sometimes a child who has nausea and vomiting may be able to tolerate only a sip or two every few minutes. The best liquids to give a child with excessive fluid loss are commercial electrolyte solutions (available from your pharmacist), which supply necessary salts and sugar. Other good liquids are gelatin desserts (liquid or gelled), weak tea with sugar, fruit juices, and carbonated drinks, such as ginger ale and colas. Plain water is less helpful. Milk products should be avoided.

PRECAUTIONS

■ Do not give milk or milk products to a child who is losing fluids.

■ If symptoms of dehydration develop, contact your doctor. The younger the child, the more urgent the situation. Diarrhea in infants can be very serious.

■ The amount of urine output is not an indication of dehydration in a diabetic child.

MEDICAL TREATMENT

Your doctor will diagnose and treat the condition that is causing dehydration. Your child may be admitted to a hospital to be given intravenous fluids and salts. The child may be tested for the amounts of salts and minerals in the body.

RELATED TOPICS: Asthma; Bronchiolitis; Diabetes mellitus; Diarrhea in older children; Diarrhea in young children; Fever; Vomiting

Diabetes mellitus

Diabetes mellitus is a condition in which the body does not properly process carbohydrates (sugars and starches). In children, it occurs when the pancreas does not produce enough insulin (a hormone that is essential for processing carbohydrates). Sugars and starches are the body's main sources of energy. When the body cannot properly turn sugars and starches into energy, abnormally high amounts of unused sugars are found in the blood and urine. Also, because the body must burn more fats for energy in place of sugars, ketone bodies (chemical compounds that are an end product of that process) are found in the urine.

Diabetes can occur at any age. It appears in one in 2,500 children by the age of 15. The disease usually runs in families. The parents may or may not be diabetic. There may be other family members who are diabetic, or there may have been diabetes in the family in the past.

SIGNS AND SYMPTOMS

The earliest signs of diabetes are increased hunger, increased thirst, and increased urination. The child will both urinate more often and produce greater amounts of urine. Other symptoms then appear, including weight loss, fatigue, and irritability. Most cases are detected by this stage. If diabetes is not detected and corrected, deep, rapid breathing followed by unconsciousness (diabetic coma) eventually develops. If you notice any of these symptoms, see your doctor. An exact diagnosis can be made only through laboratory tests.

HOME CARE

Do not try to treat a diabetic child on your own. Your doctor must diagnose diabetes and prescribe treatment. The doctor will tailor the treatment to your child's exact needs. Then you must carefully follow the doctor's instructions for caring for the child at home.

You and your child must learn as much as possible about diabetes. The doctor will give instructions for making necessary changes in the child's diet, giving insulin, and testing the urine. You will learn how to recognize and treat insulin shock (caused by too little sugar in the blood) and diabetic coma (caused by too much sugar in the blood).

PRECAUTIONS

■ Bed-wetting that suddenly occurs regularly after a child has been toilet-trained for some time may be a sign of developing diabetes. The child's urine should be tested for diabetes (and urinary tract infection) if bed-wetting continues.

■ If there is diabetes in your family background, try to keep your children from becoming overweight. If a child already has an inherited tendency toward diabetes, being overweight increases the possibility that diabetes will develop as the child grows older.

■ Untreated and uncontrolled diabetes may lead to dehydration (a serious loss of body fluids) caused by increased urination. Complicating this situation is the fact that the amount of urine output is not a reliable sign of dehydration in a diabetic child.

MEDICAL TREATMENT

To properly diagnose diabetes, the doctor will order several laboratory tests. A urinalysis will test for extra sugar and ketone bodies in the urine. A blood test can detect unusually high amounts of sugar in the blood. In a glucose tolerance test, the child drinks a known amount of glucose (a form of sugar); the level of glucose in the blood is then measured from time to time over several hours.

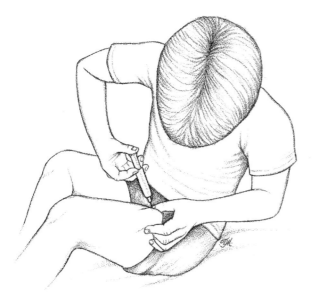

Most diabetic children require insulin injections and can be taught, from as early as four years of age, how to give themselves injections.

If diabetes is found, your doctor may hospitalize your child to regulate the diet and determine the amount of insulin the child will need to take. If the child is dehydrated or has ketone bodies in the blood and urine, these conditions will also be treated in the hospital. Before discharging your child, your doctor will make certain that you and the child understand how insulin should be given and how the child's diet should be changed. Most diabetic children require insulin daily and are instructed—from as early as four years of age—to give themselves injections.

RELATED TOPICS: Bed-wetting; Dehydration

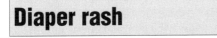

Diaper rash

Diaper rash is an irritation of the skin in the diaper area. Almost all babies get diaper rash in one form or another. Diaper rash may be caused by moisture, urine, or irritating chemicals in the diapers or by an allergic reaction.

SIGNS AND SYMPTOMS

Rashes in the diaper area can usually be identified by their appearance, their location, and other typical symptoms.

Simple diaper rashes are red, slightly rough, and scaly. The rash may appear over the whole area touched by the diaper. The skin may be irritated by chemicals in products used to launder cloth diapers (detergent, bleach, whitener, water softener, or soap). Plastic or rubber pants worn over cloth diapers sometimes affect the skin. The skin may also react to chemicals used in manufacturing disposable diapers or to the plastic outer layer on disposable diapers.

Ammonia rash is a form of diaper rash caused by the urine itself. The skin is burned by ammonia that is formed when urine is decomposed by bacteria that are normally found on the skin. Ammonia rash is worse after the child has been asleep for long periods of time without a diaper change. It is identified by an ammonia smell that can be noticed when changing the diaper.

Besides these basic diaper rashes, a variety of other rashes may appear in the diaper area, including rashes caused by an allergy to a food or drug, by a skin infection, or by contagious diseases (such as chicken pox and measles).

If your child develops a rash in the diaper area, look for the signs that indicate these different types of rashes. The appearance and location of the rash, an ammonia odor, or a rash elsewhere on the body are all clues. Have you recently changed to a different kind of diaper or changed your way of laundering cloth diapers? Has the child recently been given a new food or drug that could be causing an allergic reaction? Noting these factors can help you and your doctor find the cause of the rash.

HOME CARE

Keep your baby as dry as possible and change diapers frequently.

For simple diaper rash, apply a protective ointment (petroleum jelly, zinc oxide, vitamin A & D ointment, or an ointment combining zinc oxide, cod liver oil, petrolatum, and lanolin). Try changing your brand of soap or your method of washing cloth diapers.

If the rash seems to be caused by ammonia, avoid using an airtight outer covering over the diapers. Wash the diaper area frequently with clear water.

If you think that the rash may be an allergic reaction, stop giving the child any new foods or beverages started in the previous month. If the rash improves, reintroduce one of these items every week and watch for any change in the condition. This may help determine if a food or beverage is causing the rash. Ask your doctor if perhaps a recently prescribed medication might be causing an allergic reaction. However, do not discontinue use of any medication without your doctor's permission.

If your doctor has identified the rash as being caused by an infection or contagious disease, frequently wash the area with soap and water and apply an antibiotic ointment, such as bacitracin or neomycin. If the rash is caused by yeast, keep the area dry and apply any antiyeast cream that your doctor may have prescribed.

If the rash is spreading or severe, or if the child has a fever, irritability, or loss of appetite, see your doctor.

PRECAUTIONS

■ If the rash gets worse, even after only two days of home treatment, see your doctor.
■ Do not use more than one type of ointment (such as an antibiotic and a fungicide) at any one time unless the doctor prescribed both.
■ If your child has any other symptoms of illness, see your doctor.

MEDICAL TREATMENT

Your doctor may be able to identify the rash by its appearance or may culture the rash to identify bacteria or fungi. Changes in methods of laundering diapers, diet, and medications may be suggested. A medicated ointment may be prescribed.

RELATED TOPICS: Chicken pox; Cradle cap; Eczema; Food allergies; Impetigo; Measles; Rash

Diarrhea in older children

Diarrhea refers to looseness of the stools—not to the frequency of bowel movements. (Having frequent bowel movements with stools of normal consistency is not considered diarrhea.) The number of loose stools per day reflects the seriousness of the diarrhea.

Diarrhea in children over the age of five years differs in several ways from diarrhea in younger children. Diarrhea is less likely to cause dehydration (a serious loss of body fluids) in older children. The older and larger the child becomes, the less the chance of dehydration. Serious dehydration is unlikely past six years of age—unless diarrhea is combined with vomiting, which keeps the child from drinking enough liquids.

Viruses in the intestine are the most common cause of diarrhea in older children. Dysentery bacteria and parasites in the intestine are the next most common causes. Respiratory viruses and reactions to certain foods are the least likely causes of diarrhea in older children.

Other diseases may cause long-term, frequent diarrhea in older children (these disorders are rare or unknown in infants). *Ulcerative colitis* is a condition in which ulcers appear in the colon (large intestine). *Regional enteritis* (Crohn's disease) is a recurring inflammation in the small intestine. *Cystic fibrosis* is an inherited disease that affects the lungs, pancreas, sweat glands, and sometimes the liver and other organs. It often causes frequent diarrhea with foul-smelling stools.

SIGNS AND SYMPTOMS

The major symptom is loose, watery stools. There may be mucus or flecks of red blood in the stools. The child may have cramps, fever, loss of appetite, vomiting, and weight loss, depending on the cause of the diarrhea.

HOME CARE

If the child has both diarrhea and vomiting, treat the vomiting first, by restricting the child's diet to clear liquids. When the vomiting has stopped, treat the diarrhea by limiting or not reintroducing solid foods—especially butter, fatty meats, peanut butter, whole-grain cereals, vegetables, and most fruits (apples and bananas are OK). Do not give the child milk, which may further aggravate diarrhea.

Encourage the child to drink plenty of clear liquids; tea, water, flavored gelatin water, and commercial electrolyte solutions (available from your pharmacist) are best.

PRECAUTIONS

■ Do not give antidiarrheal medications to children, since side effects are common and can be dangerous.

■ Isolate an infant from children who are vomiting or who have diarrhea.

■ If there is blood in the stools, high fever, prostration (extreme weakness or collapse), or severe or prolonged diarrhea (lasting more than two to three days), call your doctor. Dysentery may be the cause.

■ Report frequent, repeated diarrhea to your doctor. It may be a symptom of colitis, enteritis, or cystic fibrosis, especially if there is weight loss.

MEDICAL TREATMENT

Your doctor may order blood tests, X-ray studies of the large and small intestines, and sigmoidoscopy (examination of the large intestine with a special lighted instrument). In severe cases, hospitalization may be necessary.

RELATED TOPICS: Botulism; Constipation; Cystic fibrosis; Dehydration; Diarrhea in young children; Dysentery; Food allergies; Food poisoning; Gastroenteritis, acute; Shock; Viral infections; Vomiting

Diarrhea in young children

Diarrhea is a condition in which the stools are loose and watery. Diarrhea is judged by the looseness of the stools, not by the frequency of bowel movements. (Having frequent bowel movements with stools of normal consistency is not considered diarrhea.) Any bowel movement that is partially or completely runny is diarrhea. The frequency and amount of loose stools indicate the severity of the diarrhea.

Diarrhea in infants and young children (under the age of five years) is potentially dangerous. Diarrhea can lead to dehydration (a serious loss of body fluids). The younger the child, the greater the possibility of dehydration.

Common causes of diarrhea in infants are infections of the digestive tract and reactions to certain foods and drugs. In infants, infections may be caused by respiratory viruses, intestinal viruses, bacteria, and parasites. Some foods tend to cause diarrhea in most infants (corn kernels and large quantities of prunes, for example). Other foods may cause diarrhea in some infants but not in others. Some infants are allergic to certain foods. Many antibiotics may cause diarrhea in infants.

SIGNS AND SYMPTOMS

The looseness of the stools is the major symptom. The relatively fluid, watery stools often contain mucus and sometimes flecks of red blood. A child with diarrhea may have cramps and sometimes fever, loss of appetite, vomiting, and weight loss. There may be as few as one or as many as 20 loose bowel movements a day. However, if having only one or two loose bowel movements is followed by a return to normal, the diarrhea is probably not serious.

In looking for the cause of diarrhea, consider whether a new food has recently been added to the child's diet and whether the child has recently been given antibiotics. If other children in your family are ill, your infant may be suffering from the same illness.

HOME CARE

If an infant or young child has both diarrhea and vomiting, treat the vomiting first, by restricting the child's diet to clear liquids only. When the vomiting has stopped, treat the diarrhea. Eliminate all newly introduced foods and beverages and eliminate foods with roughage, including all vegetables and fruits (except bananas and apples). Do not give the child cow's milk or cow's-milk-based formula. Do not discontinue use of antibiotics unless authorized by your doctor. Encourage the child to drink clear liquids to ward off dehydration; tea, flavored gelatin water, and commercial electrolyte solutions (available from your pharmacist) are best. Continue treatment for diarrhea until the child has had no stools or normal stools for 24 to 48 hours.

PRECAUTIONS

■ Do not give antidiarrheal medications to infants. These are of no use and can cause severe problems.

■ Solid foods aggravate diarrhea and can be avoided for many days without any danger to the child's general health. It is most important that the child drink plenty of liquids.

■ Watch for symptoms of dehydration (infrequent urination, decrease in urine output, dark-colored urine that has a strong odor, dryness in the mouth, sunken eyes, tearless crying, drowsiness, rapid or slow breathing, sunken soft spot on the top of an infant's head). If any symptoms of dehydration appear, call your doctor.

■ Improperly prepared and improperly refrigerated formulas are a common cause of serious diarrhea in infants. Be especially careful when normal refrigeration and cooking facilities are not available (picnics, camping, traveling, power outages).

MEDICAL TREATMENT

If there are signs of dehydration, your doctor will determine the degree of seriousness. (The loss of five percent of a baby's weight indicates serious dehydration.) Stools may be cultured for bacteria. If necessary, your child may be placed in the hospital to be given intravenous fluids or to determine if the intestines are functioning properly.

RELATED TOPICS: Botulism; Constipation; Dehydration; Diarrhea in older children; Dysentery; Food allergies; Food poisoning; Gastroenteritis, acute; Shock; Viral infections; Vomiting

Diphtheria

Diphtheria is a frequently fatal disease caused by a specific bacterium, (*Corynebacterium diphtheriae*). Diphtheria is contracted by exposure to a person with the disease or to a carrier of the disease. (A carrier is a person who has the bacteria in his or her body but is healthy.) Symptoms of diphtheria may develop within two to four days after exposure to the bacteria.

The diphtheria germ causes inflammation of the nose, throat, tonsils, and lymph nodes of the neck. The germ kills by destroying tissue and by producing a toxin (poison) that causes heart damage and paralysis. Croup and pneumonia are common complications of diphtheria.

The protective immunization against diphtheria has been available for over 40 years. It is among the safest, cheapest, and most effective of all known vaccines. Even though this safe vaccine is available, diphtheria still exists throughout the world because many persons are not immunized.

SIGNS AND SYMPTOMS

The major symptom of diphtheria is a persistent, severe sore throat. The infected throat develops pus and a gray membrane that looks similar to that seen in strep throat and

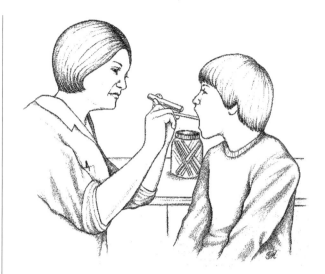

Diphtheria must be diagnosed by a doctor. The doctor will examine the child's throat and order a special nose and throat culture.

mononucleosis. Other symptoms include fever, cough, and troubled breathing.

The diagnosis of diphtheria must be made by a doctor. Diphtheria is difficult to diagnose for several reasons. First, many doctors in the United States have never seen a case of diphtheria. Second, diphtheria closely resembles mononucleosis, strep throat, and various forms of croup. Third, the doctor may not suspect diphtheria and therefore will not test for it. Routine throat cultures taken in a doctor's office to detect strep bacteria do not show diphtheria bacteria; the only way to detect diphtheria is by a nose and throat culture that is specifically designed to identify the diphtheria bacteria. Therefore, if a patient happens to have both diphtheria and a strep infection of the throat but the doctor does not consider the possibility of diphtheria and performs only a routine throat culture, the strep infection will be identified but the diphtheria will be missed. That is why it is so important to let your doctor know if your child has not been fully immunized against diphtheria.

HOME CARE

There is no home treatment for diphtheria. It is a serious (possibly fatal) disease, and treatment must be handled by a doctor. If your child has a severe sore throat, see your doctor. If your child has not been immunized or has not had the necessary boosters, you must report this so that the doctor knows to look for diphtheria as well as strep throat.

The best step parents can take is to prevent diphtheria through proper immunization. It is essential that infants be routinely immunized for diphtheria. Three shots are required during the first six months of life. Routine boosters are required at 18 months of age and again at four to six years of age. Boosters are required every ten years thereafter for a lifetime. If your child has not been immunized, every cough, sore throat, or case of croup should be suspected of being the beginning of diphtheria.

PRECAUTIONS

■ If your child's diphtheria immunization status is not up to date, be sure to inform the doctor treating your child. Diphtheria may be the furthest thought from your doctor's mind.
■ If a child is having any trouble breathing, **do not** attempt to look in the child's throat.
■ Do not give cough medicine to a child who is having any trouble breathing.
■ Remember that a child who has not been immunized can contract diphtheria from a well child or adult who is a carrier.
■ Never travel to an underdeveloped country where diphtheria is common without proper immunization or booster shots.

MEDICAL TREATMENT

If your doctor suspects diphtheria, the disease can be diagnosed and treated. Diphtheria antitoxin and large doses of penicillin or erythromycin are effective if started early enough. A tracheotomy (a surgical procedure in which an opening to the windpipe is made through the neck) may be necessary if the condition is severe.

RELATED TOPICS: Coughs; Croup; Immunizations; Infectious mononucleosis; Pneumonia; Sore throat; Strep infections

Dislocated elbow

A luxation, or dislocation, of a joint occurs when the bones are out of their proper place in the joint. When an elbow is dislocated, the bones are not completely out of place; therefore, it is more properly called a subluxation, or partial dislocation. It is the only common dislocation in young children. It frequently occurs between the ages of one and three years; it is rare beyond the age of four.

The elbow contains two separate joints. The larger is a hinge joint that allows the forearm to bend and to straighten in relation to the upper arm. The smaller, less obvious joint of the elbow is between the upper ends of the radius and ulna (the two bones of the forearm). This smaller joint allows the forearm to rotate in order to turn the palm up and down. It is this smaller joint (the radioulnar joint) that is partially dislocated when there is a sudden yank on a child's hand or wrist. It may occur when a parent tries to save the child from a stumble or fall. It may also occur when a child is swung around by the wrists in a game or when the child tries to grab a handhold to prevent falling.

SIGNS AND SYMPTOMS

When an accident causes a dislocated elbow, there is immediate pain. The pain may be felt anywhere from the elbow to the wrist. The child refuses to use the affected arm, clutching it against the side with the other arm. The child holds the affected arm with the palm of the hand facing backward. Attempts to turn the palm forward cause pain. Swelling of the wrist and hand develops several hours later.

If you know that the arm has been yanked and the child holds the arm with the palm facing backward, a dislocated elbow is a likely cause. However, if you do not know that the arm has been pulled, you may not realize the cause of the problem. A dislocated elbow is commonly mistaken for an injured wrist.

HOME CARE

As soon as you suspect that your child has a dislocated elbow, see your doctor.

Dislocation of the elbow tends to recur. There is a simple procedure for correcting a dislocated elbow, which your doctor may teach you if your child's elbow becomes dislocated often. (**Caution:** Do not attempt to correct a dislocated elbow unless you have been taught the proper procedure by a doctor.) If this maneuver is done within a few hours of the accident, a sharp snap or click will be heard and felt near the elbow. The child is relieved of pain and soon can use the arm freely.

PRECAUTIONS

■ **Do not** use the procedure for correcting a dislocated elbow unless the symptoms exactly fit the description and you are sure that the arm has been yanked. A fracture (break) of a forearm bone can produce similar symptoms.

■ A dislocated elbow should be treated as soon as possible. If the elbow has been dislocated for more than a few hours, correcting it may be more difficult because of the swelling; also, the arm may be sore and not fully usable for one to two days after correction.

■ Even after a dislocated elbow has been corrected, the joint remains susceptible to dislocation for three to four weeks. Be careful.

■ Do not lift a child by pulling on the hands, wrists, or arms.

MEDICAL TREATMENT

Your doctor will determine if the elbow has been dislocated. An X-ray examination may be ordered to be sure that there are no broken bones. (Sometimes, positioning the arm for the examination returns the dislocated bone to its proper place.) When the diagnosis is certain, your doctor will correct the dislocation using the standard procedure mentioned.

RELATED TOPICS: Fractures; Sprains and dislocations

Dislocated hips

Dislocation of the hip occurs when the thigh bone is out of its proper place in the hip socket. Before or after birth, a baby's hip socket may develop too shallowly. Eventually, the femur (thigh bone) becomes dislocated from the socket, either before or at the time when the child begins to stand and walk. The condition may occur on one side or on both sides. The cause is not certain; in some cases the condition seems to be inherited, while in others the problem seems to have been caused by an abnormal position of the infant's legs while still in the uterus.

If improper development of the hip socket is not diagnosed until after dislocation has occurred, correcting the problem will be more difficult. If it is not corrected before the child walks, the child will limp (if only one hip is dislocated) or waddle (if both hips are dislocated).

SIGNS AND SYMPTOMS

If only one hip is dislocated, parents may notice that the infant moves one leg more than the other. The folds of the buttocks or the creases on the sides of the groin may not match. A child who is already walking may limp or waddle.

HOME CARE

There is no home treatment until the condition has been identified by a doctor. Dislocation of the hip is a disabling condition if not treated early and properly. If you see any signs of hip problems, see your doctor as soon as possible.

PRECAUTIONS

■ Be sure that your baby is thoroughly examined (while completely undressed) at regular "well baby" visits to the doctor. Your doctor should examine the hips at each visit until the baby is older than one year.

■ If the child's legs are not the same (in size, shape, position, or movement), tell your doctor.

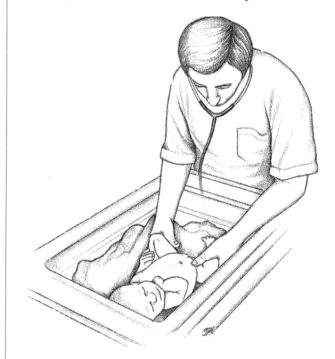

A baby's hips should be examined at birth and again at regular intervals so that dislocation of the hips can be detected early.

MEDICAL TREATMENT

Your baby should be carefully examined for dislocated hips during each checkup. A doctor will suspect dislocation if any of the early signs and symptoms appear. The doctor will then check the ability of the thighs to be rotated outward. The doctor will also listen for the "clunking" sound that a dislocated hip makes when put through a certain series of movements. Your doctor will order an X-ray examination of both hips if the disorder is suspected.

The diagnosis is not usually made at birth, but the condition becomes more obvious with the passing months. As soon as the diagnosis has been made, you should consult an orthopedic specialist. If the hip is not yet dislocated, the doctor may recommend the use of a special pillow positioned to keep the thighs spread or may apply a body splint or cast. If the hip is already dislocated, surgery may be required.

If both you and your doctor are alert, the problem can be noticed early. Early diagnosis is the key to easier treatment and optimal, permanent results.

RELATED TOPIC: Sprains and dislocations

Dizziness

Dizziness (vertigo) is the sensation that one is rotating or that one's surroundings are spinning around. It can be experienced normally by twirling rapidly in one spot until the room seems to be reeling. Dizziness makes it difficult for a person to keep balanced. If dizziness continues, it may cause nausea and vomiting.

If possible, try to find out exactly what a child means when complaining of dizziness. Children often use the word "dizzy" to describe faintness, light-headedness, nausea, and vision problems. Each of these problems can have many causes.

True dizziness has few causes. The most common cause is Meniere's disease. No one knows the cause of Meniere's disease, although some doctors think that it's an infection of the fluid in the semicircular canals. This condition usually is harmless and clears up without treatment, but it may last for weeks.

Dizziness may also accompany middle-ear infections, concussions, and fractures of the base of the skull. Dizziness occurs with tumors that involve the eighth cranial nerve or the cerebellum (a part of the brain). It may also occur in cases of meningitis and encephalitis.

SIGNS AND SYMPTOMS

If your child complains about feeling dizzy, ask him or her to describe the feeling as clearly as possible. Be sure the child is describing a spinning sensation and not some other sensation (faintness, light-headedness, nausea, or vision problems). Look at the child to see if there is a loss of balance. Also look for jerking motions of the eyes when they are turned to one side or the other (this is another sign of true dizziness).

A long period of dizziness may cause nausea and vomiting.

HOME CARE

Have a dizzy child sit down with the head lowered to the knees. Place your hand on the back of the child's head and have the child push up slightly against your hand. If the dizziness is not relieved, have the child lie down to rest, with the feet raised higher than the head. If rest does not relieve the dizziness, the cause must be determined by a doctor for proper treatment.

PRECAUTIONS

■ Try to be sure that the child is describing a sense of rotation before reporting the condition to your doctor.
■ See your doctor if dizziness occurs often or if dizziness lasts longer than one or two hours.

MEDICAL TREATMENT

The doctor will perform careful physical and neurologic (nervous system) examinations. Blood tests may be required. An ear, nose, and throat specialist may be asked to test the functioning of the inner ear, as well as the child's hearing. Your doctor may also consult a neurologist (a specialist in diseases of the nervous system). A computed tomographic (CT) scan and an electroencephalogram (EEG) may be necessary. Most often, no cause is found and the symptoms go away with time.

RELATED TOPICS: Concussion; Earaches; Encephalitis; Fainting; Meningitis; Vomiting

Draining ear

When any abnormal discharge or fluid comes out of the ear canal, the ear is said to be draining. The only material that normally comes from the ear canal is cerumen (earwax). Earwax is ordinarily brown, although it may be beige or yellowish if mixed with water when bathing, showering, or swimming. Normally, earwax has only a mild odor, contains no blood, and does not flow out in large amounts.

Discharge of any other material from the ear canal signals a potentially serious condition. It may be a symptom of a middle-ear infection, a boil in the ear canal, swimmer's ear (infection of the ear canal), rupture (break or tear) of the eardrum by injury or infection, a foreign object in the ear canal, cholesteatoma (a tumor of the middle ear), or a fracture of the base of the skull.

SIGNS AND SYMPTOMS

Abnormal discharge from the ear may be thin and watery, bloody, odorous, cheesy, green, yellow, or white.

HOME CARE

Any drainage from the ear canal other than ordinary earwax should be considered abnormal. Do not try to treat a draining ear at home. It should be seen promptly by a physician.

While the child is waiting to see the doctor, pain accompanying a draining ear may be temporarily treated with acetaminophen.

PRECAUTIONS

■ A draining ear should be examined by a doctor within 12 to 24 hours.
■ Do not pack cotton into a draining ear. Packing the canal may force the discharge back into the middle ear.
■ Do not use a cotton swab or any other object to remove material from the canal.
■ Do not attempt to wash out a draining ear, since the eardrum may be broken or torn.

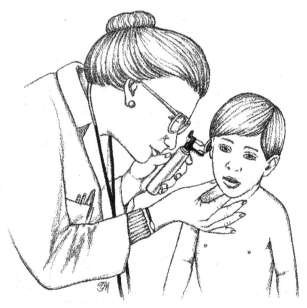

A draining ear should be examined by a doctor within 12 to 24 hours.

MEDICAL TREATMENT

Your doctor will gently clean your child's ear, inspect it, and diagnose the cause of the prob-

lem. Depending on what is found in the ear canal, treatment may include oral antibiotics, medicated eardrops, removal of a foreign body, an X-ray examination of the child's skull or mastoid bone, or surgery for cholesteatoma. In the case of a ruptured eardrum, antibiotics may be required for a long time, until the eardrum has healed and hearing has returned to normal.

RELATED TOPICS: Deafness; Earaches; Swimmer's ear

Drug and alcohol use

No child in our society can grow up without seeing drug and alcohol use daily. Ads promote the use of cigarettes and alcohol as a means to social success and happiness. Many children see their parents and friends use these addicting substance every day. Expecting our children never to use cigarettes, alcohol, or other drugs is probably unrealistic. Parents should strive to educate children so that they will be able to make well-informed decisions.

Children are using drugs at younger ages. By age 13, 30 percent of boys and 20 percent of girls have tried alcohol; by age 18, those figures rise to 93 percent of boys and 73 percent of girls. Most alcohol and drug users have tried it before the tenth grade. The same is true for cigarette use. Over 20 percent of high schoolers smoke regularly. Most smokers started in their early teens.

SIGNS AND SYMPTOMS

There are few behavioral changes in the early stages of drug use. However, you may notice some subtle changes in your child's behavior that become more common as the drug use progresses. Your child may become withdrawn and solitary, spending more and more time alone. He or she may stay out later in the evening, neglecting household chores and schoolwork, resulting in falling or even failing grades. Communication with family, teachers, and old friends lessens, with more arguments occurring. You may notice a change in your child's personal hygiene and choice of clothing. He or she may sleep more or may want to sleep during the day and be out late at night.

You may notice physical changes such as bloodshot eyes, an unusual number of headaches, "the flu," and stomach pain. Frequent nosebleeds and sniffling accompany the use of certain drugs.

If your child is smoking, the most common give-away is the odor of nicotine in the clothing and hair. The child may have "cigarette" breath, ash holes in clothing, or tobacco pieces in clothing pockets.

HOME CARE

If your child appears to be quite ill from drug use, withdrawal, or overdose, then immediate care is required. People do die from acute alcohol poisoning or alcohol withdrawal.

If you suspect a drug problem, then your child needs medical attention. Not all doctors are attuned to alcohol and drug abuse, and some are not comfortable discussing it. If your child's doctor doesn't deal with this medical problem, find one who does. There are many clinics and programs, both inpatient and outpatient, that specialize in the treatment of addiction problems.

Alcohol and drug addiction can affect any family, so don't think it can't happen to your children. A family history of abuse and dependency problems increases the chances your children will have them also.

Open and frank discussion about alcohol, drugs, and nicotine is an important first step. Many parents tell their teenage children that, if the child is in a situation where help is needed, they can always call their parent—no questions asked. Such nonjudgmental support is important.

PRECAUTIONS

■ None

MEDICAL TREATMENT

There has been an increase in the awareness of the medical profession about alcohol and drug dependency. Many doctors, called addictionologists, specialize in this area. Acceptance that the problem exists is the first step toward a cure. The best treatment plan is the twelve-step approach offered by Alcoholics Anonymous (A.A.), Narcotics Anonymous (N.A.), and other groups. The best treatment for families and friends of chemically dependent people is Alanon.

Some chemically addicted people require an inpatient program to help them get on the road to recovery. Others do well with intensive outpatient programs. Many alcoholics and drug abusers are able to begin their recovery by attending A.A. or N.A. meetings, while others need the more intensive treatment offered by inpatient or outpatient programs. Successful treatment usually requires the involvement of the entire family.

You need to understand that it isn't the addict's "fault" that he or she is addicted. And remember that recovery is an ongoing process. A chemically dependent person is never "cured" but is always working on his or her recovery.

Dysentery

In popular usage, dysentery is taken to mean any severe form of diarrhea. More accurately, dysentery is an infection of the intestinal tract caused by one of several specific organisms. Dysentery causes diarrhea, but dysentery is a distinct disease.

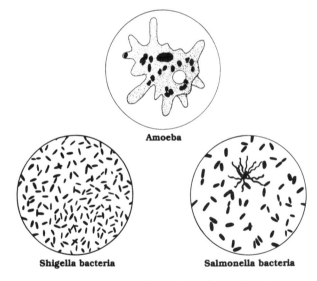

Amoeba

Shigella bacteria   Salmonella bacteria

Dysentery is an infection of the intestinal tract that is caused either by salmonella or shigella bacteria or by amoebas.

The germs that cause dysentery are salmonella and shigella bacteria. (Typhoid fever is caused by a type of salmonella bacteria.) Dysentery may also be caused by one-celled organisms called amoebas. Some doctors consider cholera to be a form of dysentery.

Dysentery is the result of eating or drinking food, milk, or water that is contaminated with these specific bacteria or amoebas. It also may be contracted from someone who has the disease or is a carrier of dysentery. (A carrier is a person who has the germ in his or her body but is healthy.) Complications that may develop from dysentery include arthritis, meningitis, and intestinal perforations (ulcers).

SIGNS AND SYMPTOMS

The major symptom of dysentery is diarrhea. The diarrhea is often severe and is commonly bloody. The child may have a prolonged high fever (103°F to 105°F). The child may also be extremely weak and exhausted. Any persistent diarrhea should be suspected of being dysentery, especially if it is severe or bloody.

HOME CARE

Do not attempt to treat dysentery on your own. Whenever diarrhea is severe or bloody, see your doctor. Dysentery must be diagnosed by a doctor and often requires treatment with specific medications.

While waiting to see the doctor, give the child plenty of clear liquids. Liquids are needed to replace those being lost because of the diarrhea. Extra liquids will help prevent dehydration (a serious loss of body fluids). Clear liquids that are the most helpful include commercial electrolyte solutions (available from your pharmacist), tea, and flavored gelatin water.

Limit or eliminate solid foods from the child's diet. Especially avoid butter, fatty meats, peanut butter, whole-grain cereals, vegetables, and most fruits (apples and bananas are OK). Do not give cow's milk or cow's-milk-based formula, since it may aggravate diarrhea.

PRECAUTIONS

■ Always report severe or bloody diarrhea to your doctor.
■ If diarrhea lasts more than two or three days, call your doctor.
■ The younger the child, the more easily dehydration can occur with diarrhea. Infants can become dehydrated rapidly (within 12 to 24 hours after diarrhea begins).
■ Do not give antidiarrheal medications to children, since side effects are common and can be dangerous.
■ When traveling, carefully choose sources of food and water, being alert to the possibility of poor sanitation.
■ If you suspect dysentery, isolate the child and dispose of stools carefully.
■ Practice good hygiene in your home. Wash hands after treating an ill member of the family. Always wash hands carefully before cooking and eating.

MEDICAL TREATMENT

A culture of the stools (with microscopic examination for amoebas and other parasites) confirms the diagnosis. Cultures of the blood and urine are sometimes performed, as well as tests for specific antibodies in the blood.

If dysentery is diagnosed, your doctor may hospitalize your child for treatment and isolation. Specific antibiotics for treating dysentery are available, although they are not always necessary. Diagnosed cases of dysentery must be reported to health authorities.

RELATED TOPICS: Arthritis; Dehydration; Diarrhea in older children; Diarrhea in young children; Meningitis

Dyslexia

Dyslexia is a type of learning disability that affects a child's ability to read. It is more common in boys than in girls. It is not known exactly what causes the problem. Dyslexia often runs in families, but no specific genetic defect has been found to account for it. Some children with dyslexia may have had an accident that caused an undetected brain injury, but others have no such history. It is known, however, that dyslexia is not a form of mental retardation and that dyslexia is *not* related to low intelligence, physical handicaps, cultural disadvantages, low social or economic status, or congenital brain damage.

A child with dyslexia often has no difficulties until entering school. Then the child finds that he or she cannot do things that other children can do easily. This experience can be embarrassing and painful. The child often finds it impossible to explain the problem and may become so frustrated that he or she either disrupts classes or becomes overly quiet and withdrawn. Other children may brand the dyslexic child as stupid; teachers and parents may consider the child lazy or unmotivated. The dyslexic child may, in fact, be very intelligent and may be trying extremely hard to learn to read. Pressure from teachers and parents to work harder can be confusing and frustrating and can lead to anger and rebellion. Some children with dyslexia find other activities that they can do well, such as sports or music. This may help them to adjust and feel more comfortable.

SIGNS AND SYMPTOMS

Dyslexia varies in severity. Some of the problems dyslexics may have include the following: confusion about whether they are right-handed or left-handed; difficulty in learning to tell time or remembering the order of days, months, or seasons; hyperactivity; problems with language; difficulty in telling left from right and up from down; coordination and balance problems; problems with memory; and seeing letters and numbers reversed.

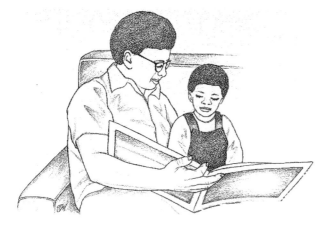

While a dyslexic child should not be overprotected, he or she will need special support and help from other family members.

Dyslexia is diagnosed by a series of tests of visual perception, memory, and space and time perception and by medical and psychological evaluations. A child who has the symptoms of dyslexia may have a disorder or disease of the central nervous system, problems with hearing or vision, or emotional problems, rather than a learning disability. The possibility of a physical or psychological cause for the problem must be ruled out before a diagnosis can be made.

HOME CARE

A child with dyslexia needs special support and help from the family. However, the child does not need to be overprotected. The child should be challenged as well as encouraged, but finding a balance is not an easy job. The child's teachers and doctor may be able to help parents work with a dyslexic child. The situation can be hard on the whole family, so parents need to be sensitive to how the problem may affect the dyslexic child's brothers or sisters, who may need extra attention or professional help.

PRECAUTIONS

■ If your child seems to be intelligent but has unexpected problems with reading, the child may have dyslexia. The sooner the problem is identified, the easier it will be for the child. Get professional help as soon as possible.
■ Do not consider the child a failure—instead, encourage him or her to develop new skills.

MEDICAL TREATMENT

There is no cure for dyslexia. If the child has physical or emotional problems as well as dyslexia, these will probably be treated first. A treatment plan will then be made to work on the reading problem. The plan may be developed by a team of educational professionals, in consultation with the child and the child's parents, doctor, and teachers. The plan will include special education and training for the child based on his or her particular problems and strengths.

RELATED TOPIC: Hyperactivity

Earaches

An earache is any pain or ache in the ear. Earaches may occur at any age from infancy on; however, they usually occur less and less often after the age of eight.

The most common cause of an earache is blockage of the eustachian tube (which connects the nose with the middle ear). This tube may become blocked as a result of a nasal allergy, a head cold, infected adenoids (lymph nodes in the passage between the nose and the throat), swimming in fresh or chlorinated water, or flying in an airplane. This blockage creates a vacuum in the middle ear, changes the pressure on the eardrum, and causes secretion of fluid into the middle ear. If obstruction of the eustachian tube continues, an infection of the middle ear (called *otitis media*) may rapidly develop. If the eardrum ruptures (breaks), discharge begins to drain out of the ear.

An earache may also result from the presence of foreign objects in the ear canal, a buildup of earwax, pain in the jaw or molar teeth, or boils in the ear canal. Boils can be caused by scratching or digging in the ear with hairpins, fingernails, or cotton swabs.

Complications of untreated middle-ear infections include mastoiditis (infection of the bone behind the ear), meningitis, perforated eardrum, and draining ear. Both middle- and outer-ear infections can cause swollen, tender lymph nodes.

SIGNS AND SYMPTOMS

Earaches may be mild or extremely painful. The pain may be constant, may come and go, or may occur only with chewing, burping, or nose blowing. Earaches may or may not be accompanied by fever or signs of a cold. They may or may not affect hearing. Progression to otitis media usually causes intense, often throbbing pain. If the eardrum ruptures, pain quickly lessens. If there is a boil, a foreign body, a buildup of earwax, or an infection in the ear canal, the pain is mild at first and gradually builds. Gentle pressure on the earlobe aggravates the pain.

If your child is too young to tell you where the pain is, prolonged crying should be considered a possible sign of an earache. An earache is especially likely if a crying child also has a head cold or congested nose, pulls on the ear, or has recently been swimming or flown in an airplane.

HOME CARE

Ear pain can usually be temporarily relieved by acetaminophen. Gentle heat applied to the ear may relieve pain but occasionally worsens it. Anesthetic eardrops must penetrate to the eardrum, and some ear, nose, and throat doctors prefer that these drops not be used. Nose drops and oral decongestants may unblock the eustachian tube to relieve an earache accompanied by nasal congestion or allergy.

PRECAUTIONS

■ A child with a severe earache or an earache that lasts more than a few hours should be seen by a doctor.
■ A child with a congested nose should not go swimming.
■ When flying in an airplane, give your child something to drink as the plane takes off and lands. Breast-feeding or giving a baby a bottle lessens the ear pain that occurs during take-off and landing.
■ Early treatment of head colds and nasal allergies with nose drops and oral decongestants may prevent some ear problems.

■ Preventive eardrops should be used at the end of each swimming day in children who tend to get swimmer's ear.
■ Never put any object (including cotton swabs) in your child's ear canal for any reason.

MEDICAL TREATMENT

To determine the cause of pain, the doctor will carefully inspect your child's ears, nose, throat, and neck. For otitis media, your doctor may prescribe antibiotics. Nose drops, oral decongestants, and antiallergy medications also may be prescribed. Surgical treatment may be recommended if there is evidence of chronic (long-standing) changes in the ear or of hearing loss.

RELATED TOPICS: Boils; Common cold; Deafness; Draining ear; Glands, swollen; Hay fever and other allergies; Meningitis; Swimmer's ear

Earring problems

Pierced ears frequently cause problems involving the earlobes. These problems are not only annoying but also occasionally serious. Three common earring problems are infection, eczema, and injury. Problems may occur if the ear piercer does not give proper instructions for care of the ears or if the instructions are not properly followed.

Infection of the earlobes immediately after piercing may be caused by lack of proper sterile technique during the piercing. Infection occurring weeks later is usually from failure to leave training earrings in place or to care for the pierced earlobes adequately.

Infections that occur after the first month are most likely the result of improperly inserting the earrings. One common error is inserting earrings with posts that are too short for the earlobes. Another common error is pushing the guards in too far along the posts. Both of these mistakes cause pressure on the earlobes and injury to the skin; infection quickly sets in. Pulling down the lobe to insert the post can also cause an infection—when the normally straight channel is curved by pulling, the inside of the channel can be scratched by the end of the post; this wound can then become infected. Sometimes infection is caused simply by inserting unclean earrings.

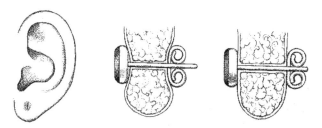

One common cause of earlobe infections is pushing an earring guard too far along the posts, which causes pressure on the earlobe and injury to the skin.

Eczema is a skin irritation. Eczema may develop on the earlobe if a person is sensitive or allergic to the metals used in inexpensive earrings. The skin of the earlobe becomes red, scaly, itchy, and sometimes infected.

The most common injury occurs when hoop earrings are worn during athletics or dancing. If a hoop is accidentally pulled or gets caught, it can tear the earlobe.

SIGNS AND SYMPTOMS

Signs of eczema are redness, irritation, itching, and scaliness of the skin of the earlobe. Signs of infection are swelling, redness, lumps in the earlobes, tenderness, discharge, and rawness around the openings.

HOME CARE

At the first sign of any earlobe problem, remove the earrings. Leave them out until the condition has been corrected. If the infection is severe, the opening may heal closed and require repiercing.

After removing the earrings, soak the earlobes in warm water and then apply antibiotic ointment to the front and back of each lobe.

If the irritation is severe, if the irritation does not clear up with treatment, or if there are signs of infection, see your doctor.

PRECAUTIONS

■ Ask the ear piercer for detailed instructions for care of newly pierced ears.
■ Leave training earrings in for one month after piercing. Turn them daily, and splash the fronts and backs with alcohol.

MEDICAL TREATMENT

Oral antibiotics may be required to cure infection. If the earlobe is badly cut or torn, plastic surgery may be necessary. The doctor may prescribe a steroid ointment for eczema.

RELATED TOPICS: Eczema; Rashes

Eczema

Eczema is a common, noncontagious rash in children. Generally, it starts between one month and two years of age, but sometimes it begins later. Eczema may disappear after two years of age, or it may appear off and on throughout childhood.

The cause of eczema has yet to be determined, but the condition is usually inherited. Eczema may be a form of atopic dermatitis (any inflammation of the skin that is a result of an allergy). Children who have eczema often later develop other allergies, such as hay fever, asthma, and eye allergies.

Eczema sometimes is an allergic reaction to foods, beverages, and medications (including vitamin supplements). It also may be an allergic reaction to substances that come in contact with the skin. In some children, environmental conditions (such as heat and cold) or emotions (such as anger) may cause itching and scaliness of the skin all over the body.

Skin affected by eczema can easily become infected, especially if the skin is scratched. Common complications of eczema include impetigo and infections with herpes simplex virus and vaccinia virus.

SIGNS AND SYMPTOMS

The eczema rash is dry, slightly scaly, pink, and itchy. The rash becomes red from rubbing and scratching. There is no fever or other symptoms, except when scratching causes an infection.

Eczema often begins on the cheeks ("clown" eczema) and around the mouth. It may also crop up on the buttocks or elsewhere. The most common location is behind the knees and in the folds of the elbows. Eczema rarely covers the entire body. It sometimes takes the form of round, coinlike patches scattered on the body (nummular eczema). When it appears in this round patchy form, eczema may be confused with ringworm and pityriasis rosea. Often eczema occurs in combination with seborrhea (cradle cap).

HOME CARE

Home treatment of eczema is often successful, except in severe or infected cases.

The first step is to stop any new foods and beverages that have been added to the child's diet within a month of the appearance of the rash. (It is important to consult your doctor before making any dietary changes, however, because of the risk of creating nutritional deficiencies.) Also, ask your physician if any medication your child has recently received could be causing the problem. (Do not discontinue any medication without your doctor's permission.) In addition, look for and remove irritating substances that may be coming in contact with the child's skin. (See the tables that follow for lists of these foods and substances likely to cause eczema.)

FOODS LIKELY TO CAUSE ECZEMA IN INFANTS UNDER ONE YEAR OF AGE

Cow's milk
Milk products
Wheat flour
Eggs
Citrus fruits and juices
Chocolate
Nuts
Peanut butter
Fish
Shellfish
Tomatoes and tomato juice
Tropical fruit drinks and desserts

FOODS LIKELY TO CAUSE ECZEMA IN CHILDREN ONE YEAR OF AGE AND OLDER

Citrus fruits and juices
Chocolate
Nuts
Peanut butter
Fish
Shellfish
Tomatoes and tomato juice
Tropical fruit drinks and desserts
Candies
Ice cream
Spices (except salt)
Corn
Berries

SUBSTANCES LIKELY TO CAUSE ECZEMA

Soaps
Detergents
Fabric softeners (especially sheets for the dryer)
Wool
Synthetic fabrics
Stretch-cotton fabrics
Fabric dyes (particularly red and blue)
Water softeners
Cosmetics
Metals
Plastics

If stopping these new items does not improve the rash in four to seven days in a child under one year of age, ask your doctor if you should stop giving all foods and beverages that are likely to cause eczema.

Ointments that contain coal-tar derivatives are safe to use, but their use can obscure the physician's initial evaluation of the condition. Bathe the child sparingly, using a mild soap. To further avoid drying of the skin, use a humidifier to moisten dry air. (Be sure to keep it meticulously clean, however. Otherwise, it can become a source of infection if microorganisms are allowed to grow in it.)

If following this procedure clears up the eczema, try gradually returning the discontinued foods to the child's diet one at a time. Reintroducing only one food each week should help detect the foods that cause a reaction. Those foods should then be avoided.

PRECAUTIONS

■ As new foods are added to your infant's diet, watch carefully for any sign of rash.
■ If your infant is allergic to soy formula as well as cow's milk, your doctor will recommend a nonsoy, nonmilk formula.
■ Coal-tar ointments increase sensitivity to sunburn. When using these ointments, keep the child out of the sun as much as possible.

MEDICAL TREATMENT

Help your doctor find the cause of eczema by trying home treatment first and noting what doesn't work and what seems to help. Inform your doctor, too, of any similar cases that have occurred in your older children. Your doctor may prescribe steroid creams, ointments, or lotions to relieve the rash. Oral steroids will not be prescribed unless eczema is severe, and then they will be given for only a brief period. Oral antibiotics may be prescribed if eczema is infected.

RELATED TOPICS: Asthma; Cradle cap; Eye allergies; Food allergies; Hay fever and other nasal allergies; Herpes simplex; Impetigo; Pityriasis rosea; Rashes; Ringworm

Encephalitis

Encephalitis is an inflammation of the brain. The causes are many, including poisons, bacteria, vaccines, and parasites. Most cases are caused by viruses, many of which cause such familiar diseases as mumps, measles, rubella, chicken pox, herpes, mononucleosis, hepatitis, and influenza. The whooping cough bacterium can cause encephalitis, as can the vaccines used to prevent whooping cough, measles, influenza, rabies, yellow fever, and typhoid. The vaccines are far less likely to cause encephalitis, however, than are the illnesses they prevent. Lead, mercury, and other poisons also may cause encephalitis.

SIGNS AND SYMPTOMS

Encephalitis may start with the symptoms of a common cold. The child usually has a mild to high fever and a headache, vomits, and is disoriented (confused) and sleepy. Occasionally, convulsions and unconsciousness may occur.

A child with encephalitis will usually be unable to bend his neck forward to touch the chin to the chest while the mouth is closed. Sometimes the child cannot sit up without supporting the trunk with both hands bracing him from behind (in a tripod fashion). **This is a life-threatening situation.**

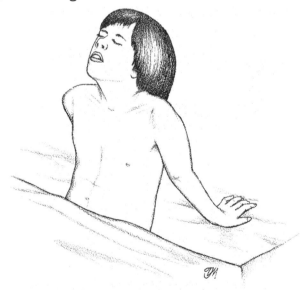

One of the symptoms of encephalitis is inability to sit up unassisted without supporting the trunk with both hands braced behind the body.

HOME CARE

None. See your doctor immediately if your child shows any symptoms of encephalitis.

PRECAUTION

■ If your child has had a severe reaction to the whooping cough, measles, influenza, rabies, yellow fever, or typhoid vaccine, be sure to tell your doctor before a booster of the vaccine is given.

MEDICAL TREATMENT

Since encephalitis may be a complication of another disease (such as measles, mumps, or whooping cough), a child with such a disease and symptoms of encephalitis will probably be examined for encephalitis. Knowing that the child has been exposed to poisons may also lead the doctor to suspect encephalitis.

A definite diagnosis is based on the child's medical history; blood tests; a spinal tap; identification of the infecting organism in the spinal fluid, nose, throat, or stools; and the presence of antibodies (protective substances made by the body to fight infecting organisms) in the patient's blood.

If encephalitis is diagnosed, hospitalization may be required. There is specific treatment for only a few types of encephalitis, since most viral infections are difficult to treat. There is no medication that can kill the invading virus after it has caused the infection. Usually, however, treatment to ease the symptoms and to help the patient withstand the disease until it has run its course leads to recovery.

RELATED TOPICS: Chicken pox; Common cold; Convulsions with fever; Hepatitis; Herpes simplex; Immunizations; Infectious mononucleosis; Influenza; Lead poisoning; Measles; Mumps; Poisoning; Rubella; Whooping cough

Eye allergies

Allergic reactions of the eyes may affect the conjunctiva (the transparent covering over the whites of the eyes and the insides of the eyelids), as well as the skin on the eyelids and around the eyes.

Eye allergies are caused by a wide variety of substances carried to the eyes in the air or by the hands. Seasonal airborne materials are pollens from trees, grass, ragweed, and other plants. Nonseasonal airborne materials include house dust, feathers, molds, and animal dander (tiny scales from the skin of an animal). Many irritants may be carried to the eyes by the hands, including nail polish, household cleaning products, materials from stuffed toys, and finger paints.

SIGNS AND SYMPTOMS

The whites of the eyes become red and itchy. The eyes water, but no pus is formed. Occasionally, the whites become visibly swollen with clear, jellylike material. The eyelids become swollen and red. The skin of the eyelids may be smooth or rough and scaly. The pouches beneath the eyes may become swollen and bluish.

Certain clues can distinguish eye allergies from several other conditions that also cause reddened eyes (such as conjunctivitis, viral infections, foreign bodies in the eyes, styes, and glaucoma). Eye allergies cause itching and tearing but almost never pain or pus. Swelling of the whites of the eyes is a key sign of an eye allergy.

HOME CARE

Oral antihistamines usually help. Your doctor may recommend the use of eyedrops containing phenylephrine or ephedrine, which often bring temporary relief. Applying cold compresses to the eyes may also ease the discomfort. Identifying and avoiding the irritating substance, if possible, is clearly the best solution.

PRECAUTIONS

■ If there is pus or pain in the eyes, the condition is almost certainly not an allergy.
■ If the pupils of the eyes are dilated (enlarged) and slow to respond to light, see your doctor.
■ If home treatment is not effective in 24 hours, see your doctor.
■ If vision is affected, see your doctor.

MEDICAL TREATMENT

Your doctor will examine the outsides and insides of your child's eyes. Medicated eyedrops are usually effective but are safe only after a doctor's examination. Skin tests may be suggested to help identify the substances causing the allergic reaction. As a rule, desensitization shots over an extended period are rarely recommended.

RELATED TOPICS: Conjunctivitis; Eye, blocked tear duct; Eye injuries; Styes; Viral infections

Eye, blocked tear duct

Tears form in the tear glands that lie above the eyeballs within the bony eye sockets. These tear glands continuously produce fluid that flows across the eyeballs and down the slender tear ducts that connect each eye with the nose (the nasolacrimal ducts). The pinpoint opening to each tear duct can be seen near the corner of the eye next to the nose. Each tear duct leads to a lacrimal sac between the corner of the eye and the side of the nose, where tears collect and from which they drain into the nose.

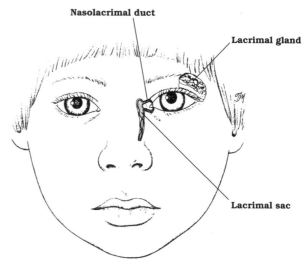

Tears form in the lacrimal glands (tear glands), which lie above each eyeball. The tears continuously flow across the eyeballs and into the nasolacrimal ducts (tear ducts) through the pinpoint-size openings that can be seen at the inner edges of the upper and lower eyelids. The ducts lead into the lacrimal sac, where the tears collect and then drain down the nose.

In newborns, the openings into the tear ducts are often too small. These openings may be further blocked by the silver nitrate or other drops placed in the eyes at birth to prevent eye infections. Blockage of these openings may cause tears to flow out of the outer corner of the baby's eye, even when the infant is not crying. Occasionally, instead of normal eye fluid, green or yellow pus will collect in the eye. This discharge will further block the tiny tear ducts.

If the nasolacrimal duct becomes blocked inside the nose, tearing and infection may occur. Such blockage may be present at birth, or it may be caused by congestion from a cold or an allergy. In such a case, the nasolacrimal sac may swell with fluid and be visible as a distinct lump the size of a green pea.

SIGNS AND SYMPTOMS

In infants, simple tearing in one or both eyes is so common (and harmless) as to be considered normal. However, if there is pus in the eye, redness and rawness at the outer corners of the eyelids, or swelling of the lacrimal sac (with or without redness), treatment may be needed.

HOME CARE

Simple tearing needs no treatment. The tears can be wiped away and the eyelids cleaned by wiping with a cotton ball dipped in sterile water. Call the doctor if the eye is red, pus is present, or the tear duct is swollen. Redness of the skin at the outer corner of the eye, redness of the eye itself, or the presence of pus may be treated with antibiotic eyedrops prescribed by the doctor, often over the telephone. If the lacrimal sac is swollen, your doctor may teach you how to gently massage it. (Do not attempt to massage the lacrimal sac without a doctor's instructions.)

PRECAUTIONS

■ With home treatment, the eyes should improve within 24 hours. If there is no improvement, notify your doctor.

■ If improvement is prompt, continue treatment until the eye has been clear for at least two days.

■ Repeated problems of eye tearing are common in infants. Save the eyedrops for possible future use, but check the expiration date on the label before reusing.

MEDICAL TREATMENT

Your doctor can demonstrate the proper method of massaging the lacrimal sac, if needed. If the condition continues past the age of eight months to one year, your doctor may refer your child to an ophthalmologist (a physician who specializes in disorders of the eyes), who may surgically enlarge the nasolacrimal duct with the child under general anesthesia.

RELATED TOPICS: Conjunctivitis; Eye allergies

Eye injuries

The eyeball is a fragile, hollow sphere with a wall that is less than one-eighth inch thick. Within the eyeball, there are many complex and delicate structures. Fortunately, the eyeball is well protected by its bony socket and the eyelids. Even so, the eye can be injured by small objects like sand or metallic splinters that land on or become embedded in the surface or that penetrate to the inside of the eye. Sharp objects, such as fingernails, knives, and fishhooks, can scratch the surface and penetrate the eye. Dull objects, such as balls and baseball bats, can jar the eye and dislodge its internal structures. A tiny speck may settle on the surface of the eyeball or hide under the eyelid. The eye may also be injured by harmful liquids or powders (acids, alkalis, gasoline) that come in contact with the eye.

SIGNS AND SYMPTOMS

If the child cannot easily open the eye, **do not** try to force it open to look in the eye. See your doctor promptly.

If the child can easily open the eye, you can examine it for signs of damage. Look carefully for all of the following signs of injury: Is there any free blood coming from the eyeball? (Do not be misled by blood from a cut near the eye that may have run into the eye.) Are there any differences in the size or color of the pupils? Are there any differences in the color or position of the irises? Is there any sign of collapse of the eyeball? Is there any puddling of red blood in front of the iris? Is there any blurring of vision? If none of these symptoms is present, you may safely look for foreign objects on the surface of the eyeball or lodged under the eyelid.

HOME CARE

Do not attempt to treat an eye injury at home if the child cannot easily open the eye. Place a soft bandage over the eye, and see your doctor as soon as possible.

Do not attempt to treat at home if the child has any of the following symptoms: bleeding from or in the eyeball; differences in the size or color of the pupils; differences in the color or position of the irises; any collapse of the eyeball; blurring of vision. If any of these symptoms appears, place a soft bandage over the eye, and see your doctor promptly.

Do not attempt to remove a fishhook or any other object that has penetrated the eye. Go directly to the nearest emergency room.

If a harmful liquid or powder (such as an acid, alkali, or gasoline) has entered the eye, **immediate action is essential**. Seconds count! Hold the eye open, and flush it with several pints of cool water. Pour the water over the eyeball from the inside corner, allowing it to run out of the eye from the outer corner. Do not allow the water to run from the affected eye into the unaffected eye. If possible, put the child into a cool shower, clothes and all, and wash out the eye. Then immediately take the child to your doctor for further care.

If none of the above signs is present and you see a speck on the eyeball or under the lid (and the child is cooperative), you may try to remove the speck with gentle strokes of a cotton swab. If the speck does not immediately come off, stop. The object may be embedded. See a doctor immediately.

PRECAUTIONS

■ Be cautious about treating eye injuries yourself.

■ Some golf balls explode if they are unwound and can cause eye injuries. Do not let young children play with golf balls, and do not allow anyone to unwind them.

■ Aerosol spray cans and carbon dioxide cartridges explode violently in fires or in extreme heat. Be sure that your child knows this.

■ Machine sanders, paint removers, grindstones, and similar types of machines throw off particles that can injure the eyes. Everyone should wear protective glasses around these machines. Keep children far away from such machines.

MEDICAL TREATMENT

A doctor can easily anesthetize the eye and examine it internally and externally without pain or damage. The doctor may stain the eyeball with drops to make small injuries and foreign objects readily visible. Areas inside and outside the eye can be examined with a special microscope.

RELATED TOPICS: Eye allergies; Vision problems

Fainting

Fainting is a temporary loss of consciousness, usually due to an insufficient amount of blood in the brain. Fainting can be brought on by pain, physical fatigue, low blood sugar level, or emotional stress.

Fainting is not uncommon in preadolescent children and adolescents. It often occurs after the child has gone without eating for an extended period of time. A partial faint (light-headedness without loss of consciousness) or a complete faint is also common when a teenager abruptly changes position (for example, after jumping up from a reclining or sitting position). It also can occur in a dentist's chair as a result of pain, anxiety, and turning the head sharply to one side (which places pressure on the carotid artery in the neck). Excessive exercise in hot weather may cause fainting.

SIGNS AND SYMPTOMS

Just before losing consciousness, the child experiences light-headedness, blurred vision, and sometimes mild nausea. The skin may feel clammy (cold and moist) and become pale or take on a greenish tinge. An observer may notice a glazed look in the eyes before the child loses consciousness. Rarely will the child lose control of the urine or stools. Consciousness will be recovered within a few minutes, and the child will probably not remember fainting.

The pulse at the wrist may be feeble and slow or not present at all. The heartbeat (which can be measured by placing your ear against the child's chest) is slow, usually 50 beats per minute or less.

Consider the circumstances under which the child fainted. If the situation was one in which fainting typically can occur, and if the child rapidly and completely recovers, this suggests nothing more serious than an isolated spell.

HOME CARE

The only danger in fainting is possible injury from falling. Try to catch the child before the fall; it is especially important to protect the child's head from hitting the ground. Place the child flat on his or her back, raising the legs to increase blood flow to the head. Cool air from an open window or air conditioner may help. Keep the child lying down for five to ten minutes after consciousness has returned.

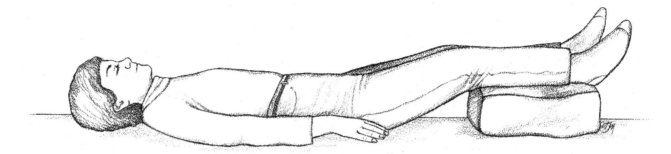

Place a child who has fainted flat on his back with his feet raised higher than his head.

If a child feels a faint coming on but has not yet lost consciousness, have the child sit with the head between the knees. Place your hand on the back of the child's head, and have the child push the head up slightly against your hand. This maneuver forces extra blood into the head.

PRECAUTIONS

■ Sometimes a first convulsion is mistaken for fainting. If fainting occurs often, or if there are any signs of epilepsy, see your doctor.
■ If the child's skin turns bluish during an apparent faint, or if your child is not completely well before and after fainting, consult your doctor. Extremely rare heart conditions sometimes resemble fainting.
■ Smelling salts are not necessary and are not always helpful. There is also a danger of burning the membranes inside the nose if they are held too near the nose or held under the nose for too long.

MEDICAL TREATMENT

If there is any question about the cause of the fainting, the doctor will examine the child for various causes of unconsciousness. Your doctor may order an electrocardiogram, an electroencephalogram, blood tests, or a chest X-ray examination.

RELATED TOPICS: Convulsions without fever; Dizziness

Fifth disease

Fifth disease (*erythema infectiosum*) is a moderately contagious childhood disease. It is thought to be caused by a virus that has not yet been identified. Symptoms may appear an average of two weeks after being exposed to a person with the disease (although they may appear anywhere from one week to four weeks after exposure). Epidemics of fifth disease often occur in schools and neighborhoods.

SIGNS AND SYMPTOMS

Usually the child has little or no fever and feels only slightly or not at all ill. The disease is identified by the sudden appearance of a bright red rash on the cheeks, making it look as though the child had been slapped. A pink rash forming a pattern like a lace tablecloth appears on the trunk and limbs. The rash can last 2 to 40 days and may itch. In older children and young adults, headache, sore throat, runny nose, loss of appetite, and nausea may occur.

Fifth disease usually is obvious from the typical appearance of the rash, especially if an epidemic is occurring in the neighborhood or school. Fifth disease is occasionally confused with rashes caused by medications, rubella, and other viral rashes. On rare occasions, the condition is confused with scarlet fever.

HOME CARE

No treatment is required. The child need not be isolated. Public health authorities have stated that a child with fifth disease can attend school if there is no fever and the child feels well enough. Itching can be treated with antihistamines.

PRECAUTIONS

■ None

MEDICAL TREATMENT

There are no laboratory tests to diagnose the disease. The doctor will confirm the diagnosis from the appearance of the rash, after ruling out other possible causes.

RELATED TOPICS: Rashes; Rubella

Flatfoot

Flatfoot is a condition in which the arches of the feet are flattened so that the entire sole of the foot touches the ground.

A normal newborn does not have arches in the feet. (The normal condition of a child's feet before arches develop is sometimes called "physiological flatfoot.") The arches don't start to develop until the child begins to walk unaided. They are not fully formed until the child is three to four years old. Arches are formed by the exertion of forces by the developing leg muscles on the bones and ligaments of the feet.

SIGNS AND SYMPTOMS

With true flatfoot, there are no arches when a child stands. The child walks on the inner edges of the feet. This wears down the inner edges of the heels and soles of the shoes. The child may complain of painful feet after brief exercise.

The presence or absence of an arch at any age can best be judged when a child stands on the tips of the toes. After age three or four, your child should no longer wear out the inner edges of the shoes.

HOME CARE

If a child under three or four years of age wears out the inner edges of the heels before the shoes are outgrown, buy shoes with a stronger counter.

PRECAUTIONS

■ Do not use orthopedic shoes or devices without competent professional advice. Thomas heels, scaphoid pads ("cookies"), and orthopedic shoes are expensive, and if not needed, they may actually harm normal feet. They are rarely prescribed.
■ Pain in the feet after excessive use and exercise is not abnormal.

MEDICAL TREATMENT

Your doctor will examine your child's feet carefully while the child stands, sits, stands on tiptoes, and walks. The doctor will conduct tests of the movement of the foot joints, the strength of the foot muscles, and the strength of the tendons. Worn shoes will also be examined. Rarely will X-ray examination of the feet be ordered. After considering these factors, as well as the child's age, the doctor may prescribe orthotic shoe inserts or orthopedic shoes.

Food allergies

A food allergy is an unusual reaction or sensitivity to a specific food or beverage. Food allergies are more likely to occur in infants than in older children. Symptoms include vomiting, diarrhea, and abdominal cramps, which may occur from minutes to hours after the child has consumed certain foods or beverages. Cow's milk is the most common cause of food allergy, but eggs, wheat, soybean formulas, orange juice, tomatoes, chocolate, fish, berries, and melons may also be responsible.

If there's a family history of food allergies or intolerances, it's best to delay adding those foods to your baby's diet. The longer you delay their introduction, the less likely that the allergy will develop.

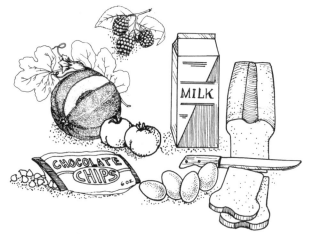

Nonpasteurized cow's milk, eggs, wheat, tomatoes, chocolate, berries, and melons may all cause a food allergy.

A malabsorption syndrome, which occurs when the digestive system lacks certain natural chemicals to digest food, may produce symptoms similar to those of a food allergy. Normally, the body produces natural chemicals called enzymes that break down starches, fats, proteins, and sugars into forms that the body can use. In a malabsorption syndrome, an enzyme is missing, which means that the child cannot digest certain foods. For example, a condition called celiac disease interferes with the digestion of gluten (a starch found in wheat and rye), and the disease cystic fibrosis hampers the digestion of fats and proteins.

SIGNS AND SYMPTOMS

Hives, eczema, runny nose, and asthma may all be signs of food allergy. Sometimes blood appears in the baby's stools. If a particular food brings on abdominal cramps and diarrhea (with or without vomiting), a food allergy can be suspected. By changing the diet and observing your child's reactions, you may be able to identify the problem. Often, however, specific and complex tests are required to diagnose a food allergy. If the child does not seem to tolerate several kinds of foods and is not doing well generally, the cause may be a malabsorption syndrome.

HOME CARE

If your infant vomits or has cramps or diarrhea after the introduction of a new food into the diet, withdraw the food promptly. This does not necessarily indicate a food allergy, but you should wait (two to four weeks) before reintroducing the food. Add new foods to the child's diet one at a time, and allow several days between each introduction so that you can be sure that no problems are occurring.

PRECAUTIONS

■ Persistent diarrhea is a clue to a malabsorption syndrome or an allergic problem; consult your child's doctor if your child suffers from persistent diarrhea.
■ If diarrhea persists, ask your doctor if you should temporarily remove milk and milk products from the child's diet and substitute clear liquids.
■ Symptoms of malabsorption call for a sweat test to rule out cystic fibrosis.

MEDICAL TREATMENT

The doctor diagnoses a food allergy or malabsorption syndrome on the basis of the following: changes in the child's diet; culture and examination of stools for blood, fat, and starch; analysis of digestive enzymes; biopsy of the intestinal lining; sugar tolerance tests; sweat test; chest X-ray examination; and other factors. Treatment involves a controlled diet, sometimes including digestive enzyme supplements.

RELATED TOPICS: Asthma; Cystic fibrosis; Diarrhea in young children; Eczema; Gastroenteritis, acute; G6PD deficiency; Hives

Food poisoning

Food poisoning is a disorder of the stomach and intestines caused by bacteria or chemicals in foods. The classic form of food poisoning is caused by staphylococci ("staph" bacteria), the same germs that cause boils and impetigo. The germs enter the food during its preparation. If the food is not properly refrigerated, the germs multiply rapidly, contaminating the food with a toxin (poison) produced by the germs. The foods in which staph germs grow best are pastries and other starchy foods ordinarily served cold, salads, cold chicken, ham and beef in gelatin, whipped cream, and custards. Since staph germs and their toxins are odorless and tasteless, the contaminated food smells and tastes normal.

A variety of organisms other than staph germs can cause food poisoning of a milder nature. Two more serious conditions that are sometimes classified as food poisoning are botulism and dysentery.

SIGNS AND SYMPTOMS

Food poisoning causes vomiting, abdominal cramps, and diarrhea usually within one to six hours after the contaminated food was eaten. Sometimes symptoms may not appear for 24 hours or longer after the tainted food was eaten. The child may or may not have a fever. Symptoms last 12 to 24 hours.

Food poisoning is usually considered when a number of people who have eaten the same food become ill within hours of one another. Food poisoning can occur after picnics, parties, or eating in a cafeteria or restaurant where foods have been prepared in advance and improperly stored.

HOME CARE

When a child has both diarrhea and vomiting, treat vomiting first by restricting the child's diet to clear liquids only. Once the vomiting has stopped, treat the diarrhea by limiting or not reintroducing solid foods—especially butter, fatty meats, peanut butter, whole-grain cereals, vegetables, and most fruits (apples and bananas are OK). Do not give the child cow's milk or cow's-milk-based formula, since cow's milk may further aggravate diarrhea.

Encourage the child to drink plenty of clear liquids, such as tea, water, flavored gelatin water, and commercial electrolyte solutions (available from your pharmacist).

PRECAUTIONS

■ Do not prepare food that requires refrigeration for your child's lunch box or for a picnic if refrigeration will not be available.

■ A child with diarrhea and vomiting needs plenty of clear liquids to avoid dehydration (a serious loss of body fluids).

■ Do not give antidiarrheal medications to children, since side effects are common and can be dangerous.

■ Isolate an infant from children who are ill with vomiting and diarrhea.

■ If there is blood in the stools, high fever, prostration (extreme weakness or collapse), or severe or prolonged diarrhea (more than 12 to 24 hours for a young infant or more than two to three days for an older child), call your doctor.

MEDICAL TREATMENT

In severe cases, hospitalization may be required so that the child can be given intravenous fluids. Local health departments can investigate food poisoning outbreaks and trace the source of food poisoning by testing suspected foods.

RELATED TOPICS: Botulism; Dehydration; Diarrhea in older children; Diarrhea in young children; Dysentery; Stomachache, acute; Vomiting

Fractures

A fracture is another name for a broken bone. Since children's bones are still growing, their fractures (especially those in very young children) are different in some ways from fractures in adults. For example, broken bones heal more quickly in children than in adults. Also, any fracture that heals in a poor position may cause deformity of the fractured bone, but in a child such deformity is sometimes corrected as the bone continues to grow. (However, if poor positioning of the bone during healing shortens or rotates the bone, further growth of the bone will not correct the deformity.) Certain types of fractures in children (such as fractures through the growing areas of cartilage near both ends of the long bones in the arms and legs) may stop growth of the bone and cause major deformities.

SIGNS AND SYMPTOMS

Deformity of the bone that can be seen or felt is the most obvious sign of a fracture. In many fractures, however, there is no visible deformity. Then you must look for other symptoms of a fracture. There is pain in the area of the fracture, which is aggravated by attempts to move the broken bone. There is tenderness to pressure, which is most severe at the point of the fracture. The fractured part does not function or move normally. There is swelling at the fracture site. Bruising often develops, but sometimes not until days later and often in areas many inches from the fracture.

HOME CARE

If you think that your child may have a fractured bone, see your doctor. If a fracture is found, the doctor will treat it and give you instructions for caring for the child at home.

Of course, you must take certain precautions immediately after the injury occurs. Protect the injured part of the body and keep it from moving. If the arm or shoulder is fractured, the child will usually hold the arm in the most comfortable position with the other arm. If a leg fracture is suspected, prevent your child from putting weight on the leg. If splinting is required for your child's arm or leg, a thick newspaper tied around or under the affected area is often the best splint. Once you have immobilized the fractured bone in a comfortable position, take the child to your doctor.

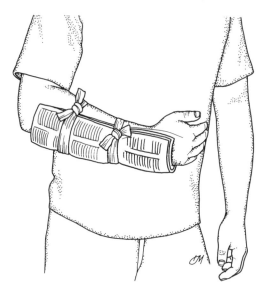

If you think your child may have a fractured bone, protect the injured part of the body and keep it from moving.

If there is any possibility that the spine or neck may be fractured, do not move the child. Call for an ambulance and allow professionals to take the child to an emergency room.

PRECAUTIONS

■ Do not move an injured limb when applying a splint. Splint a possible fracture in the position in which you found it; do not try to straighten it out to make it conform to the splint.

■ Always have a doctor treat possible fractures.

MEDICAL TREATMENT

Your doctor will examine the injury and order X-ray studies. Treatment will depend largely on which bone is fractured and what the X-ray films show. If necessary, the doctor will return the fractured bone to its normal position for proper healing. A cast or mechanical pins may be used to hold the bone in position while healing takes place.

RELATED TOPICS: Dislocated elbow; Sprains and dislocations

Frequent illness

Parents often become concerned that their children are ill too frequently. Sometimes the parents are right, and the child does have some underlying medical problem. Normally, however, having many illnesses is not due to any particular problem in the child. How often a child becomes ill usually depends on the number of children in the family and the number of diseases to which each child is exposed.

Except for accidents and allergies, 95 percent of all illnesses are caused by germs that live exclusively in humans. Most children's illnesses are caught from other children. Whether a child will catch a disease depends on two factors: whether the child is exposed to the germ and how strong the child's resistance is.

If your child is frequently ill with different minor illnesses, the illnesses are usually due simply to exposure to many people. As soon as a child begins going to day care or school, the child is exposed to other children with illnesses. The number of children in a household also is a factor. Mathematically, a four-child family could have 16 times as many childhood illnesses as a one-child family.

A child who is frequently ill with the same illness may have a defect of local resistance (a lowered resistance to disease in one area of the body). For example, repeated pneumonia in the same part of a lung suggests an abnormality in that area.

A child with frequent major illnesses or frequent complications of minor sicknesses may have a general lack of resistance. This occurs with immune mechanism defects, which hinder the child's ability to fight infectious diseases. For instance, colds that always end up as croup, bronchiolitis, bronchitis, or pneumonia may indicate an underlying allergy or other immune system defect.

SIGNS AND SYMPTOMS

The first step is to decide whether a child is actually ill more often than most other children. Some reports show that the average normal child between 1 and 12 years of age may have as many as eight illnesses per year. Other figures show that a first child will seldom be ill during the first year, but will have increasingly frequent illnesses as he or she begins to play with other children and attend school. An infant with older brothers or sisters will be ill the first year as often as other children are. To decide if your child is ill too frequently, compare the number and seriousness of the illnesses with those of the child's brothers, sisters, and friends.

HOME CARE

How much your child is exposed to illnesses depends somewhat on you and your circumstances. Being overprotected and isolated from other children can lead to emotional problems that could be harder to treat than physical problems. On the other hand, overexposure to other children who may be ill can lead to an almost unbroken string of minor illnesses, especially in very young children. Keep older children who are ill—yours and your neighbors'—away from infants. Isolate any ill child from your other children as much as is practical.

PRECAUTIONS

■ Frequent illnesses that could interfere with normal growth must be investigated. If the child stops gaining height or weight or begins to lose weight, see your doctor.

■ Repeated pneumonia in the same part of a lung must be evaluated by your doctor.

■ Frequent lower respiratory tract infections

with a prolonged cough can be a sign of cystic fibrosis or asthma.

MEDICAL TREATMENT

Your doctor will help you decide whether your child is ill more often than others of the same age and under similar circumstances. If it appears that he or she is, your doctor will seek the cause through a variety of diagnostic studies, such as a sweat test, measurement of immune globulins and other blood tests, X-ray examination of the chest and sinuses, nose and throat cultures, and allergy tests. You may be referred to a specialist in disorders of the immune system; to an allergist; or to an ear, nose, and throat specialist.

RELATED TOPICS: Asthma; Common cold; Cystic fibrosis; Pneumonia

Frostbite

Frostbite is the freezing of skin tissue caused by exposure to the cold. It can occur anywhere on the body, but most commonly affected are the toes, feet, fingers, ears, nose, and cheeks—areas that are frequently exposed to the cold and that have the lowest degree of circulation. The very young and the very old are particularly susceptible to frostbite.

Frostbite can have serious consequences. If the frostbite is severe enough to cause the death of skin tissue, surgery may be necessary to remove the dead tissue. Muscles, tendons, and nerves may be damaged. Severe frostbite can also cause blood clots to form in small blood vessels in the affected area, in turn causing death of deeper tissues because of reduced blood supply. Gangrene can result, necessitating the amputation of the affected parts.

Prolonged exposure to the cold is the most frequent cause of frostbite, but even a short exposure can freeze skin tissue if the cold is severe enough. Obviously, inadequate or inappropriate clothing can increase the risk of frostbite. Strong winds can intensify the effect of cold air on the skin.

SIGNS AND SYMPTOMS

Frostbite occurs in stages. As with burns, there are three stages of frostbite.

In *first-degree frostbite*, the skin becomes whitish or slightly yellow. This discoloration is accompanied by a burning or itching sensation. If the affected areas are warmed promptly, the child should recover completely. If exposure to the cold continues, the child will lose sensation in the affected area and will feel no pain. This loss of sensation is a danger signal that should be heeded.

Second-degree frostbite is characterized by reddening and swelling of the tissues involved. Rewarming the area may produce blisters and peeling of the skin.

In *third-degree frostbite*, the skin becomes waxy white and hard throughout, which indicates that skin tissue has died. The affected parts may swell up with edema (collection of fluid in the tissues).

HOME CARE

The best treatment is prevention. Be sure that your child is adequately dressed on cold days, and be aware of the warning signs of frostbite.

If the child does get frostbitten, first aid is important. However, it is just as important to know what *not* to do. Do not rub the affected part with snow. In fact, do not rub the area at all, since this can cause further damage to frozen tissue. Do not let the child exercise the frostbitten part or walk on frostbitten feet.

Take the child indoors as soon as possible, and rewarm the frostbitten area. Rapid rewarming produces pain, redness, and perhaps blisters, but it also reduces tissue loss and helps prevent complications. Do not expose the affected area to the direct heat of a radiator, stove, or fire. Instead, immerse the frostbitten area in water at a temperature of 100°F to 110°F. Be sure that the temperature does not exceed 110°F, since higher temperatures can cause a burn in skin that lacks sensation. If you do not have a thermometer, try to make the water lukewarm (neither hot nor cold). Pat the skin dry carefully.

If the child is outdoors, the affected areas can be warmed by placing them in contact with warm areas of the body (for example, under the arms or between the thighs) until shelter can be reached. Frostbitten toes can be wrapped in a warm, dry blanket. Warm drinks (not alcohol) may be helpful. The affected areas should be kept clean.

After the frozen areas have thawed, elevate them to improve blood circulation. Keep the frostbitten skin at room temperature, and do not rub it. Consult your doctor about all cases of frostbite.

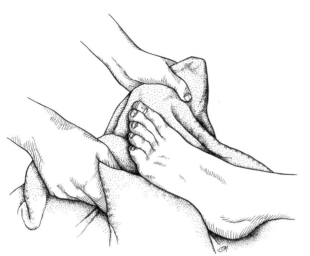

Do not rub frostbite, but rewarm the frostbitten area as quickly as possible. If a child is outdoors, a warm dry blanket may be used.

PRECAUTIONS

■ Be watchful for the signs of frostbite. Even brief exposure to extreme cold can cause frostbite.

■ Strong winds can intensify the effect of cold air on the skin.

■ **Do not** rub frostbitten areas.

■ **Do not** let the child walk on frostbitten feet or exercise frostbitten parts of the body.

■ **Do not** expose frostbitten areas to the direct heat of a radiator, stove, or fire.

■ **Do not** give alcoholic drinks to a person with frostbite.

■ Loss of sensation in the affected areas is a danger signal.

■ Frostbite can have serious consequences, including gangrene, which may necessitate amputation of the affected part.

MEDICAL TREATMENT

The doctor may prescribe medications to ward off infection or drugs to prevent the formation of clots in the blood vessels.

RELATED TOPIC: Blisters

Funnel chest

Funnel chest is a condition in which the breastbone is depressed or sunken in.

The breastbone connects the front ends of the ribs. The diaphragm (a band of muscle separating the chest and abdominal cavities) attaches in front to the lower ribs and to the

bottom of the breastbone. In children, the ribs are made of tough elastic tissue called cartilage, which gradually hardens into bone as the child grows. Since cartilage is not as strong as bone, the ribs of a baby are delicate. The diaphragm, however, is relatively strong, and when some babies breathe in, the diaphragm pulls in the lower half of the breastbone, causing a hollow (like a funnel) in the center of the chest. A true funnel chest exists if the breastbone is depressed when the child breathes out as well, even while the child is at rest.

Depression of the breastbone may be exaggerated when a child is making a greater effort to breathe (for example, if the child is choking or suffering from bronchitis, bronchiolitis, or pneumonia). This mechanism, called *retracting*, is a sign of breathing difficulty. If retracting occurs only when a child has difficulty in breathing, the child is not considered to have a true funnel chest.

If the condition is mild or moderate, a funnel chest will cause no harm and will gradually correct itself over the years as the child's ribs grow heavier and stronger. If funnel chest is severe, it may not correct itself and may interfere with breathing. Rarely is it severe enough to affect the position or functioning of the heart.

SIGNS AND SYMPTOMS

If the breastbone appears to be sunken in, forming a hollow in the center of the chest, whenever a child breathes out, this may be a sign of true funnel chest.

HOME CARE

A true funnel chest cannot be treated at home. Bring it to the attention of your doctor.

PRECAUTIONS

■ Don't be alarmed by persistent mild to moderate depression of the breastbone in an infant or young child.

■ Do not restrict your child's activities.

■ If a child has not previously shown signs of a funnel chest, retractions of the lower portion of the breastbone are an important sign of breathing difficulty.

MEDICAL TREATMENT

Your doctor will determine if the child has a true funnel chest or if the child is having temporary difficulty in breathing. X-ray studies, an electrocardiogram, and measurements of the lung capacity may be performed to evaluate the severity of the condition and its effect, if any, on the heart and lungs.

If funnel chest is severe and persists without gradual improvement, the condition may require surgery. Surgery may be performed if there are signs of limited heart or lung function or for cosmetic reasons.

RELATED TOPICS: Bronchiolitis; Bronchitis; Choking; Hyperventilation; Pneumonia; Shortness of breath

Gastroenteritis, acute

Acute gastroenteritis is a highly contagious infection of the digestive tract. In some cases it is probably caused by viruses, only a few of which have been identified. There is evidence that the disease may also be caused by some types of *Escherichia coli* bacteria. These bacteria are normally found in the human intestines, and most types of the bacteria are known to be harmless or even beneficial. Inadequately cooked meat may contain *Escherichia coli.*

This disease is readily transmitted from person to person. Symptoms may begin within one to four days after exposure to the germ. The disease is not generally serious except in young babies, who may suffer dehydration (a serious loss of body fluids). Though sometimes referred to as "stomach flu," acute gastroenteritis has no relationship to true influenza (a disease of the respiratory tract).

SIGNS AND SYMPTOMS

Acute gastroenteritis causes sudden vomiting or diarrhea and cramps. The disease may last one to three days or as long as a week. Fever may be high (104°F), low (101°F), or absent. Bloody diarrhea is rare. Occasionally, if vomiting is severe, there are small amounts of blood in the vomit, and petechiae (red spots) may appear on the face.

Acute gastroenteritis is more easily identified if there are other cases in the family or neighborhood. It occasionally may be confused with dysentery or food poisoning.

HOME CARE

Treat both vomiting and diarrhea by limiting food intake to clear liquids until the illness subsides. To avoid dehydration, give the child plenty of clear liquids, such as tea, flavored gelatin water, and commercial electrolyte solutions (available from your pharmacist). Do not give the child cow's milk or cow's-milk-based formula.

Acetaminophen is better for relief of fever than aspirin is; aspirin may aggravate vomiting in some children.

PRECAUTIONS

■ Practice good hygiene. Be sure to wash your hands before going from the ill child to other children in the house. Wash your hands carefully before preparing food.
■ If a young child develops the disease, watch carefully for signs of dehydration (infrequent urination, dryness in the mouth, sunken eyes, drowsiness, rapid or slow breathing, tearless crying, sunken soft spot at the top of the head). If any of the symptoms of dehydration appears, call your doctor.
■ Do not give antidiarrheal medications to children, since side effects are common and can be dangerous.
■ If there is blood in the stools, high fever, prostration (extreme weakness or collapse), or diarrhea that is severe or prolonged (for more than 12 to 24 hours for a young infant or more than two to three days for an older child), call your doctor. Dysentery may be the cause.

MEDICAL TREATMENT

Your doctor will confirm the diagnosis by knowledge of what illnesses are occurring in the community, by the circumstances of the child's illness, and by the absence of other physical findings on examination. Blood studies and a stool culture might be required if the diagnosis is in doubt. If there is evidence of dehydration in an infant, hospitalization will be necessary to administer intravenous fluids.

RELATED TOPICS: Appendicitis; Botulism; Dehydration; Diarrhea in older children; Diarrhea in young children; Dysentery; Food poisoning; Influenza; Stomachache, acute; Vomiting

Geographic tongue

Geographic tongue is a common, harmless patterning of the tongue. It is seen in five to ten percent of all infants and children. The cause is unknown. There are no other symptoms or discomfort of any sort.

The surface of the tongue is made up of closely packed papillae (taste buds). The smooth, red areas of changing shape on a geographic tongue appear because papillae have shrunk or temporarily disappeared.

SIGNS AND SYMPTOMS

Geographic tongue is easily identified by the typical appearance of the tongue. No other condition resembles geographic tongue.

One or more smooth, bright red patches appear on the surface of the tongue. In the course of several days, these patches change size, shape, and location. The general appearance is that of a slowly changing map (hence, the name). The condition lasts for months to years and may recur during upper respiratory tract infections.

Although the condition involves changes in the taste buds, there are no noticeable changes in the sense of taste, and there is no pain.

HOME CARE

No treatment is necessary.

PRECAUTIONS

■ Geographic tongue does not indicate a vitamin deficiency, a reaction to toothpaste, or any other problem.
■ Do not try any home treatment.
■ Reassure your child that there is no need to be concerned about geographic tongue.

MEDICAL TREATMENT

Your doctor will identify the condition and reassure you and your child that geographic tongue is not a cause for concern. No other treatment is necessary.

Glands, swollen

The term *swollen glands* is often used to refer to swelling of the lymph nodes. Lymph nodes are sometimes called lymph glands, although they are not true glands. Lymph nodes are widely distributed throughout the body, and in their normal state are an eighth-inch to a quarter-inch in size.

Many lymph nodes lie just beneath the skin. These lymph nodes are located in front of the ears, behind the ears, at the base of the skull,

under the chin, down the sides of the neck, in the armpits, in the folds of the elbows, and above and below the creases in the groin. Lymph nodes are also found within the chest and abdomen, but these lie too deeply within the body to be felt.

The lymph nodes lie along thin-walled tubes called lymphatic vessels. These vessels resemble and roughly follow the course of the veins in the body. They do not contain blood, however. They carry a thin, clear, slightly sticky liquid called lymph, which resembles the clear, watery fluid that oozes from a scrape or that forms within a blister caused by friction.

Lymph nodes are important in helping the body fight infections and disease. When lymph nodes become swollen, it is a sign that they are fighting an illness or infection. The lymph nodes throughout the body may be swollen, or nodes may be swollen in only one area of the body.

When all the lymph nodes or the lymph nodes in many areas are swollen, this usually indicates a general illness or widespread infection affecting the entire body.

When lymph nodes are swollen in only one location, this is a sign of an infection in the area of the body guarded by those nodes. Swollen lymph nodes in one area might be caused by a variety of local infections. The appearance of red streaks under the skin (which typically indicates blood poisoning) is caused by infection traveling along the lymphatic vessels in that area.

In some cases, an infection may become too severe for the lymph nodes to handle. In such a case, the lymph node itself may become infected.

SIGNS AND SYMPTOMS

Swollen or tender lymph nodes are a symptom of illness or infection. If lymph nodes continue to swell, become painful, and redden the overlying skin, the nodes themselves may have become infected. If the node is destroyed by the infection, it breaks down into pus, which may erupt through the skin like a deep-seated boil.

HOME CARE

Mildly swollen lymph nodes usually require treatment only for the disease or infection causing the swelling. If lymph nodes are greatly enlarged, very tender, or red, see your doctor.

PRECAUTIONS

■ In infants, swollen lymph nodes in the neck (and sometimes in other locations) require a doctor's attention because infants have limited resistance to diseases.

■ Any lymph node that continues to increase in size or tenderness or that becomes reddened should be called to a doctor's attention.

■ Swollen lymph nodes are a sign of infection or illness, ranging in severity from the common cold to more serious conditions, such as leukemia. Always consult your doctor about persistent or recurring lymph-node enlargement.

■ Healthy children may have visible lymph nodes the size of fresh peas or smaller in the sides of the neck, which may become especially noticeable when the child turns the head. This is normal.

MEDICAL TREATMENT

Your doctor will seek the cause of swollen lymph nodes by conducting a complete examination of all sites of nodes as well as the spleen and liver. The doctor may also order blood studies and, in severe cases, X-ray examinations of the chest and kidneys. Your doctor will treat the disease causing the swollen lymph nodes and may treat the nodes themselves by prescribing antibiotics. An infected lymph node may be opened and drained or removed, either as treatment or for a biopsy (removal of a tissue sample for diagnostic purposes).

RELATED TOPICS: Blood poisoning; Boils; Burns; Cat scratch fever; Chicken pox; Common cold; Cuts; Impetigo; Infectious mononucleosis; Insect bites and stings; Leukemia; Rubella; Scabies; Scrapes; Sinusitis; Tonsillitis; Toothache

Goiter

A goiter is an enlargement of the thyroid gland, which causes a swelling in the front of the neck. The thyroid gland lies just below and to either side of the larynx (voice box). The thyroid gland produces hormones that control the body's metabolic rate (the rate at which food is used for energy and growth). A normal thyroid is barely visible (if at all) and can hardly be felt.

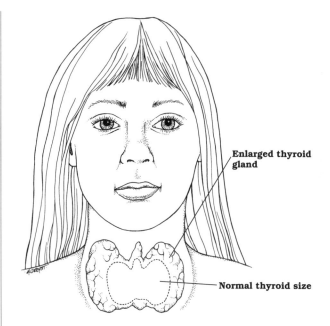

Enlarged thyroid gland

Normal thyroid size

Goiter is a swelling in the neck caused by enlargement of the thyroid gland.

A goiter may be present in a newborn infant, especially if the pregnant mother was taking certain medications (such as anti-asthma and cough medicines that contain iodides). Insufficient iodine in your child's diet also can cause a goiter. Although this disorder was once common, it is now rare because of general use of iodized table salt and more widespread eating of seafood. (Seafood is naturally high in iodine.)

Goiter is most common between the ages of 6 and 16 years and affects girls more often than boys. It may be due to Hashimoto's thyroiditis, an autoimmune disorder of unknown cause. (An autoimmune disorder is one in which the body's defense system reacts against some of its own tissue and produces antibodies to destroy it.) Enlargement of the thyroid is rarely due to malignancy. A goiter may be hyperactive (producing too much hormone) or hypoactive (producing too little hormone), but usually it is neither.

SIGNS AND SYMPTOMS

A goiter can be seen and felt as a swelling in the front of the neck. This swelling usually appears just below and to either side of the larynx. Often the swelling is noticed when a shirt collar or neck jewelry no longer fits. Generally, there are no other symptoms.

HOME TREATMENT

No home treatment should be attempted. Goiter must be diagnosed by a doctor. The cause cannot be identified without laboratory tests.

PRECAUTION

■ During pregnancy, do not take any medications (even over-the-counter drugs) without your doctor's approval. Some drugs taken by a pregnant woman can interfere with synthesis of thyroid hormone in the fetus, causing congenital (present at birth) goiter.

MEDICAL TREATMENT

Blood tests, often requiring complicated laboratory work, are used to find the cause of a goiter. The treatment for a goiter depends on the cause but may include long-term drug therapy. Surgery is not necessary except in rare cases of malignancy or obstruction of breathing.

RELATED TOPIC: Thyroid disorders

Gonorrhea

Gonorrhea is an infection caused by a specific gonococcus bacterium, which is usually sexually transmitted.

In the days before antibiotics, infants born to mothers who had gonorrhea commonly contracted gonorrhea infections of the eyes, which caused blindness. Now the use of antibiotics and the mandatory placement of silver nitrate solution into the eyes of all newborns have almost eliminated this cause of blindness.

Today, venereal (sexually transmitted) gonorrhea in adolescent and younger boys and girls is being seen with increasing and alarming frequency. One of the dangers of genital gonorrhea is that often a girl who has gonorrhea will show no symptoms; therefore, the infection may not be detected and treated. Serious consequences, including sterility, may result from untreated gonorrhea in females.

Another disease caused by gonococcus bacteria is now being recognized in adolescents and even in younger children who have been sexually abused. It causes sore throat and anal infection, with or without fever.

SIGNS AND SYMPTOMS

Gonorrhea of the genitals in boys causes burning during urination and a discharge from the penis. In girls, gonorrhea may cause vaginal discharge and abdominal pain, but frequently there are no symptoms at all.

HOME CARE

There is no home treatment. Gonorrhea must be diagnosed and treated by a doctor. Diagnosis requires special culture techniques, with microscopic examination of discharges from the vagina or penis.

PRECAUTIONS

■ Be aware that the disease still exists and that it exists in children of all ages.
■ Provide sex education for your children.
■ Many physicians advocate the practice of taking periodic vaginal cultures at the time of routine school and annual examinations of sexually active girls.

MEDICAL TREATMENT

Your doctor will diagnose gonorrhea by smear and special culture techniques. If gonorrhea is diagnosed, antibiotics will be prescribed. Although some gonococcus germs are now resistant to penicillin (that is, not destroyed by it), other new antibiotics are reliably effective. By law, cases of gonorrhea must be reported to health departments. Most cases are diagnosed by tracing the sexual contacts of the individuals with known cases of gonorrhea. Treatment of minors is confidential; parental consent is not required.

RELATED TOPICS: Sore throat; Vaginal discharge

Growing pains

The concept of "growing pains" is half truth and half myth. Growing children do have normal pains, particularly in their legs and feet. These pains, however, are caused, not by growing, but by excessive use of young muscles and joints that are not yet completely developed. Young children are extremely active, and this extra activity places stress on their still-developing muscles and joints.

SIGNS AND SYMPTOMS

Growing pains generally occur in different parts of the thighs, calves, and feet. The pains can be severe enough to awaken a child from sleep.

A key symptom of growing pains is that they occur only when the child is at rest, usually at night or during naps. They never occur when the child is active. This fact distinguishes growing pains from pains caused by diseases or abnormalities, which are typically worse when the child is active. Growing pains do not interfere with or interrupt a child's daily play or routine and are never accompanied by fever or other symptoms of general illness.

HOME CARE

Apply heat to painful muscles. Massaging the muscles also helps. Giving the child aspirin or acetaminophen may relieve pain. Having the child wear sturdier shoes may reduce the frequency and severity of growing pains. Since the pain can be quite severe, sympathy and understanding are important in comforting the child.

PRECAUTION

■ One rare bone disease, osteoid osteoma, causes severe bone pain that occurs almost exclusively at nighttime. If your child complains of frequent pain *in the same spot* at night, the cause must be checked by your doctor.

MEDICAL TREATMENT

Your doctor will perform a careful examination to rule out other diseases. X-ray studies may be necessary on more than one occasion to check for osteoid osteoma.

RELATED TOPICS: Arthritis; Fractures; Sprains and dislocations

G6PD deficiency

Glucose 6-phosphate dehydrogenase (G6PD) is an enzyme. (An enzyme is a type of protein produced by the body that participates in digestion and other chemical functions in the body.) G6PD deficiency is an inherited disorder in which there is not enough of this enzyme in the body.

It is possible for a person from any ethnic or racial group to have G6PD deficiency. However, it is most common in ethnic groups from around the Mediterranean Sea and in Oriental and black persons.

G6PD deficiency is less common in females, because a female who inherits the gene for G6PD will often have a second, normal gene that causes the body to produce normal G6PD, so that she may never have symptoms of the disorder. However, if a female inherits two defective genes, the disorder will be the same as it would be in a male.

When a person with the deficiency has an infection, takes certain drugs, or eats certain foods, his or her red blood cells break up. This causes anemia (a shortage of red blood cells). Some of the substances that can cause a G6PD reaction are drugs for treating malaria; sulfa drugs and nitrofuran drugs, which are antibacterial agents; aspirin and other pain-relievers; poison antidotes, such as methylene blue and dimercaprol; and fava beans. Infections that can cause a reaction include hepatitis, infectious mononucleosis, bacterial pneumonia, and viral infections, such as colds and flu.

SIGNS AND SYMPTOMS

The symptoms of G6PD deficiency include paleness, jaundice (yellowing of the skin and the whites of the eyes), dark-colored urine, and back pain. In extreme cases, anemia can become severe enough to cause shock and even death. Between attacks, there are usually no symptoms, but occasionally a person with G6PD deficiency will have long-term anemia and jaundice and also an enlarged spleen. Infants with the disorder may be born with jaundice; this is most common in babies of Mediterranean ancestry, Oriental babies, and premature black babies.

G6PD deficiency is diagnosed through blood tests. The enzymes in the red blood cells are analyzed to see if normal amounts of G6PD are present. The problem may be difficult to detect in black persons during an attack, because in the form of the disorder that is most common in the black population, the red cells are affected suddenly and then quickly replaced with normal cells. In other forms of the disorder, defective red cells remain in the blood for a longer period. Screening tests for the deficiency may be given to members of families that have a history of the disorder. Many doctors routinely screen all Oriental and black male children for G6PD deficiency. Otherwise, the problem may not be discovered until a child has a sudden attack of anemia.

HOME CARE

If your child has the symptoms of G6PD deficiency, especially during an infection or after taking a drug, consult your doctor.

PRECAUTIONS

■ If your child has G6PD deficiency, avoid giving aspirin to the child.
■ Be sure that any doctor who is prescribing drugs for the child knows that the child has this disorder.
■ If fava beans cause a reaction in your child, do not include them in the child's diet.
■ If you are breast-feeding a baby who has this disorder, be careful about what you eat and what drugs you take. Some drugs and foods pass into the breast milk and can cause a reaction in the baby.

MEDICAL TREATMENT

There is no cure for G6PD deficiency. The only treatment is to try to avoid the foods and drugs that cause the problem. In mild cases, no other treatment is necessary, even during an attack. In severe cases, a child may have to be hospitalized during an attack and treated for severe anemia and possibly shock.

RELATED TOPICS: Anemia; Common cold; Food allergies; Hepatitis; Infectious mononucleosis; Influenza; Jaundice in children; Jaundice in newborns; Pneumonia; Poisoning; Shock

Gumboils

A gumboil is an abscess (a collection of pus in inflamed tissue) in the gum at the base of a decayed tooth. It is caused by infection reaching the root canal and traveling to the tip of the root. Gumboils are common after a cavity in a tooth has been repaired and filled. They are also common in untreated decayed or injured teeth.

SIGNS AND SYMPTOMS

Gumboils can be recognized by their typical appearance. Inflammation or swelling that comes to a point, like a tender pimple, appears where the lip meets the gum at the base of a decayed tooth. The area is sometimes painful. Eventually, the gumboil discharges yellow pus. Usually, the associated tooth is obviously injured (fractured or discolored) or has an untreated or recently filled cavity. The tooth may be tender when tapped or may be slightly loose. A gumboil is not usually accompanied by fever.

A gumboil may be confused with a canker sore. However, a canker sore is ulcerated (looks as if it has been dug out); it does not protrude like a gumboil.

HOME CARE

Give aspirin or acetaminophen for pain. Warm soaks or warm saltwater rinses will help the inflammation and promote drainage of the boil. (Use one-half teaspoon of table salt in about four ounces of warm water.) If the associated tooth is about to fall out naturally, a gumboil can be left untreated. The loss of the tooth will allow the pus to drain and the gumboil to heal.

PRECAUTIONS

■ If a young child has a gumboil, consult a dentist.
■ **Never** apply aspirin directly on a gumboil or the surrounding area. (This practice can cause a chemical burn.)
■ Some dentists feel that a gumboil on a baby tooth endangers the permanent tooth that has not yet emerged.
■ Premature loss of first-year or second-year molars (or permanent six-year molars) can cause later problems in spacing and positioning of the permanent teeth.

MEDICAL TREATMENT

Your dentist will decide whether to leave the tooth in, pull it, replace it with a space retainer, or save the tooth by performing root-canal work. It is seldom necessary to give the child antibiotics or to open and drain the gumboil.

RELATED TOPICS: Herpes simplex; Toothache

Gynecomastia

Gynecomastia is the name given to development of breasts in a boy. Normal males have undeveloped breast tissue that can become enlarged by estrogens (female hormones) and, rarely, by androgens (male hormones). A boy with tumors of the testes or adrenal glands may develop breasts. Also, the breasts may develop after taking a medication that contains sex hormones or after eating poultry fattened by hormones.

Normal adolescent boys commonly develop small breasts on one or both sides. These generally persist for 2 to 24 months. They may be tender and are often an embarrassment. The breasts may become quite pronounced and may remain so for years, but this is very rare.

Overweight boys may develop large accumulations of fat that resemble breasts but contain no true breast tissue. This condition is known as pseudogynecomastia.

Marijuana use sometimes causes breast enlargement, but usually of only one breast. Another common cause is repeatedly rubbing, pulling, pinching, or hitting the breast.

SIGNS AND SYMPTOMS

The development of breasts is obvious except when the boy tries to hide the condition out of embarrassment. If this happens, his parents may not be aware of the problem.

HOME CARE

It is very important to be understanding and to reassure the child that the condition will disappear. In more obvious cases, the boy may need to be excused from activities that require undressing or showering with other boys.

PRECAUTIONS

■ Ninety-eight percent of all cases of gynecomastia will disappear on their own.
■ Your doctor should examine your boy if the condition persists.
■ Take steps to ensure that the boy is not subjected to taunting by other children.

MEDICAL TREATMENT

Your doctor will examine your boy carefully. The doctor will check for the presence or absence of true breast tissue; check the coloration of the areolae (the circular areas around the nipples); and examine the boy's abdomen, testes, and body hair. The doctor will consider whether any drugs or foods could be causing the problem. If other causes of the condition are ruled out, the doctor can usually only recommend that you patiently support and counsel the child. Hormonal studies or chromosome studies are rarely needed. In severe or prolonged cases, a plastic surgeon can remove the extra breast tissue without visible scarring.

Hand, foot, and mouth disease

Hand, foot, and mouth disease is a common contagious illness caused by the Coxsackie

viruses. The disease is common during warm weather. It is transmitted by mouth-to-mouth contact with someone who has the disease or by eating something that has been contaminated with feces. Symptoms of the disease may appear within three to five days after exposure to the virus.

SIGNS AND SYMPTOMS

The disease is easily identified. Blisters and sores (resembling canker sores) appear inside the mouth, on the tongue, and inside the cheeks, lips, and throat. Small clear blisters (one-sixteenth to one-eighth inch in diameter) appear on the fingers, hands, toes, and feet. The child will generally have a low fever (about 101°F). The illness lasts three to seven days. Other types of Coxsackie viral illnesses in the family or among your child's friends are another clue to the disease.

HOME CARE

Give the child acetaminophen for fever and soreness of the mouth. Avoid giving the child foods that sting the mouth, such as citrus juices, ginger ale, and spices. Popsicles are soothing and a good source of fluids. Check with your doctor before giving the child nonprescription antihistamines for the itchiness of the blisters.

PRECAUTIONS

■ Occasionally this disease can be dangerous for young infants. Isolate babies from older children who are ill with this disease.
■ If your infant contracts this disease, call your doctor.
■ Children occasionally become dehydrated if they refuse all fluids because of mouth pain.

MEDICAL TREATMENT

Your doctor will rule out other possible causes. In rare cases, a seriously ill infant may need to be hospitalized.

RELATED TOPICS: Dehydration; Rashes; Viral infections

Hay fever and other nasal allergies

Allergic reactions of the membranes of the nose are often responses to substances inhaled from the air. When such a response occurs only during a particular time of the year, it is usually hay fever, a seasonal allergy to pollens of trees, grasses, or weeds. (Pollens of flowers are usually too heavy to be airborne or inhaled.)

When a nasal allergy is present year-round, it may be caused by house dust, molds, and feathers from pillows, comforters, or pet birds. A nasal allergy may also be a reaction to animal dander (tiny scales from the skin of an animal) from a cat, dog, horse, or cow. (Horse or cow dander may be present in felt carpet padding that contains horse or cow hair.) Nasal allergies are not usually caused by dander from guinea pigs, hamsters, gerbils, or mice. Nasal allergies are rarely a reaction to foods, beverages, or medications.

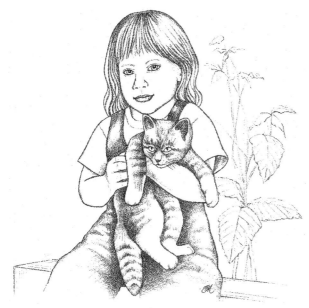

A nasal allergy may be a reaction to animal dander, such as that from cats.

SIGNS AND SYMPTOMS

The major symptoms are nasal congestion, sneezing, clear nasal discharge, and itching of the nose. The child frequently rubs and wrinkles his or her nose. The membranes inside the nose are pale or white instead of the normal pink.

The eyes may also be affected. Congestion in the sinuses may cause a headache. The ears feel blocked and are sometimes painful. The child may not hear as well as usual if there is congestion in the eustachian tubes, which connect the nose with the ears. The child may have bluish circles under the eyes, called "allergic

shiners," which may be due to obstruction of blood flow in the area by swollen mucous membranes. The child may snore and complain of fatigue. A child with allergies also displays the "allergic salute"—swiping of the hands across the base of the nose while sniffling.

If oral antihistamines recommended by your doctor quickly relieve the symptoms, this is often a clue that the nasal congestion is due to an allergy rather than to some other illness.

Secondary (additional) bacterial infections are common complications of hay fever. Symptoms of a secondary bacterial infection include fever, moderate to severe earache, swollen lymph nodes in the neck, and opaque (green, yellow, or milky) nasal discharge.

HOME CARE

Consult your doctor before giving a child medications for hay fever and other nasal allergies. The most commonly used medications are oral antihistamines. Decongestants containing ephedrine, pseudoephedrine, or phenyl-propanolamine may provide added relief.

Whenever possible, try to avoid exposing the child to substances that seem to cause nasal allergic reactions. (The dander of a cat or dog allowed in the house only once can remain in the home for four to six weeks.) Keep the windows closed against pollens, and use an air conditioner if possible. Hot-air ducts should have filters at room inlets to reduce the amount of dust in the air. Use nonallergenic pillows, and keep the house as dry and free of humidity as possible.

PRECAUTIONS

■ Foam-rubber pillows are considered nonallergenic; however, mold may breed in them as they age.
■ Avoid the repeated use of decongestant nose drops and nasal sprays. These can cause worse congestion after the initial brief period of relief.

MEDICAL TREATMENT

The doctor will confirm the diagnosis by examining the child's nose and by testing nasal secretions for specific white blood cells called eosinophils. The doctor may be able to identify the offending substances by investigating the child's medical history or may recommend allergy skin testing. A program of desensitization shots to decrease the child's sensitivity to the allergy-causing substances may be useful in some cases.

RELATED TOPICS: Asthma; Common cold; Earaches; Eye allergies; Glands, swollen; Headaches; Sinusitis

Headaches

Headaches are probably as common in children as in adults and have as many different causes. Fever and strong emotions (anxiety, fear, excitement, sadness, and worry) probably account for about 95 percent of all headaches in children. Less common causes of childhood headaches are high blood pressure, head injuries and concussions, tumors and inflammation of the brain (such as meningitis and encephalitis), bleeding inside the skull, sinusitis, eye strain, and psychiatric problems.

SIGNS AND SYMPTOMS

Pain, ache, and throbbing in any area of the head are obvious signs of a headache. The type of headache experienced depends somewhat on the cause. Some clues to the cause are the location of the pain, how long the pain lasts, the time of day at which it occurs, the circumstances leading to the pain, other accompanying symptoms, and the effect medications have on the pain. In general, a headache is not serious if it can be relieved by aspirin or acetaminophen, rest, or comforting attention to the child.

Migraine. A child that has migraine headaches usually has a strong family history of the condition. A migraine headache is often on one side of the head. It is generally accompanied by nausea and vomiting ("sick headache"). Sometimes it is preceded by an aura (seeing light flashes or having double vision). A migraine lasts for hours and usually cannot be relieved by aspirin or acetaminophen.

High blood pressure. A throbbing pain occurs with a headache caused by high blood pressure. The child may sweat and turn pale or become flushed. The heart pounds, and the pulse throbs. Aspirin or acetaminophen does not relieve this type of headache.

Concussion. A headache caused by concussion follows an injury to the head.

Tumors, infections, or bleeding within the head. Headaches associated with these conditions gradually become more severe and more frequent. The child starts to vomit and to show other signs of disorders of the nervous system, such as a stiff neck, vision problems, confusion, loss of balance, and sometimes fever.

Sinusitis. When headache is caused by sinusitis, the nose is congested or runny.

Eye strain. A headache from eye strain usually follows reading or watching television.

Psychiatric problems. Behavior problems occur along with a headache that is caused by psychiatric problems. The headache is frequently at the top of the head, or it may affect the entire head, which is unusual with other forms of headache.

HOME CARE

Try aspirin or acetaminophen to relieve the pain. Cold compresses on the forehead may offer relief. If the child has nasal congestion, warm compresses on the forehead, antihistamines, or nose drops may help both the congestion and the headache. Have the child lie down in a darkened room. Comforting and cuddling the child often helps, since many headaches have an emotional basis. Do whatever you can to remove stress. If the headache persists, see your doctor.

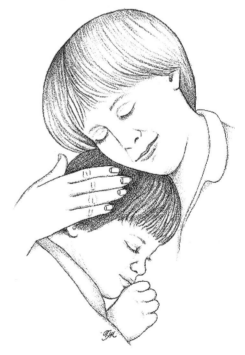

Comforting and cuddling the child may relieve headaches since many have an emotional basis.

PRECAUTIONS

■ Sudden, severe headache may be a true **emergency**—especially if the child also has fever, extreme weakness or collapse, violent vomiting, disorientation (confusion), vision problems, or a stiff neck. **Get medical help immediately.**

■ Repeated headaches that become more frequent and severe may be serious. See your doctor.

MEDICAL TREATMENT

Your doctor will perform a complete physical examination on your child, including measuring the blood pressure and examining the eyes, as well as a neurologic (nervous system) examination. Laboratory tests may be ordered. To discover if the headache is a migraine, your doctor may prescribe the drug ergotamine for a trial period, since this drug relieves only migraine headaches.

The doctor may have you consult a neurologist (a specialist in disorders of the nervous system); an allergist; an ear, nose, and throat specialist; or a psychiatrist.

RELATED TOPICS: Concussion; Encephalitis; High blood pressure; Meningitis; Sinusitis; Vision problems

Head lice

Head lice are tiny parasites (less than one-eighth inch long). They are grayish-white, almost transparent, six-legged creatures that live exclusively on humans—not on pets. The lice pass easily from one person to another. Head lice live on or close to the scalp, where they bite and suck blood. Their eggs, which are called nits, are milk-white and about the size of a flake of dandruff. During the past few years, infestation with head lice has become common among school-age children.

SIGNS AND SYMPTOMS

Head lice cause itching of the scalp and sometimes a red, scaly rash on the back of the neck at the hairline. Scratching may cause sores on the scalp. The lymph nodes at the base of the skull may be enlarged.

Unless hundreds are present, it is difficult to see lice in a child's hair. Look for the small but easily visible nits attached to the shafts of the hairs. Although nits are about the same color and size as flakes of dandruff, they can be easily distinguished from dandruff: Flakes of dandruff can be blown or brushed away; nits can be removed with the fingernails only with difficulty.

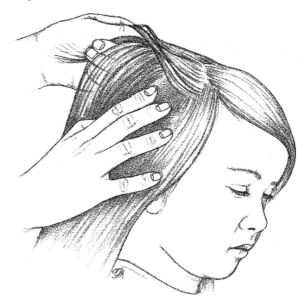

Check your child's scalp on a regular basis if he or she has been exposed to head lice in school or day care.

HOME CARE

Apply the recommended amount of a one-percent gamma benzene hexachloride shampoo (which your doctor will prescribe) to your child's dry hair. Work it into a lather, and leave it on for four minutes. Then rinse well with water. Be very careful not to get this shampoo into the child's eyes or mouth. After rinsing, comb the child's hair with a fine-tooth comb to remove the nits. If necessary, use a vinegar rinse to loosen the nits before combing. Repeat the shampoo and combing only once, four to seven days later. This procedure kills both the lice and the eggs. Clean combs and hairbrushes with the gamma benzene hexachloride shampoo. To kill stray lice, clean hats and pillowcases by washing and ironing or by dry cleaning.

Lice can also be killed by using one of several special shampoos containing pyrethrins. These shampoos are available without a prescription. Always follow the package instructions carefully.

PRECAUTIONS

■ Gamma benzene hexachloride is lindane, a white powder used chiefly as an insecticide. It is *poisonous* if swallowed or absorbed through the skin. It can also harm the eyes. Do not let it come in contact with the eyes or mouth. Do not leave it within your child's reach. Do not apply it more than twice.

■ If one person has head lice, all family members except infants and pregnant women should be treated with the shampoo.

■ If the lice are accompanied by infected sores on the scalp or enlarged, tender lymph nodes at the base of the skull, consult your doctor.

■ Children should be discouraged from sharing hats, combs, and other such items.

MEDICAL TREATMENT

If there are infected sores or infected lymph nodes, your doctor may culture the sores and prescribe an oral antibiotic for five to ten days.

RELATED TOPICS: Glands, swollen; Scabies

Heart murmurs, innocent

A heart murmur is an extra sound made by the heart as it pumps. A heart murmur may indicate abnormalities in the heart, or it may simply be a normal sound caused by turbulence as the blood rushes through the heart. The sounds that do *not* indicate heart disease or abnormalities may be called "innocent murmurs," "insignificant murmurs," or "functional murmurs." They are perfectly normal.

Some experts believe that almost every healthy child has at least one innocent murmur, and if the child will stay still long enough in a quiet room a doctor will eventually be able to hear it. Other experts put the figure lower, at half of all normal children. As the child grows, the extra sounds usually become increasingly hard to hear. By the time the child is a teenager, the murmur usually has disappeared or become so quiet that it cannot be detected. Only 15 to 20 percent of innocent murmurs continue into adolescence or adulthood.

SIGNS AND SYMPTOMS

When the child is born and then again at periodic checkups, the doctor will listen to the child's heartbeat with a stethoscope. The doctor is checking to see if the heartbeat is regular and strong, as well as to detect heart murmurs. Ordinarily, the doctor will hear the noise made by the ventricles (the lower chambers of the

heart) as the heart muscle contracts. Also, the valves that regulate the flow of blood through the heart can be heard as they shut. Any unexpected sounds that the heart makes are called "murmurs." The doctor can usually identify the innocent murmurs.

If any murmur is found, however, the doctor may recommend a complete examination of the child's heart, to make sure that the heart and circulation are normal and healthy. This will involve taking a detailed medical history, making a complete physical examination, and possibly performing some special studies, such as an electrocardiogram, a chest X-ray examination, and an echocardiogram, in which sound waves bounced off the heart are recorded to form a visual image.

HOME CARE

An innocent murmur is completely normal and does not require any treatment or extra care. Treat the child as the normal, healthy child that he or she is.

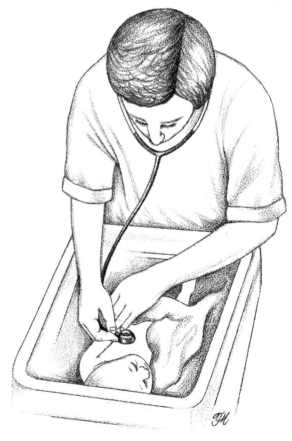

At periodic checkups, the doctor listens to the child's heart to see if the heartbeat is regular and to detect heart murmurs.

PRECAUTIONS

■ No precautions are needed. Sometimes parents are frightened by the idea of a heart murmur and overprotect a child whose heart is quite normal. This is not good for the child.

■ If your doctor diagnoses an innocent murmur, do not be alarmed by the complicated names for innocent murmurs or by the tests your child may have.

MEDICAL TREATMENT

No medical treatment is necessary for an innocent murmur. The doctor may listen for the murmur at routine checkups to see if the sound can still be heard, but it really doesn't matter whether the murmur continues or not. Occasionally, an innocent murmur will sound like another type of murmur. If this happens, the doctor may wish to check the child's heart again after a few years to be sure that the original diagnosis was correct.

Heat rash

Heat rash is a mild skin condition caused by temporary blockage of the sweat gland openings on the skin. Heat rash, also known as prickly heat and miliaria, is the most common of all rashes in children. Almost all babies get heat rash during hot weather. However, heat rash can occur even in cold weather if your child is overdressed either during the daytime or the nighttime. Fair-skinned children (redheads and blonds) get heat rash more frequently than other children, and they suffer the most from it.

SIGNS AND SYMPTOMS

Heat rash consists of hundreds of tiny, pinhead-sized eruptions, each surrounding a skin pore. These eruptions may look like small pink or red bumps or like tiny water blisters. They are moderately itchy and may show scratch marks. If you look at the rash with a magnifying glass in good light, each dot of heat rash can be seen at the mouth of a pore from a sweat gland.

The rash usually appears on the cheeks, neck, and shoulders; in skin creases; and in the diaper area. It frequently appears if the child has been overdressed, perspiring, or wearing a wet bathing suit or if the weather has been hot and humid.

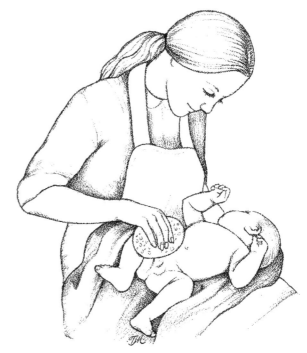

A cool sponge bath may help relieve heat rash.

HOME CARE

Infants and children are safest from heat rash in an air-conditioned environment. Keep a child with heat rash as cool as possible. Cool baths and baby powder or cornstarch, applied lightly with a powder puff, help ease the condition. If the heat rash is on your baby's face, rest the baby's face on an absorbent pad in the crib. During warm weather, using prickly heat powders may give some relief.

PRECAUTIONS

■ Be careful with baby powder. If a baby inhales it, inflammation of the lungs can occur.

■ Detergents and bleaches used on laundry may aggravate heat rash.

■ Bubble baths, water softeners, and oily lotions should be avoided.

■ Do not overdress your baby. He or she needs to be dressed no more warmly than you would dress yourself on any given occasion.

MEDICAL TREATMENT

A doctor's treatment is usually not necessary. Heat rash can generally be adequately and safely treated at home. However, if the rash is persistent or other symptoms develop, consult your doctor.

RELATED TOPICS: Diaper rash; Rashes

Heatstroke

Heatstroke is caused by a sudden, uncontrolled rise in body temperature. Heatstroke occurs when the body is exposed to excessive heat but cannot replace the body fluids lost through perspiration. If the lost fluids are not replaced, dehydration (depletion of body fluids) occurs and leads to a decrease in blood volume. At this point the body has to decide whether to supply the diminished amount of blood to the internal organs or to the skin; since the internal organs take priority, they will receive the blood. At the same time, the body loses its ability to sweat. The situation becomes critical for two reasons: the body cannot produce enough sweat, so the normal cooling mechanism of evaporation of sweat from the skin is lost; and the skin is deprived of the blood supply that normally ensures that excess heat can be released through the skin.

If heatstroke is not treated quickly and correctly, it can cause permanent brain damage or death. When there is loss of blood volume, which can mean that there is not enough blood to circulate through the body, the victim goes into shock. Also, at high temperatures, the blood cannot clot properly, which can result in leakage of blood from the vessels into body organs.

Heatstroke most often strikes athletes and other people who do strenuous work in hot weather. People who have had heatstroke once are more likely to suffer another attack if they return to strenuous exercise within a week. Lack of water, excessive sweating, vomiting, and diarrhea all increase the body's susceptibility to heatstroke.

SIGNS AND SYMPTOMS

The onset of heatstroke is signaled by a feeling that the lungs and muscles are "on fire." The child may have a dry mouth and blurred vision and may experience dizziness, nausea, and difficulty in breathing. However, the most characteristic signs of heatstroke are extremely hot, flushed, dry skin; high fever; and the complete absence of sweating, which usually leads to unconsciousness.

HOME CARE

If you suspect that your child has heatstroke, call immediately for emergency help and then

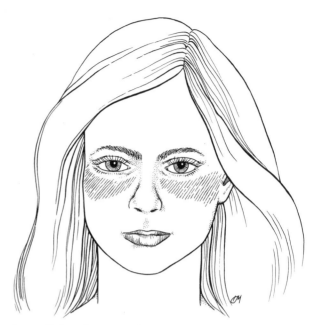

One of the characteristic signs of heatstroke is hot (but dry) flushed skin.

begin first aid. Remove the child's clothing and place him or her in a shady area. Place the child in a reclining position with the feet higher than the head. Pour cold water over the child, rub the body with ice, and then fan the child to promote evaporation, which will lower the body temperature. Continue this treatment until the child is conscious and the body temperature is back to normal. Then give fruit juices, which will replace minerals as well as fluids lost during dehydration. Watch the child carefully; if the symptoms recur, repeat the treatment.

PRECAUTIONS

■ Heatstroke can cause brain damage or death if not treated correctly and promptly. A child with heatstroke who does not revive within minutes requires professional emergency care immediately.
■ Heatstroke occurs most often when both temperature and humidity are high.
■ Strenuous exercise within one week of an attack of heatstroke may lead to another attack.
■ Lack of water, excessive sweating, vomiting, and diarrhea increase the child's susceptibility to heatstroke.
■ Taking salt tablets can increase rather than lessen a person's risk of getting heatstroke.

MEDICAL TREATMENT

If a child who is suffering from heatstroke does not revive within minutes of losing consciousness, then injections of special intravenous fluids will be necessary.

RELATED TOPICS: Dehydration; Shock

Henoch-Schönlein purpura

Henoch-Schönlein purpura is a disorder that affects the skin, the kidneys, the digestive tract, and the joints. It is characterized by a rash that is caused by bleeding from tiny blood vessels just below the surface of the skin.

The cause of Henoch-Schönlein purpura is not known, but some experts believe that it is an allergic reaction. It often appears as a child is recovering from a viral infection. The disorder usually lasts about six weeks. In a few children, it reappears several times over the next few months, or even over several years. In rare cases, the condition leads to complications, but usually the symptoms disappear and leave no lasting effects.

SIGNS AND SYMPTOMS

If you press a clear drinking glass against the rash and the rash remains visible, it is purpura. Other types of rashes are on the skin surface and will not show under a glass. Purpura may look like tiny purplish spots or a purple bruise. The other symptoms of this disorder are abdominal pain, blood in the urine, and pain and swelling in the joints. The disorder can be identified from this unique combination of symptoms. The doctor may have the child's urine and bowel movements tested for

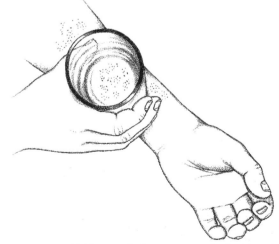

One way to tell if a rash is purpura is to press a glass against the skin. If the rash remains visible, it is purpura.

blood to confirm the diagnosis and learn if the digestive tract is involved.

HOME CARE

A child with this disorder should be under a doctor's care. Ask the doctor about ways to make the child more comfortable if there is pain in the joints or abdomen.

PRECAUTIONS

■ If you notice a rash on your child that looks like large bruises or tiny purple dots, contact the doctor at once. Purpura does not always indicate Henoch-Schönlein purpura. It can be a sign of a serious blood disease.

■ Henoch-Schönlein purpura can lead to intestinal damage. Watch a child with this disorder for severe abdominal pain or passage of a large amount of blood in the stools. These symptoms may indicate that the wall of the intestine is perforated or that it has telescoped into itself. Report such symptoms to the doctor at once.

■ It is possible for a child who has recovered from Henoch-Schönlein purpura to later suffer kidney complications, such as nephritis. To detect kidney involvement before it leads to kidney damage and possibly kidney failure, the child should have checkups and urine and kidney tests for up to six months after recovery.

MEDICAL TREATMENT

There is no specific treatment for this disorder. Routine blood tests are usually done to make sure that the rash is not caused by a serious blood disorder. The doctor will want to test the child's urine and bowel movements for blood several times to detect complications early. The child will also be tested for strep throat, because strep infection can be associated with Henoch-Schönlein purpura. If a strep infection is found, the doctor will probably prescribe an antibiotic.

To guard against complications in some cases, the child may be hospitalized when the condition is at its worst.

RELATED TOPICS: Arthritis; Nephritis; Rashes; Stomachache, acute; Strep infections

Hepatitis

Hepatitis is an infection of the liver (an organ of the digestive system, located in the abdominal cavity), usually caused by a virus. Hepatitis A virus causes infectious hepatitis. Hepatitis B virus causes serum hepatitis. (There are other types of hepatitis, including C and D, that are also viral; less is known about them. Another form of hepatitis can occur as a complication of infectious mononucleosis.) Serious, acute complications and long-term progressive (continually worsening) liver disease may occur as a result of hepatitis.

Hepatitis A is contracted from the stools or blood of a person with the disease. The virus is also present in contaminated water and food (for example, shellfish). Symptoms may appear within 15 to 45 days after exposure to the virus. The patient is contagious from three weeks before the onset of jaundice until one week after onset.

Hepatitis B is contracted in one of two ways: either by close mouth-to-mouth contact or from the blood of a patient or carrier (someone who carries the virus without having the disease). It is usually transmitted by a blood transfusion or by an injection with a contaminated needle (as in drug addiction and tattooing). It can also be passed by a pregnant woman to her fetus. Symptoms may appear six weeks to six months after exposure to the virus. Hepatitis B is con-

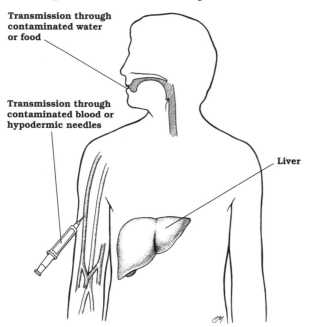

Transmission through contaminated water or food

Transmission through contaminated blood or hypodermic needles

Liver

Hepatitis A can be transmitted through the digestive system by contaminated water or food. Hepatitis B is transmitted most often through blood transfusions or use of contaminated hypodermic needles.

tagious during the incubation period (the time between exposure to the virus and the onset of symptoms), and possibly for months or years thereafter. The symptoms are similar to those of hepatitis A, but often come on more gradually and are milder. Joint pain and rashes are often associated with hepatitis B.

SIGNS AND SYMPTOMS

The first symptoms are fever, malaise (body discomfort), headache, and sometimes signs of a common cold. The key symptoms are a marked loss of appetite (often with nausea, vomiting, and upper abdominal pain) and the onset of jaundice (characterized by yellowed skin, yellowed whites of the eyes, dark-amber urine, and light-colored stools). Jaundice lasts two to four weeks, followed by one to two months of diminishing fatigue. The liver often is enlarged and tender. Specific diagnosis (A type or B type) depends on blood test results and must be made by a doctor.

HOME CARE

If symptoms of hepatitis appear, isolate your child to lessen the chance of spreading the disease. Then call your doctor. Hepatitis must be diagnosed and treated by a doctor. Your doctor will give you specific instructions for caring for the child at home and will probably recommend rest, liquids, and a low-fat diet that is easy to digest.

PRECAUTIONS

■ If your child has been exposed to hepatitis, call your doctor. The child and other family members should be given preventive gamma globulin or hepatitis B immune globulin injections as soon after exposure as is practical and before symptoms appear.

■ If you are caring for a child with hepatitis B, remember that this form is now known to be contagious (contrary to past beliefs). Practice good hygiene, particularly careful hand washing, to avoid spreading the disease.

MEDICAL TREATMENT

The doctor may hospitalize your child for treatment. Tests are also available to determine when hepatitis B is no longer contagious.

RELATED TOPICS: Arthritis; G6PD deficiency; Infectious mononucleosis; Jaundice in children; Jaundice in newborns; Rashes

Hernia

A hernia (or rupture) is a protrusion of tissue through the wall of a body cavity. It might be compared to the protrusion of an inner tube through a hole in a bicycle tire.

The most common hernia in a child is an *indirect inguinal* hernia, which is present at birth but may or may not be recognized immediately. In fact, this type of hernia is not usually noticed until later. The hernia begins as a bulge just above the midpoint of the crease of the groin. It then enlarges toward the middle of the body until it reaches and enters the scrotum (the pouch containing the testes) of a boy or the labia majora (the outer folds of the external genitalia) of a girl. The bulge is actually a pouchlike sac underneath the skin made of peritoneum (the membrane that lines the abdominal cavity). The sac usually contains either a portion of the veil-like apron that overlies the intestines or a loop of the small intestine. Less often, it contains a loop of the large intestine, part of the urinary bladder, or an ovary.

More rarely seen in children is a *femoral hernia*, which appears below the crease of the groin, near where the pulse of the main artery to the leg can be felt.

Occasionally, a *ventral hernia* appears in the midline of the abdomen, above or below the navel.

In infants, an *umbilical hernia* often appears at the umbilicus (the navel). This is not a true hernia, however, because it contains no sac. An umbilical hernia usually disappears without treatment before the child reaches five years of age. They rarely need any treatment other than time. Umbilical hernias are the most common type of hernia seen in infants.

SIGNS AND SYMPTOMS

The key sign of a hernia is a bulge in one of the typical locations: just above or below the crease of the groin, at the navel, just above or below the navel, in the scrotum of a boy, or in the labia majora of a girl.

A hernia in any of these locations is called a *simple hernia* if the contents of the sac can be reduced (pushed gently back into the abdominal cavity). If a hernia cannot be reduced, it is called an *incarcerated hernia*. Simple and incar-

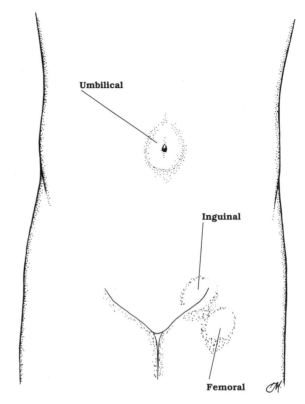

Some of the possible locations of hernias in children are shown here.

cerated hernias often produce no discomfort or pain; they may merely cause a sense of heaviness. If the blood supply to the contents of the hernia is cut off, it is said to be a *strangulated hernia*. Such a hernia causes intense pain and swelling.

HOME CARE

If there is any sign of a hernia, see your doctor. A simple hernia can be temporarily reduced by gentle pressure while the child is relaxed—in a tub of warm water if necessary. Trusses and belts to keep a hernia reduced are useless and may be harmful or even dangerous. Strapping an umbilical hernia is of no benefit.

PRECAUTIONS

■ A strangulated hernia is a **medical emergency** that requires immediate (within hours) surgical correction. Signs that a hernia has become strangulated are swelling, severe pain, and sometimes nausea, vomiting, and extreme weakness or collapse. If any signs of a strangulated hernia appear, take your child to a doctor or emergency room **immediately**.

■ Never attempt to reduce a strangulated hernia.

MEDICAL TREATMENT

Surgical repair is required for all except umbilical hernias. An umbilical hernia usually cures itself. Since inguinal hernias often appear on both sides, the surgeon may correct both sides even though only one side is visibly herniated.

RELATED TOPICS: Testis, torsion of; Testis, undescended

Herpes simplex

Herpes simplex is a highly contagious viral disease caused by *Herpesvirus hominis*, types 1 and 2. The infection is transmitted by direct contact with an infected person. The disease is recurrent. After the symptoms of the initial attack have cleared up, the virus continues to live in the body in a latent (inactive) state, usually for the person's lifetime. When the person's resistance is lowered (for instance, by fever, sunburn, exhaustion, or emotional stress), the "sleeping" virus is reactivated. This recurrent condition is contagious each time it appears.

Infection by the type 1 virus may occur as *oral herpes* (popularly known as *canker sores* when evidence of infection is seen inside the mouth and *fever blisters* when it appears on the mouth) or may affect the eyes. Type 1 infection is common before the age of four but can occur at any age. An attack usually lasts seven to ten days.

Genital herpes is usually an infection by the type 2 virus. It is most often transmitted sexually when the lesions (blisters) are present on the genitalia. A baby born to a mother with genital herpes can contract the disease while passing through the birth canal during delivery; in such a case, there is about a 50 percent chance that the infant will have a severe birth defect or die.

SIGNS AND SYMPTOMS

Oral herpes causes multiple painful ulcers of the mucous membranes and skin in the mouth area (lips, cheeks, tongue, and soft palate). Accompanying signs are red, swollen gums and swollen lymph nodes in the neck. The child's fever may climb to 105°F. Canker sores have a distinctive appearance and are easily distinguished from other mouth sores, such as gumboils: Canker sores are open, red ulcers with a scooped-out appearance, unlike gumboils, which

protrude above the surface of the membranes. When oral herpes appears as fever blisters, the blisters may be mistaken for impetigo (fever blisters are usually more painful, however). Fever blisters may also become infected with impetigo. Type 1 infection may also cause painful ulcers on the eyeballs. Genital herpes causes painful ulcers and blisters on the genitalia.

HOME CARE

For oral herpes, give acetaminophen to relieve the pain. Have the child eat bland, soothing foods such as ice cream, gelatin desserts, puddings, and milk. Encourage an older child to rinse the mouth with a mild solution of table salt. Canker sores can be treated in older children with triamcinolone in dental ointment form or with thick solutions of local anesthetic available from the pharmacy. Antibiotic ointment applied to fever blisters may prevent painful cracking and lessen the chance that impetigo will develop. Liquid diphenhydramine is a topical anesthetic; dabbing a small amount on the lesions helps to lessen the pain.

For genital herpes, warm soaks help relieve inflammation and pain. There is a drug that has been used by adults to lessen the severity of recurring attacks, but this drug has not been tested in children.

PRECAUTIONS

■ Herpes simplex of the eyeball is a serious condition and requires the immediate attention of an eye doctor.
■ Herpes can be severe in an infant. Adults and children with herpes should be kept away from a baby. If a baby contracts herpes, consult a doctor.
■ There is no cure for recurrent herpes.

MEDICAL TREATMENT

The doctor will probably prescribe eyedrops to treat herpes of the eyeball. If a child with herpes has a severely ulcerated mouth, hospitalization may be necessary so that intravenous fluids can be given until the child can swallow normally again.

A cesarean section (surgical delivery of an infant) may be performed in the case of a pregnant woman with genital herpes because the baby might be exposed to the disease during a vaginal delivery.

RELATED TOPICS: Gumboils; Impetigo

High blood pressure

It has been known for decades that high blood pressure, or hypertension, occurs in infants and children as well as in adults. A baby's blood pressure at birth is normally about 80/40. The blood pressure then rises gradually until, by the time the child is a teenager, it is about 120/80. If the blood pressure is substantially higher than that, a child is considered to have high blood pressure.

The most common cause of transient (temporary) high blood pressure in children is emotion (for example, fear or worry). Persistent high blood pressure can be caused by kidney disease (tumors, obstructions, infections, or nephritis), adrenal and testicular tumors, defects of the heart or of a major artery, an overactive thyroid gland, certain medications (for example, steroids and ephedrine), and extreme overweight. Essential hypertension, the most common type of high blood pressure in adults, may be hereditary and has no known cause.

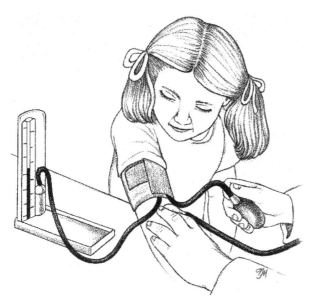

Be sure that your doctor checks your child's blood pressure during each checkup.

SIGNS AND SYMPTOMS

High blood pressure has been called the "silent disease" because it often has no symptoms. Symptoms, if they occur, can include headaches, pounding heartbeat, shortness of breath during exercise, and flushing of the face.

Accurate diagnosis can be made only by taking careful blood pressure measurements with instruments that are the correct size for use on your child. If the blood pressure is high on the first reading, the doctor will check it several times at return visits to make sure that the first reading was accurate.

HOME CARE

There is no home treatment for high blood pressure. The condition must be diagnosed and treated by a doctor. All children should have an annual physical examination. High blood pressure in childhood is curable, but it can be dangerous if it is not treated.

PRECAUTION

■ Be sure the doctor checks your child's blood pressure during each checkup.

MEDICAL TREATMENT

The doctor will give your child a complete physical examination, including measuring the blood pressure, feeling the arteries in the groin, and examining the eyes for changes in the blood vessels in the backs of the eyes (where the effects of high blood pressure may be recognized early). The doctor will also examine the child's heart, abdomen, and genitalia.

It takes complicated diagnostic evaluation to check for all of the many possible causes of high blood pressure. Except in rare cases, all the causes of high blood pressure can be successfully treated or cured by medications, changes in diet, or surgery. However, it is frequently necessary for the child to be hospitalized for tests and determination of treatment.

RELATED TOPICS: Nephritis; Thyroid disorders

Hip problems

Children are susceptible to joint pains, most of which come and go and are not serious—for example, sprains and growing pains. Occasionally children get arthritis, which may affect the hips. Dislocated hips sometimes occur in infants and toddlers. There are also three specific causes of hip pain that occur commonly in children.

Acute synovitis of the hip can be described as a bruise of the inside of the hip joint. Usually it is associated with a viral illness and is nearly always a harmless condition that disappears by itself. It can occur at any age, but most frequently between the ages of two and six years.

Legg-Calvé-Perthes disease is a serious condition in which the femoral head (the upper end of the thigh bone) softens and becomes deformed. No one knows why it happens, but it usually begins between the ages of four and ten years and affects boys more often than girls. If Legg-Calvé-Perthes disease is not treated, it results in a severe and permanent deformity of the hip.

Slipped capital femoral epiphysis is another condition of unknown origin, but it is possible that it is a delayed result of an injury. It occurs most often in the teen years, usually in overweight youngsters. It results in severe deformity if it is not treated.

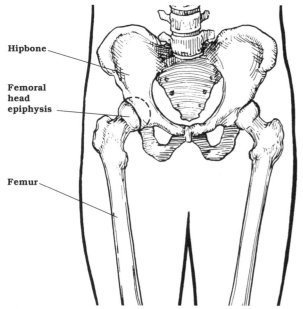

Hipbone

Femoral head epiphysis

Femur

The femoral head epiphysis (the rounded uppermost portion) of the femur (thigh bone) fits into a cup-shaped socket in the hipbone.

SIGNS AND SYMPTOMS

The three conditions described above cause pain in the hip accompanied by a limp. It is important to note, however, that pain in the knee can also indicate a hip problem. In rare cases, synovitis may be accompanied by a slight fever; the other two conditions do not produce fever. In all three conditions, the hip joint is limited in one or more of its movements—stretching and flexing, rotating inward or outward, or moving toward and away from the midline of the body.

HOME CARE

The child should stay off the legs for three or four days. (Crawling rather than walking does *not* keep weight off the hip.) If the condition does not seem to be corrected after three to four days of rest, consult the doctor.

PRECAUTIONS

■ If your child complains of pain in the knee, consider the possibility of a hip disease.
■ Marked pain, a limp, and high fever may be symptoms of a serious form of arthritis, which requires medical attention. Consult the doctor if the child's hip pain is accompanied by a fever.

MEDICAL TREATMENT

The doctor will examine the child carefully and may order X-ray studies of the hip. However, synovitis rarely shows at all on an X-ray film, and early Legg-Calvé-Perthes disease and slipped capital femoral epiphysis do not always show on X-ray studies. The doctor may suggest that the child continue bed rest, either at home or in the hospital. In the hospital, the leg may be immobilized, and X-ray studies of the hips will be performed at intervals so that the doctor can monitor the child's progress. Tests for arthritis may also be performed. Slipped capital femoral epiphysis always requires surgery. Legg-Calvé-Perthes disease is treated by having the child keep weight off the legs and not walk for a period of months until the condition heals; sometimes surgery is necessary.

RELATED TOPICS: Arthritis; Dislocated hips; Knee pains; Sprains and dislocations

Hives

Hives (also called urticaria) are an allergic reaction of the skin. About 20 percent of children have hives at least once. In about 95 percent of cases, hives are caused by foods, beverages, or medications to which the child is allergic. Among the substances most likely to trigger a reaction are citrus fruits, chocolate, nuts (including peanut butter), tomatoes, berries, spices, candies, tropical fruits and fruit juices, and artificial food flavorings.

In the small proportion of cases of hives not caused by a food or medication allergy, hives are caused by one of the following: a substance that the child has touched, such as a plant, ointment, or cosmetic, or the saliva of a dog or cat; an insect bite or sting; overexposure to sunlight or cold temperatures; or something the child has inhaled, such as pollen, mold, insecticide, animal dander, or feathers. One rarely seen form of hives, *erythema multiforme*, is caused by respiratory or other viruses, by the streptococcus bacterium, or by certain medications.

SIGNS AND SYMPTOMS

Hives appear as itchy, red, raised welts that can range in size from a quarter-inch to several inches across. Hives can involve any area of the skin. The most noticeable characteristic of hives is that they change appearance rapidly—they come and go and change in size from one hour to the next. Because no other type of rash has this characteristic, you can be fairly certain that any welts that itch and change appearance rapidly are hives.

Sometimes an insect bite looks like a hive at the point of a bite; however, it does not come and go as rapidly. Hives that are triggered by an allergic reaction to an insect bite appear at sites distant from the bite itself. Hives can also accompany allergic arthritis, which is signaled by stiff, swollen, red joints.

The form of hives known as erythema multiforme appears as welts that look like red targets of different sizes painted on the skin.

You can sometimes pinpoint the cause of your child's hives by considering his or her activities in the minutes or hours before the hives appeared.

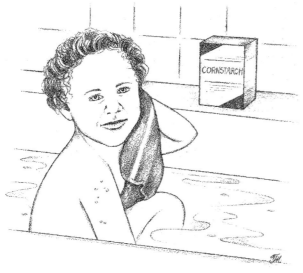

Cornstarch baths may help to make the child more comfortable.

HOME CARE

Unless the child has been given medication with instructions to take it when the hives recur, home treatment of hives should be confined to measures to relieve the itching. Cold-water compresses, calamine lotion, and cornstarch baths may help make the child more comfortable. The antihistamine diphenhydramine helps relieve allergic reactions and lessen the itching of hives. Frequent or repeated cases of hives require medical attention. Also, if the child has been given medication but the medication fails to relieve the symptoms, you should call the doctor.

PRECAUTIONS

■ **If the hives appear after an insect bite or sting, take the child to the nearest emergency room.**

■ If hives appear on the tongue, if they make the child cough, or if they cause difficulty in breathing or swallowing, see your doctor immediately.

■ If hives are accompanied by fever, see your doctor to rule out a strep infection.

■ If antihistamines do not help relieve a case of hives, call your doctor for advice.

MEDICAL TREATMENT

Your doctor may administer epinephrine to reduce the intensity of the outbreak and then prescribe antihistamines to be taken by mouth. If the hives recur and it is not possible to pinpoint the cause, the doctor may order skin tests or refer the child to an allergy specialist. The doctor may also order a throat culture to check for strep infection. If the child shows symptoms of arthritis, tests are necessary to confirm or rule out that possibility. If the hives are caused by an allergy to the venom released in an insect bite, the doctor may suggest a long-term course of injections to decrease the child's sensitivity to the venom; these shots may be given over a period of years. In the case of an allergy of this type, the doctor may prescribe a medication to be taken in the event of a bite.

RELATED TOPICS: Arthritis; Food allergies; Insect bites and stings; Rashes; Strep infections

Hoarseness

Anything that interferes with the normal vibrations of the vocal cords can cause the cords to swell and produce hoarseness—distortion or loss of the voice. In children, the most common cause of hoarseness is abuse of the voice by screaming. Hoarseness can also be caused by croup, laryngitis, or an allergy. More rarely, the condition can result from diphtheria, injury to the larynx, or a foreign body that the child has inhaled.

Extreme hoarseness can cause temporary total voice loss. Repeated hoarseness leads to the formation of tiny, wartlike growths on the vocal cords. In children, these growths are known as "screamer's nodes." (When they occur in adults, they are referred to more politely as "singer's nodes.") The presence of these nodes can cause the hoarseness to become a chronic condition.

A baby may be born with a soft, underdeveloped larynx that collapses partially each time the baby takes in a breath; the baby makes a crowing sound, and there may be a hoarse note to the cry. This condition should clear up without treatment; you do not need to be concerned about it.

SIGNS AND SYMPTOMS

Hoarseness may lead your child to speak or cry at a lower pitch than usual or to be unable to speak above a whisper. Check whether the child has other symptoms—fever, cough, difficulty in breathing, sore throat, or an obstruction of the nose—that might be responsible for the voice change. If not, and if the child has been yelling or screaming a lot, it is probably a simple case of hoarseness.

HOME CARE

A child experiencing hoarseness should rest the voice, inhale steam, and drink warm liquids. If the hoarseness is due to an allergy, and antihistamines have been prescribed for an allergic condition, the medication should relieve the hoarseness. Remember that hoarseness in a baby's cry, if it is happening because the larynx is still soft, is not a cause for concern and should disappear by the time the child is one year old.

PRECAUTIONS

■ Hoarseness in children is not usually due to any potentially dangerous cause. If no other signs of illness are present, the home care recommended should take care of the problem.
■ If the hoarseness gets more severe or persists for longer than a few days, consult your doctor.

MEDICAL TREATMENT

A doctor using a tongue blade and flashlight can see no farther than the epiglottis (a "lid" that covers the voice box above the vocal cords) and cannot examine the vocal cords. If your doctor is concerned about the hoarseness, you may be referred to an ear, nose, and throat specialist, who has the equipment necessary to perform a more complete examination. It is rarely necessary to surgically remove screamer's nodes.

RELATED TOPICS: Choking; Coughs; Croup; Diphtheria; Fever; Laryngitis; Sore throat

Hyperactivity

All healthy children are active—frequently more active than the adults in their lives wish them to be. Some children are extremely lively and always on the go. Of such children, however, only a small handful (one to ten percent) are truly hyperactive. The term is used very freely, and in common use its true medical definition is distorted. In fact, hyperactivity (also known as hyperkinesis, Attention Deficit Disorder, and Attention Deficit Hyperkinesis Disorder) is a specific clinical condition known as minimal brain dysfunction, which makes a child incapable of being quiet and still for more than a few moments. Hyperactivity may be due to late or faulty development of the brain centers that filter incoming stimuli (things that the child sees, hears, smells, touches, or tastes) and enable the child to react appropriately to these stimuli.

Sometimes children who are either neglected or raised in an overly permissive environment exhibit behavior that closely mimics hyperactivity. These children may have normally developed brain centers but may have been deprived of the social training that teaches children to control their behavior.

SIGNS AND SYMPTOMS

An extremely hyperactive child seems to be constantly in motion. The child cannot sit still (for instance, to listen to a story or watch television) for more than a few seconds or minutes. The child's behavior may be annoying or destructive, but the child is not deliberately misbehaving—he or she cannot control the hyperactive behavior. An experienced physician or neurologist (a specialist in nervous system disorders) may be able to recognize a severely overactive child at a glance. Many cases, however, are more difficult to pinpoint, and it may require a number of professionals to confirm the diagnosis.

HOME CARE

Until the hyperactive child has been professionally evaluated, home treatment cannot be undertaken. Once the diagnosis has been confirmed, the family of the hyperactive child is given specific recommendations tailored to the child's needs. Removing from the child's diet foods that contain artificial colorings, flavorings, or preservatives was once believed by some specialists to lessen the incidence of hyperactive behavior. However, others feel that the special attention given to a child whose diet is being controlled, not the diet itself, probably accounts for any improvement in behavior. Ask your doctor before you initiate any changes at home.

PRECAUTIONS

■ True hyperactivity is present from infancy. If your normally active child is more than two years old and suddenly becomes overactive, look for clues in the child's environment.
■ Never accept a diagnosis of hyperkinesis from anyone but a trained, skilled, and experienced professional.
■ Remember that an accurate diagnosis usually requires a team approach involving all those who care for the child—parents, teachers, doctors, and other professionals.
■ Don't mistake ordinary misbehavior for hyperactivity. If a child is overactive with one family member but not with the others, the child is not hyperactive.

MEDICAL TREATMENT

If hyperkinesis is suspected, your child should have a complete medical examination, including vision and hearing tests. The doctor will take a detailed account of the child's medical background, evaluate school reports, and usually recommend a series of tests to be carried out by a psychologist. The doctor may also try various medications, such as dextroamphetamine, methylphenidate, and pemoline.

Both you and the child's teachers will be asked to keep the doctor informed of changes in the child's behavior once a program of treatment has been established. The hyperkinetic child may need special educational placement. Also, because hyperkinetic children often have emotional problems resulting from poor social relationships at home and at school, counseling may be indicated.

RELATED TOPIC: Dyslexia

Hyperventilation

Hyperventilation syndrome is a condition characterized by the *sensation* of breathing difficulty, or "air hunger." The child complains, often bitterly or fearfully, of being unable to "get enough air," while at the same time taking deep breaths in and out with no apparent difficulty.

Unlike the many conditions that cause genuine difficulty in breathing (for example, asthma, bronchiolitis, diphtheria, the common cold, croup, hay fever, and pneumonia), hyperventilation syndrome is *not* a physical illness at all. There is no cough, nor is there any obstruction or abnormal sound to the breathing. The child's temperature and color are both normal.

The symptoms of hyperventilation are due to breathing that is too rapid or too deep, which causes the child to exhale too much carbon dioxide. (Although carbon dioxide is a waste product of the body—produced in the cells as a result of food usage, carried by the blood to the lungs, and then exhaled—the respiratory center in the brain requires the presence of a certain amount of carbon dioxide in the blood for breathing to continue normally.) As the concentration of carbon dioxide in the blood drops as a result of hyperventilation, the child will experience tingling and numbness in the hands and feet, followed by spasms of the muscles that control the hands, fingers, ankles, and toes. If hyperventilation continues, fainting occurs.

In most cases, the underlying cause of the abnormal breathing of hyperventilation is essentially the same as that of sighing—nervous tension, fear, anxiety, or depression. In fact, the deep breathing can often be recognized as sighing, one sigh right after another.

SIGNS AND SYMPTOMS

Close observation will determine if your child is having difficulty in breathing or is actually getting many full breaths of air in and out. Hyperventilation syndrome is not accompanied by cough or fever, and there is no abnormal sound during breathing.

Hyperventilation syndrome is more common in older children and teenagers. Children who tend to hyperventilate may have repeated attacks.

HOME CARE

It is important to remain calm and to reassure the child. Have your child breathe into a large paper bag held loosely over the mouth and nose. This will allow the child to rebreathe exhaled carbon dioxide.

If fainting occurs, recovery will follow naturally. The child will breathe normally while unconscious, allowing the carbon dioxide concentration in the blood to return to an appropriate level.

Look for such causes of hyperventilation as intolerable pressures or anxieties in the child's surroundings—at home, at school, or in relationships with friends.

PRECAUTION

■ Hyperventilation syndrome can be the result of rapid, prolonged, forced deep breathing, which is a party stunt in some circles. Encourage other kinds of games.

MEDICAL TREATMENT

Treatment of the underlying cause of hyperventilation syndrome depends on identifying possible sources of stress and emotional upset for your child. Psychiatric counseling may be recommended in severe cases.

RELATED TOPICS: Asthma; Bronchiolitis; Bronchitis; Common cold; Croup; Diphtheria; Fainting; Hay fever and other nasal allergies; Pneumonia; Shortness of breath

Impetigo

Impetigo is a highly contagious infection of the outer layers of the skin. It is caused by staphylococcus and streptococcus bacteria. The germs are transmitted by direct contact when the child touches either an infected person or something that person has been using—for example, clothing, towels, or toys. The condition appears two to five days after exposure.

SIGNS AND SYMPTOMS

Impetigo typically appears as fragile blisters containing thin, yellow pus. The initial sore often occurs at a point where the skin has been injured or irritated by an insect bite, a scrape, or a skin condition. If the child picks at the nose, the blister may appear in that area. The blister breaks easily, leaving an open, weeping sore that increases in size. The discharge hardens into a yellow crust or scab that looks like hardened honey. Impetigo spreads rapidly, and the child can aggravate this by scratching a sore and transferring the discharge on the hands to other parts of the body.

The infecting bacteria can be identified only through laboratory tests. If the culprit is the streptococcus bacterium, the doctor will watch for the possible development of a kidney condition known as glomerulonephritis.

HOME CARE

If only a few small areas are involved, scrub the crusts of the sores with soap and water.

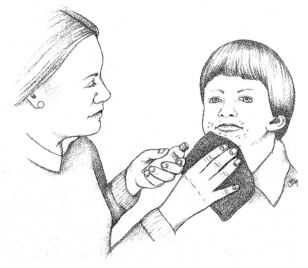

Mild impetigo can be treated by scrubbing the crusted sores with soap and water and applying antibiotic ointment several times a day.

(Streptococcal and staphylococcal infections thrive under the crusts.) Apply a nonprescription antibiotic ointment several times a day. Cover the sores with gauze to keep the ointment in place and to discourage the child from scratching and spreading the disease.

PRECAUTIONS

■ To prevent impetigo, wash minor scratches and scrapes with soap and water and cover with a sterile bandage.

■ Impetigo is highly contagious. If your child has impetigo, watch the rest of the family carefully for signs of the disease and treat cases promptly if they occur.

■ Keep the washcloth, towel, and clothing used by the child separate from items used by other family members. This will reduce the chance that the disease will spread.

■ Launder the infected child's clothing and linens frequently. Ordinary laundering sterilizes adequately.

■ If home treatment for impetigo is effective, do not discontinue the treatment until the sores have completely healed and the skin is smooth. It can take a long time to clear the condition completely.

■ If home treatment does not seem to be working within four or five days or if the sores continue to spread or multiply, see your doctor.

MEDICAL TREATMENT

Mupirocin (Bactroban) is an antibiotic ointment specifically designed for impetigo that usually cures the infection. The doctor may culture the sores to identify the causative organism. If streptococcal infection is present, a 10- to 14-day course of penicillin may be prescribed. If staphylococcal infection is found, further tests may be required to determine the most effective antibiotic medication.

RELATED TOPICS: Eczema; Insect bites and stings; Nephritis; Pityriasis rosea; Poison ivy; Rashes; Scrapes

Infectious mononucleosis

Infectious mononucleosis, or "mono," is a fairly common contagious disease. It is caused by an organism called the Epstein-Barr virus and is transmitted by secretions from the nose and throat (which is why it is also referred to as the "kissing disease"). Mono can occur at any age from infancy on but is most often seen among young people of high school or college age.

SIGNS AND SYMPTOMS

The usual symptoms of mono are general weakness and bodily discomfort accompanied by sore throat (often with pus on the tonsils), prolonged fever, and swelling and slight tenderness of the lymph nodes, particularly those of the neck. In 10 to 20 percent of cases, mono produces a mottled red rash, especially on the trunk of the body. The spleen may be enlarged.

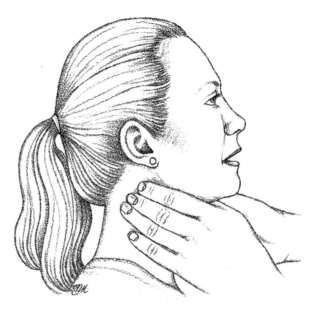

Swollen lymph nodes in the neck are one of the common symptoms of infectious mononucleosis.

The disease appears one to six weeks after exposure to the virus. A person with mono may be acutely ill for weeks, and fatigue and weakness can continue for months. In most teenagers, the acute illness lasts about two weeks and complete recovery occurs within four to six weeks.

Because the symptoms of mono are also typical of other diseases, it is rarely possible to make an accurate diagnosis without laboratory tests. Symptoms such as fever, severe sore throat, swollen lymph nodes in the neck, and rash can also be signs of a strep infection, viral pharyngitis, or diphtheria. If these symptoms do not improve with time or treatment, the doctor will suspect mono. It is also possible to have mono as well as another disease; for example, the doctor may diagnose and begin treating a case of strep throat without realizing at first that mono is also present.

The most common laboratory test for mono is the "mono spot" blood test. A positive test confirms the diagnosis of mono. However, often the mono spot does not become positive until two to three weeks into the course of the disease, and it may remain positive for up to two years after the illness.

HOME CARE

Rest, acetaminophen, and a general diet (as tolerated) are the basis of home care. Although mono is contagious, it is not necessary to isolate the child, and it is unlikely that other family members will contract the disease. The child can return to school as soon as the weakness and fatigue disappear and the child feels well enough.

If the spleen is enlarged, however, the child's activities should be restricted. An enlarged spleen protrudes beneath the ribs, which normally protect it, and is susceptible to injury or rupture. The child should not take part in contact sports or other energetic activities until the spleen has returned to its normal size. This can take weeks or months.

PRECAUTIONS

■ Do not allow a child who has had mono to return to school or other activities until weakness and fatigue have disappeared.

■ Do not allow a child with an enlarged spleen to take part in contact sports or other strenuous activities until the spleen has returned to its normal size.

MEDICAL TREATMENT

Your doctor will examine the child thoroughly, paying special attention to the lymph nodes, liver, and spleen. The doctor will also take a throat culture; if the throat culture reveals a strep infection, the child will be given penicillin or another antibiotic. Although most cases of mono can be treated at home with rest, diet, and acetaminophen, some severe cases require hospitalization. This would be the case if the child needed to be given fluids intravenously or needed other types of supportive care.

RELATED TOPICS: Diphtheria; Glands, swollen; G6PD deficiency; Hepatitis; Sore throat; Strep infections

Influenza

A child with any viral infection of the upper respiratory tract will probably be described as having the "flu," particularly if the child also has chills, fever, a cough, and muscle aches. However, true influenza is a specific, highly contagious respiratory infection that occurs in epidemics in which large numbers of persons in a community get the disease within a short period of time. It is caused by the influenza A or influenza B virus and is transmitted by droplets from nose and throat discharges of persons who have the disease. Influenza has a short incubation period (the time it takes for symptoms to develop once a person has been exposed to the virus) of one to three days and is contagious for seven days, starting before symptoms appear.

SIGNS AND SYMPTOMS

The symptoms of influenza are sudden chills, a sharp rise in temperature to 102°F to 106°F, flushing, headache, sore throat, hacking cough, redness of the eyes, and pains in the back and limbs. The symptoms come on quickly, and your child may go from feeling well to being very sick within a few hours. Young children may vomit and have diarrhea. Fever lasts three to four days and is followed by days of weakness and fatigue, during which the child is susceptible to other illnesses.

Secondary bacterial complications are responsible for many of the serious outcomes of flu. Their presence is suggested by the following: the return of high fever after the child's temperature has been normal for three or four days; progressive worsening of the cough, changing from dry and hacking to loose and productive; formation of pus in the eyes; rapid breathing and shortness of breath beyond that expected from the fever; severe earache; stiff neck; confusion; and extreme weakness, exhaustion, or collapse.

In isolated cases, flu cannot be diagnosed with certainty by physical examination. During an epidemic, the disease is diagnosed by similarity to other cases.

HOME CARE

The prescription for home care includes bed rest during the height of the fever and acetaminophen, **not aspirin**, for fever and pains. You should encourage the child to drink a lot of fluids. Keep the child isolated from the rest of the family, and do not let the child return to school until fully recovered. This will lessen the child's chances of getting another disease while his or her resistance is lowered by the influenza.

PRECAUTIONS

■ Reye's syndrome has been linked to the use of aspirin to treat influenza. Although a cause-and-effect relationship has not been established, aspirin should not be given if your child is suspected of having influenza. Watch for signs of complications, and report them to your doctor.
■ If there are no complications, the fever accompanying influenza often peaks in two cycles. The child's temperature is elevated for a day or two, normal for a day, and then elevated for a day or two. Do not misinterpret 24 hours of normal temperature as indicating a "cure," and do not allow your child to resume normal activities until the temperature has been normal for two or more days.

MEDICAL TREATMENT

If complications occur, cultures, blood tests, antibiotics, and hospitalization may be required.

Vaccines to prevent influenza are not very helpful for children. The influenza viruses have a number of different strains, which change their structures from year to year. Therefore, last year's vaccine may be useless against this year's virus. Moreover, reactions to influenza vaccines in children are frequent, although these reactions are rarely serious. At the moment, medical experts advise that only children at special risk from influenza be immunized annually. The conditions that are considered special risks are rheumatic heart disease, congenital heart disease, hypertensive heart disease, cystic fibrosis, severe asthma, tuberculosis, nephrosis, chronic nephritis, chronic diseases of the nervous system, and diabetes.

RELATED TOPICS: Asthma; Common cold; Coughs; Cystic fibrosis; Diabetes mellitus; Fever; Meningitis; Nephritis; Reye's syndrome

Ingrown toenails

Sometimes the corners and edges of toenails break the skin surrounding the nail. Once the skin is broken, infection can set in. The infection causes the tissues to swell, forcing the corner of the nail farther into the toe. This condition cannot heal as long as the ingrown portion of the nail remains within the tissues.

The initial wound may be caused by injury to the toe as a result of being stepped on or being squeezed by ill-fitting shoes. Another possibility is that the nail may have been trimmed to leave a sharp spur at the corner; this spur pierces the skin as the nail grows.

Most cases of ingrown toenails involve the big toes of older children; however, any toe can be involved, at any age. A baby can develop an ingrown toenail by digging his or her bare toes into the crib mattress or into another surface onto which the baby has been placed facedown.

SIGNS AND SYMPTOMS

The toe becomes red, painful, and tender to the touch. The wound produces a thin, watery pus that works its way under the nail. The tenderness, redness, pain, and swelling gradually get worse, eventually involving one entire side of the toenail. Often the nail becomes partly covered by raw, red tissue and a wet crust.

HOME CARE

If you discover an ingrown toenail early, you can often treat it successfully by gently cutting out the spur, or the ingrown corner of the nail, and then frequently soaking the toe in warm water for long periods. Even if the toe is so tender to the touch that you cannot release the embedded portion of the nail, prolonged soaking in a strong Epsom-salts solution (one cup to one quart of water) may cure the condition. Cover the foot with a bandage or cloth, and soak both foot and bandage in the solution. Then cover the dripping foot with plastic wrap or encase the foot in a plastic bag. In this manner, the nail can be soaked for hours with little effort on your part.

Because an infant's nails are so delicate, the ingrown toenail of an infant can often be cured by wiping the area several times a day with rubbing alcohol, and then soaking the toe in clear, warm water.

PRECAUTIONS

■ If your child repeatedly has ingrown toenails, check the child's shoes; they may be too small or too pointed.

■ Teach your child to trim the toenails straight across, without leaving sharp spurs that may cause problems.

■ An infection near the nail that lasts for more than a few days is probably the result of an ingrown nail.

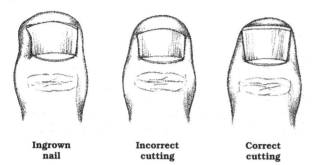

Ingrown nail **Incorrect cutting** **Correct cutting**

In most cases, correct trimming of toenails—straight across—will prevent ingrown toenails.

MEDICAL TREATMENT

If an ingrown toenail does not clear up with home treatment, your doctor can remove the embedded piece of nail. If the toe is very painful, the doctor may apply a local anesthetic before removing the ingrown area of the nail. If ingrown toenails occur frequently, your doctor may suggest minor surgery to narrow the nail and make ingrowing less likely.

Insect bites and stings

The bites and stings of most insects are only minor annoyances to most children. The only common complication is impetigo, a highly contagious skin infection that tends to occur at a point where the skin is already broken—for instance, where a child has scratched the site of an insect bite.

Some insect bites, however, can cause serious conditions.

Black widow spiders and scorpions can inject a venom (poisonous secretion) powerful enough to kill. The bite of the brown recluse spider can cause a large, open ulcer and fever. Female wood tick bites can cause paralysis and death.

Among the diseases that may result from insect bites are Rocky Mountain spotted fever, Colorado tick fever, Lyme disease, and tularemia (transmitted by certain types of ticks); rickettsialpox (mouse mites); viral encephalitis (mosquitoes); and typhus (red mites, lice, and rat fleas).

Some people are allergic to the venom contained in the stings of bees, wasps, hornets, and yellow jackets and can suffer a severe reaction if stung. This reaction can take the form of generalized hives, asthma, or circulatory collapse (insufficient blood pressure to maintain circulation of the blood) and can even lead to death.

Some children become allergic to the bites of mosquitoes, stable flies, fleas, and lice, but an allergic reaction to the bite of one of these is usually less severe than that caused by the venom of a stinging insect.

SIGNS AND SYMPTOMS

Flying insects usually bite only exposed areas of the skin. Crawling insects bite anywhere; multiple bites are common. Flea bites are most often found on the ankles and lower legs. Bedbugs often leave three to five bites spaced about an inch or two apart and arranged in a fairly straight line. Honeybees leave the stinger in the wound; bumblebees and other stinging insects do not. Ticks remain attached to the skin for long periods while they suck blood; when engorged with blood, they resemble small plump raisins.

HOME CARE

In most instances, insect bites can be treated by applying ice for a few minutes and then applying calamine lotion. A nonprescription antihistamine taken by mouth should relieve the itching and reduce the swelling. In the case of a tick bite, touching the still-hot tip of a burned-out match to the protruding portion of the insect will usually cause the tick to fall off the skin without leaving the head in the wound.

PRECAUTIONS

■ Protect children with proper clothing, mosquito netting, and insect repellents.

■ Learn about the insects in your locale and how to protect your child against the dangerous ones.

■ If your child develops hives or difficulty in breathing, speaking, or swallowing after being bitten by a scorpion or black widow spider or after being stung by a bee, wasp, or hornet, take the child immediately to the nearest emergency room.

■ If your child has had a severe reaction in the past, you should consider getting a self-injecting pen containing epinephrine, a drug that reverses the allergic reaction. Talk to your doctor about this.

■ If your child has been bitten by a tick and develops a red rash at the site, followed by headache, chills, fever, and body aches and stiffness, see your doctor. These symptoms may indicate Lyme disease.

MEDICAL TREATMENT

If your child has an allergic reaction to an insect bite or sting, the doctor will probably prescribe epinephrine, antihistamines, or steroids to inhibit the reaction. The doctor may recommend a series of injections to reduce the child's sensitivity to the insect in question. The doctor may also teach you or the child how to treat a bite or sting at home.

In the case of scorpion and black widow spider bites, the doctor will give the child an antidote that counteracts the effects of the poisonous venom. Steroid medications are also prescribed for these bites and the bite of the brown recluse spider.

Lyme disease, if caught early, can be eliminated with antibiotics. If it's not treated early, complications involving the joints, brain, and heart may occur.

RELATED TOPICS: Asthma; Encephalitis; Hives; Impetigo; Rocky Mountain spotted fever

Jaundice in children

Jaundice is characterized by yellowing of the skin and the whites of the eyes due to the accumulation in the body of a substance called bilirubin, which is released when old red blood cells are replaced by new ones. Bilirubin is normally excreted by the liver into the intestine as bile. Jaundice develops when the red blood cells are rapidly destroyed (as in sickle cell anemia and other forms of anemia); when the liver cannot transform bilirubin into bile; or when bile cannot flow through the bile ducts into the

intestine (for example, if the bile duct is blocked by stones, cysts, or a malformation).

Jaundice rarely occurs as a complication of a generalized infection, but it may be caused by some drugs and poisons. The usual cause of jaundice in children over one month of age is hepatitis, which damages the liver cells and interferes with the formation of bile.

SIGNS AND SYMPTOMS

The yellow, gold, or orange color of the skin and the whites of the eyes suggests jaundice. When a child has jaundice, all of the body fluids are stained; the tears are yellow, and the urine is dark orange. However, the diagnosis can be exceedingly complex and depends on the results of laboratory tests.

HOME CARE

Only after a clear diagnosis has been made can anything be done in the home.

PRECAUTIONS

■ Jaundice caused by a drug will disappear when the child stops taking that particular medication. However, do not discontinue any medication without your doctor's approval.

■ All other types of jaundice in children are potentially serious and require prompt medical attention.

MEDICAL TREATMENT

Laboratory tests are necessary to define the cause of the jaundice. Hospitalization is sometimes required.

RELATED TOPICS: Anemia; G6PD deficiency; Hepatitis; Jaundice in newborns; Sickle cell anemia

Jaundice in newborns

A substance known as bilirubin is released when old blood cells are replaced by new cells. The liver transforms bilirubin into bile, which is then passed into the intestine. When the liver is not functioning properly because of immaturity, injury, or abnormality, this transformation process is slowed or halted; bilirubin accumulates in the body, and jaundice results.

Approximately 60 percent of full-term infants and 80 percent of premature babies have so-called *normal jaundice* during the first week of life. This occurs because of the rapid destruction of the excess red blood cells with which all healthy babies are born. The jaundice usually begins in the second or third day of life and disappears between the fifth and tenth days. With rare exceptions, this jaundice is harmless.

The two most frequent causes of *abnormal jaundice* in the newborn are infection that has spread to the blood (blood poisoning) and erythroblastosis fetalis. Blood poisoning, a generalized infection caused by bacteria or viruses, causes jaundice in the newborn by destroying red blood cells and injuring the liver. Erythroblastosis fetalis is due to incompatibility between the child's blood and that of the mother. The mismatch may be in the Rh factor (for example, when the mother is Rh-negative and the infant is Rh-positive), in the ABO factors (for example, when the mother's blood is type O and the baby's is type A or B), or in rarer blood factors. Because of the incompatibility, the mother's blood forms antibodies (protective substances that form to fight off disease or anything the body interprets as an attacking organism) that rapidly destroy the infant's red blood cells.

Jaundice may also develop in breast-fed newborns because a substance in the mother's milk interferes with the functioning of the baby's liver. This form of jaundice usually is harmless. There are many other causes of jaundice in the newborn, including certain forms of anemia, hepatitis, and German measles, but jaundice due to these causes is rare.

Because either erythroblastosis fetalis or blood poisoning can be fatal to newborn babies if not treated immediately, a doctor's diagnosis must be made promptly. Other forms of jaundice can also be serious if the bilirubin in the blood exceeds a safe level. If jaundice is suspected, a doctor must monitor the bilirubin level closely.

SIGNS AND SYMPTOMS

The condition is recognized by the presence of a yellow tinge to the skin and the whites of the eyes. To judge the yellowness of the skin and eyes accurately, observe the baby in natural light. (Artificial light obscures the true color.) If you suspect jaundice, inform your doctor at once.

HOME CARE

The parents of a newborn should watch carefully for the development of jaundice in the first

week of the child's life at home. If jaundice develops, a doctor should see the child promptly.

PRECAUTIONS

■ Jaundice in the first 24 hours of life is abnormal. Because a newborn infant's nervous system is especially susceptible to permanent damage, jaundice during the first days of life has special significance.
■ Jaundice that develops or worsens after a baby leaves the hospital should be reported to your doctor.
■ Poor nursing, excessive drowsiness, irritability, and fever in a jaundiced baby should be reported to the doctor immediately.
■ If jaundice develops in your infant, follow your physician's directions exactly.

MEDICAL TREATMENT

Blood tests and cultures are used to identify the cause of the jaundice and to chart the progress of the condition. To lower the bilirubin level, your doctor may expose the baby to special lights or replace the infant's blood with that of a donor through transfusion.

RELATED TOPICS: Blood poisoning; G6PD deficiency; Jaundice in children

Knee pain

The knee is the most structurally complicated joint in the body. Four bones come together at that site: the femur (thighbone), the tibia (shinbone), the fibula (the small outer bone of the lower leg), and the patella (kneecap). Other important structures include two crescent-shaped pieces of cartilage (elastic, semi-hard tissue) and two crossed ligaments (the tough connective tissues that hold bones together).

Because of its complexity, the knee is subject to a wide variety of injuries and disorders—ranging from rheumatoid arthritis (the form of arthritis that occurs most commonly in children) to puncture wounds that occur during play or sports activity. The knee can also be the site of pain without being the site of the actual problem; a hip condition can show up as a pain in the knee, for instance.

Active adolescents are subject to Osgood-Schlatter disease, a painful and tender swelling of the bony prominence, called the tibial

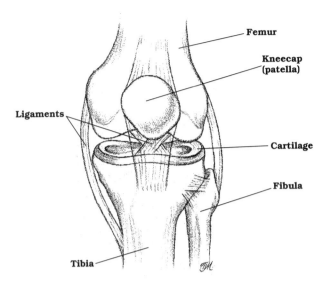

Because of its complexity, the knee is suscepti-ble to a wide variety of injuries.

tuberosity, at the upper end of the shinbone. The leg is straightened when the large muscle at the front of the thigh pulls (via the kneecap) on this tuberosity. If an injury cuts off the blood supply to the tuberosity, it becomes swollen and tender, and straightening the leg causes pain.

SIGNS AND SYMPTOMS

Tenderness without swelling at the edges of the kneecap usually indicates that the cartilage on the underside of the kneecap has been bruised and softened (a condition called chondromala-cia). Swelling of the knee joint (as evidenced by fullness on both sides of the kneecap) indicates inflammation in the joint or an internal injury. Diagnosing the cause of knee pain depends on the patient's history, the presence or absence of symptoms, and the location of pain.

HOME CARE

Treatment depends on the problem, but usually (as in Osgood-Schlatter disease and chondro-malacia) it involves limiting the child's activi-ties, particularly strenuous activities like track, trampoline, football, and soccer. For two to four weeks, or until the swelling and tenderness are gone, the knee must not be bent or extended. From the child's point of view, this rules out two-legged stair climbing, bicycling, running, and jumping. An elastic knee support can be a helpful reminder that the knee needs rest dur-ing this period of healing.

PRECAUTIONS

■ Swelling of the knee joint may be serious; it requires a doctor's attention.
■ If one knee cannot be straightened to match the opposite knee, fluid (blood or the serum that remains after blood has formed a clot) or pus has probably accumulated at the joint. The knee should be checked by a doctor.
■ The child should not put weight on a swollen knee until it has been examined by a doctor.
■ Remember that knee pain may be a sign of a hip problem.

MEDICAL TREATMENT

The doctor will make a thorough, detailed examination of each part of the knee and leg and will check the range of normal and abnor-mal movement. The doctor may order a number of different tests to better understand the cause of the knee pain. X-ray studies show if there are any bone abnormalities. CT scans and MRIs allow the doctor to "see" inside the knee joint without actually making a cut. The arthro-scope, a small tube that an orthopedist inserts inside the knee joint, can allow the doctor to see swelling, accumulation of fluid, and distor-tion or injury of parts of the joint. Certain types of injuries can be repaired through an arthro-scope, as well. The doctor may also order tests of fluid drawn from the joint. Depending on the diagnosis, treatment of knee pain may include bed rest, antibiotics, a cast, crutches, or surgery.

RELATED TOPICS: Arthritis; Hip problems; Puncture wounds; Sprains and dislocations

Laryngitis

Laryngitis is an inflammation of the larynx (voice box), which is almost always due to a respiratory virus. It is closely related to croup, but unlike croup, it is not associated with breathing difficulties. Laryngitis may last from a day to a couple of weeks.

SIGNS AND SYMPTOMS

Hoarseness; a dry, hacking cough; and a scratchy throat—but not breathing difficulty—are the signs of laryngitis. There is sometimes a low-grade (101°F) fever.

HOME CARE

Give your child warm drinks. Discourage the child from talking. Give acetaminophen for fever or pain and a nonprescription expectorant cough remedy for temporary relief of the cough.

A humidifier or vaporizer may make breathing easier. (Be sure to keep it meticulously clean, however. Otherwise, it can actually become a source of infection if microorganisms are allowed to grow in it.)

PRECAUTIONS

■ If any breathing difficulty arises, notify a doctor.

■ If your child has a climbing fever and difficulty in breathing, he or she may have an inflammation of the epiglottis (the structure in the back of the throat that prevents food from entering the larynx and windpipe). Inflammation of the epiglottis is a **medical emergency**; take your child to a doctor immediately.

MEDICAL TREATMENT

Your doctor will confirm the diagnosis and rule out other conditions by physical examination of the child. A throat culture and blood tests may be necessary. If laryngitis persists, your doctor may order X-ray studies of the child's chest and neck or may refer you to an ear, nose, and throat specialist.

RELATED TOPICS: Coughs; Croup; Hoarseness

Lazy eye

A "lazy eye" is one in which the vision is poor because the brain has suppressed the image received by that eye. Known technically as *amblyopia ex anopsia*, it is basically a loss of vision from lack of use. Most cases of lazy eye result from weakness of one or more of the six small muscles that move the eyeball. Such muscle weaknesses can cause the eyes to turn in or out in relation to each other. This can lead to the child's seeing double. If a young child learns to ignore one of the double images, a loss of vision in the unused eye results.

In other cases of lazy eye, the eye muscles are normal but the vision is poor in one eye. To compensate, the child may learn to ignore the poor image received. This can result from marked nearsightedness or farsightedness,

astigmatism, or other interference with vision in one eye. Such interference might be caused by a congenital cataract (clouding of the lens of the eye) or scars on the cornea (the transparent front part of the eye).

SIGNS AND SYMPTOMS

Lazy eye should be suspected when the eyes are not parallel all or most of the time or are parallel less and less often. See your doctor if your child's eyes are not parallel, if the pupils of the eyes are different colors, if your child is over two years old and has trouble seeing or judging distances when reaching for an object, or if your child cocks the head to one side or turns the face to see better (the child may be compensating for double vision).

HOME CARE

No home treatment for lazy eye is advised until a doctor has diagnosed the condition.

PRECAUTIONS

■ Be watchful for lazy eye so that if the condition occurs in your child, you can catch it in time for treatment to be successful.

■ Have your child's vision checked each year after the age of three or four years. Lazy eye can be treated successfully in children up to

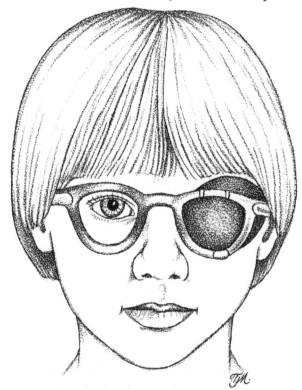

Lazy eye is corrected by blocking the good eye; this forces the child to use the lazy eye.

the age of seven years. If the condition is left untreated, however, it may become permanent.

MEDICAL TREATMENT

Your doctor will inspect the insides and outsides of both eyes and test their movements in all directions. If the child is old enough to understand directions, the doctor can check the vision, using a letter or picture chart. A younger child's vision should be checked by an ophthalmologist, who can use a system that does not require the child to follow instructions.

Lazy eye is corrected either by patching the good eye or by hindering the vision in the good eye with eyedrops or glasses. When the good eye is blocked, the child is forced to use the lazy eye. As a final resort, surgery is sometimes necessary.

RELATED TOPICS: Crossed eyes; Vision problems

Lead poisoning

Lead is a heavy, dense metal that is poisonous to the human body. Microscopic particles of lead can enter the body if a person swallows something that contains lead or inhales air contaminated with lead. The metal then accumulates in the blood and body tissues. The most serious effects of lead poisoning are on the brain and nervous system. Lead can also damage the digestive system and the kidneys.

Before 1977, lead was an ingredient in paint, plaster, and putty, and most cases of lead poisoning occur when a small child eats fragments of lead-based paint that have peeled off a wall or have been left in the soil around a house. Although house paint manufactured today no longer contains lead, the metal is found in many other places. Some of the sources of lead poisoning include artist's pigments, exhaust from cars (some gasoline contains lead), soil around buildings that were once painted with lead-based paint, and the air in cities where lead may be used in industry and where the exhaust from many cars is concentrated. Lead is also found in high-acid foods and beverages (for example, orange and tomato juice) that have been stored in lead-containing pottery that was not properly glazed.

Lead poisoning can cause permanent damage to the brain, especially in cases in which the symptoms are severe. Such damage may not occur if the problem is quickly identified and treated. However, it may take as long as a year for a child who has had lead poisoning to recover completely. Lead poisoning occurs most often in children under the age of five years. It is most dangerous if the child is less than two years old.

SIGNS AND SYMPTOMS

The symptoms of lead poisoning vary with the age of the child and the amount of lead that is in the child's body, and they are difficult to identify because they may build up gradually. Symptoms may include poor appetite, vomiting, constipation, extreme irritability, slow mental and physical development, aggressive behavior, convulsions, personality changes, clumsiness, and symptoms of anemia (paleness, tiredness, weakness, breathlessness, and fainting). In severe cases, the child may become unconscious.

A routine blood or urine test will not detect lead poisoning. Before the problem can be diagnosed, the doctor must suspect that lead may be causing the child's symptoms. Specific laboratory tests are then done to measure the lead content in the blood and urine. A serum lead level test measures a child's current lead level, while the free erythrocyte protoporphyrin and zinc protoporphyrin tests measure chronic lead levels.

HOME CARE

Be alert for changes in your child's behavior. Also, watch to see if your child has a habit of putting nonfood objects in the mouth and swallowing them; this habit, which is called pica, can result in lead poisoning. Check your home and yard for sources of lead. Have the paint and plaster in your home tested for lead content.

PRECAUTIONS

■ If you are remodeling a home—especially if you are burning, scraping, or sanding paint and plaster inside the building—you may be releasing lead into the air. Pregnant women, infants, and small children should live elsewhere until the work has been completed and the dust has been cleaned up. Consult your local health department about the proper way to remove lead from the home environment.

■ Anyone whose work involves exposure to lead should be especially careful about bringing home lead-containing dust on work clothes. Such occupations include lead smelting; storage battery manufacture, repair, and recycling; automobile assembly; and automobile body and radiator repair.

MEDICAL TREATMENT

Treatment for lead poisoning is called chelation therapy. The doctor prescribes a drug that combines with the lead in the body and draws it out of the tissues where it is stored. The lead passes out of the body in the urine. A special diet or a change in diet may also be prescribed. Of course, this treatment will not be effective if the child is still taking in lead. The source of lead must be identified and removed first.

RELATED TOPICS: Anemia; Constipation; Convulsions without fever; Vomiting

Leukemia

Leukemia is cancer of the white blood cells. Although it is rare, leukemia is one of the four types of cancer most frequently seen in children. It can afflict children at any age, but most frequently occurs between the ages of three and four years.

The disease can progress slowly or rapidly. About 25 percent of leukemia cases are diagnosed during a routine physical examination before the appearance of any symptoms of the disease.

SIGNS AND SYMPTOMS

Typical symptoms of leukemia include anemia, indicated by paleness, weakness, or fatigue; bruises that appear on the body for no apparent reason; swollen, red, and bleeding gums; a low-grade fever (101°F); swelling of the lymph nodes (although the nodes are neither red nor painful); bone pain; frequent, heavy nosebleeds; and the appearance of blood in the child's urine or stool.

It is important to remember that symptoms similar to those of leukemia can also occur in a child suffering from some other quite different (or even minor) disorder. Doctors may suspect leukemia when the typical signs and symptoms are accompanied by an enlarged spleen or liver. Suspicion is heightened when blood studies reveal malignant (cancerous) white blood cells. The diagnosis is confirmed by an examination of the bone marrow.

HOME CARE

No home care is advised until a doctor has diagnosed the condition. Leukemia is a serious condition that always requires close medical attention.

PRECAUTION

■ Leukemia is uncommon. Many illnesses imitate leukemia, however, and these illnesses are *not* uncommon; among them are infectious mononucleosis, herpes simplex infections of the mouth, vitamin C deficiency, rheumatic fever, rheumatoid arthritis, sickle cell anemia, and other diseases that cause spontaneous bruising. Do not jump to the conclusion that your child has leukemia because of the presence of any of the signs or symptoms. To ease your mind, have your child examined by a doctor.

MEDICAL TREATMENT

The survival rate for childhood leukemia has been rising over the past few years because of the use of new anticancer drugs. These drugs may result in long periods of remission (during which the illness gets no worse) and even cure. Pediatric oncologists (cancer specialists) select and supervise the treatment of leukemia.

RELATED TOPICS: Anemia; Arthritis; Bruises; Herpes simplex; Infectious mononucleosis; Sickle cell anemia

Measles

Measles (also known as rubeola) is a highly contagious disease caused by a specific virus. It affects mainly the respiratory system, the eyes, and the skin and is spread from person to person in airborne droplets of moisture from an infected person's respiratory system. The incubation period (the time it takes for symptoms to develop once the child has been exposed to the virus) is 10 to 12 days. Measles can be passed to other people between the fifth day of the incubation period and the sixth day after the appearance of the rash that is characteristic of this disease.

Measles used to be one of the more dangerous childhood diseases, but it is relatively uncommon today because a vaccine is now available to protect against it. Most children are vaccinated against measles by an injection given at the age of about 15 months. If a mother is immune to measles (because she has either had it or been vaccinated against it), her baby will receive temporary protection against the disease. This protection lasts three to six months after birth. The reason that vaccination is delayed until the baby is 12 to 15 months old (and not given as soon as the temporary immunity acquired from the mother wears off) is that the vaccination is not fully effective in a baby under 15 months. It is important to note, however, that measles is dangerous in a child under three years old; if an unvaccinated young child is exposed to the virus, you should consult the doctor at once. Measles is also likely to be serious in children who have chronic (long-term) diseases. A second dose of the vaccine is recommended between ages four and six years.

Measles is considered dangerous mainly because of the complications it can cause, among them pneumonia (infection of the lungs), middle ear infection, and encephalitis (inflammation of the brain). Encephalitis occurs in only 1 or 2 of every 1,000 cases of measles, and death from measles or its complications is now very rare.

SIGNS AND SYMPTOMS

The first symptoms of measles are a runny nose, reddish eyes, a cough, and fever. However, measles cannot be diagnosed during the earliest stages of the disease. Spots that look like grains of salt surrounded by a red rim (Koplik's spots) appear inside the cheeks near the molars. After three or four days, the fever rises to 104°F or 105°F, the cough worsens, and a heavy, splotchy, red rash develops on the neck and face. The rash quickly spreads over the trunk, arms, and legs. When the rash has erupted fully, the fever breaks, and the child gets better.

HOME CARE

With measles, prevention is better than cure; be sure that your child is properly vaccinated against this disease. A child with measles should be given acetaminophen to reduce the fever and a cough suppressant to ease a severe cough. Keep the child away from bright light; light bothers the eyes but does not injure them. Encourage your child to drink extra liquids.

PRECAUTIONS

■ If the fever and cough do not subside as the rash peaks, be alert for possible complications, such as pneumonia, encephalitis, and middle ear infection.
■ A newborn baby is immune to measles for three to six months only if the mother is immune.
■ If a child under the age of three years who has not been vaccinated against measles is exposed to the virus, call the doctor.
■ Be sure that your child is vaccinated against measles.

MEDICAL TREATMENT

If your child has not been vaccinated and has been exposed to the measles virus, your doctor can give injections of gamma globulin within six or seven days of exposure to prevent or lessen the severity of the disease.

RELATED TOPICS: Earaches; Encephalitis; Immunizations; Pneumonia

Meningitis

Meningitis is an infection of the meninges (the layers of tissue that cover and protect the brain and spinal cord). Most often, meningitis is caused by a viral infection. Bacterial meningitis is usually caused by one of three types of bacteria: meningococcus, pneumococcus, or *Hemophilus influenzae.*

Meningitis is seldom spread by a person who has the disease. It is usually contracted by direct contact with a healthy carrier (a person who has no symptoms of the disease but can pass it on to others) or by inhaling airborne droplets of moisture from that person's respiratory system.

Meningitis may be a complication of a skull fracture if the fracture has extended into the nose, middle ear, or nasal sinuses. Meningitis can also follow an upper respiratory tract infection or middle ear infection.

SIGNS AND SYMPTOMS

The characteristic symptoms of meningitis are moderate to high fever, headache, vomiting, exhaustion or collapse, convulsions, and a stiff neck (the child cannot touch his or her chin to the chest with the mouth closed). The combination of fever and the presence of purplish red spots (called petechiae) scattered over the body may indicate one form of meningococcal infection. The diagnosis of meningitis can be made with certainty only by testing a sample of spinal fluid obtained by a spinal tap.

HOME CARE

Meningitis is a **medical emergency** in which hours, if not minutes, count. Do not attempt any home treatment. See a doctor at once.

PRECAUTIONS

■ A child who is suffering from exhaustion or extreme weakness and who has a fever and a stiff neck is in danger and should be taken to a medical facility immediately.

■ The unnecessary use of antibiotics to treat an upper respiratory tract infection may mask the onset of meningitis.

■ Inform your doctor immediately if you discover that your child has been in contact with a person who has meningitis.

MEDICAL TREATMENT

Your doctor will take the child's complete medical history and perform a thorough examination. If the doctor suspects meningitis, he or she will then order a spinal tap. Spinal fluid will be examined for cells, bacteria, and abnormal chemical components. This is the only way to differentiate between meningitis and encephalitis (inflammation of the brain), which is also a life-threatening disease. Cultures of the spinal fluid, blood, and nose and throat mucus will also be performed.

Immediately after the spinal tap and cultures, the doctor will administer intravenous fluids and antibiotics. If the infecting organism is unknown, the doctor may prescribe two antibiotics to be taken at the same time. If the meningitis is found to be caused by a virus, no antibiotics will be used, since viruses do not respond to antibiotics.

A vaccine is now available to protect against *Hemophilus influenzae* infection. It is recommended that all children receive the vaccine at 2 months, 4 months, 6 months, and 12 to 15 months of age.

A vaccine against pneumococcal infection is available, but it is recommended for use only in children in certain high-risk groups. A vaccine against meningococcal infection is still in the experimental stage and is used only in specific cases.

RELATED TOPICS: Bruises; Earaches; Encephalitis

Menstrual irregularities

Most girls in the United States begin to menstruate sometime between 9 and 17 years of age. The average age is 12. Following menarche (the onset of menstruation), it may take from several months to five years for the hormones to balance and produce regular menstrual periods. Menstrual irregularity during this time is to be expected and is not necessarily abnormal.

SIGNS AND SYMPTOMS

For about five percent of adolescent girls, abdominal cramps and backaches lasting one or two days at the start of a menstrual period may be severe enough to interfere with normal activities. In many instances, cramps and backaches are related to emotional factors such as tension and anxiety. They also may be due to a hormonal imbalance or pelvic disease. Some women experience pain in the middle of the cycle, when they are ovulating. This pain, called Mittelschmerz pain, doesn't mean anything is wrong.

Because the range of normal is so wide, it is difficult to judge whether a menstrual abnormality exists. Symptoms that warrant investigation include: menstruation before the age of nine, failure to menstruate by the age of 17, absence of menstrual periods for six months (or for one month in a sexually active teenager, in whom the failure to menstruate may indicate pregnancy), repeated excessive bleeding, and pain severe enough to interfere with normal activities.

HOME CARE

Give aspirin, ibuprofen, naproxen, or acetaminophen to relieve mild pain. Hot baths or hot soaks may help relieve discomfort. Encourage your daughter to maintain her normal activities during her menstrual period.

PRECAUTIONS

■ Explain the process of menstruation to your preteen daughter; in this way, you can counteract any "old wives' tales" she may have heard from others and prepare her for this important part of growing up.

■ There are good books available (for both parents and teenagers) that can help explain the process of menstruation and provide accurate information.

MEDICAL TREATMENT

If a girl is having menstrual problems, the doctor should conduct a complete physical examination that includes rectal and limited pelvic examinations. Chromosome and hormone studies may also be necessary. In some cases, the doctor will order blood tests or tests of thyroid function. (The thyroid gland, located at the front of the throat, regulates the body's temperature, energy production, growth, and fertility.) If the girl is sexually active and has missed a period, a pregnancy test will be performed. Your doctor may well find no abnormality, and no treatment will be necessary. In some cases, the doctor will prescribe hormone medications to be taken over a period of several months. In other cases, an iron supplement or a thyroid medication may be prescribed.

RELATED TOPIC: Vaginal bleeding

Moles

Moles are benign (noncancerous) growths on the skin. They can be flat, dome-shaped, or protruding. They vary in color from tan or brown to blue or black and in size from one-sixteenth to one-half inch or larger. Moles are rarely present at birth; they develop during childhood. No child is totally free of moles, and some children have hundreds of them.

It is very unlikely that any mole will become cancerous (malignant). However, one exception to this statement is a type of mole called a pigmented nevus. This mole, which is present at birth, is extremely large (several inches wide) and dark.

SIGNS AND SYMPTOMS

Moles are easily recognizable, but if the doctor is in any doubt about a growth on the skin, a laboratory examination of part of the growth may be necessary. Examination of an entire mole under the microscope may be needed.

HOME CARE

If a mole requires any kind of treatment, it must be medical, not home, care.

PRECAUTION

■ A mole should be seen by a doctor if it has been partly removed by accident; if it is bleeding, crusting, changing color, or growing rapidly; or if the pigment (color) is moving into the surrounding skin.

MEDICAL TREATMENT

If removal of a mole is necessary (or desired, for cosmetic reasons), it must be performed by a doctor. Any pigmented nevus probably should be removed surgically because of the possibility of malignancy.

Surgical excision (complete removal with a scalpel) will leave a scar of some sort. Moles cannot be safely removed by a procedure called electrocautery or with the use of acids, dry ice, or liquid nitrogen.

Molluscum contagiosum

The condition known medically as molluscum contagiosum is often mistaken for an outbreak of warts or pimples. In fact, it is a common, chronic infection of the skin, caused by a specific virus.

The disease is spread by direct contact with an infected person or by contact with articles used by that person. The virus has a long incubation period (the time it takes for symptoms to develop once the child has been exposed to the virus) of two to seven weeks. Scratching can cause the eruptions, or molluscum papules, to become infected. Molluscum contagiosum has no other symptoms.

SIGNS AND SYMPTOMS

Each molluscum papule is a plump, round, slightly waxy-looking, pimplelike eruption that grows to a diameter of one-quarter inch or more. They later become flatter with a small central depression. In the course of months, molluscum papules may spread and number in the hundreds.

The diagnosis is based on the appearance of the pimplelike eruptions. The indentation in the center of each molluscum papule can be easily seen on close inspection in good light.

HOME CARE

Molluscum contagiosum requires medical treatment. Call the doctor, who will give directions for home care.

PRECAUTION

■ The condition readily spreads among members of a family. Keep the infected child's clothing, linen, and towels separate from those used by other family members. Ordinary laundering with soap or detergent kills the virus.

MEDICAL TREATMENT

The doctor will give specific instructions about treatment of this condition. The first recommendation may be a special cream to be applied to the molluscum papules, which are then buffed with a rough pad. If this does not work, the doctor may use a pointed scalpel to open each molluscum papule and remove the hard, white, pearl-like center. (Do not attempt this treatment at home.)

Motion sickness

Car sickness, airsickness, and seasickness are all forms of motion sickness. Prolonged rhythmic motion up and down or from side to side will make most children nauseated, presumably because the movement affects the balance mechanism of the inner ears. Some children are more susceptible to motion sickness than others; young infants are apparently immune. Motion sickness is not deliberately brought on by the child, nor can the child control it. Susceptible children will have repeated attacks.

SIGNS AND SYMPTOMS

Motion sickness is fairly easy to recognize. A motion-sick child becomes nauseated, greenish or pale, and anxious. The child may perspire and vomit.

HOME CARE

If your child suffers from motion sickness, ask your doctor to recommend an antinausea medication. Give your child the antinauseant as directed before and during the trip. Dimenhydrinate, available in tablet and liquid forms, is a highly effective and safe antinauseant. It is also helpful to keep the child cool and on a light diet (for example, bland foods and carbonated drinks, but no dairy products) before and during the trip. Having the child look out the car window, especially the front window, will often eliminate motion sickness. Distracting the child with a game during the trip can also be useful.

PRECAUTION

■ Prolonged motion sickness (over a period of hours) that causes excessive vomiting can lead to dehydration, which requires medical attention.

MEDICAL TREATMENT

Your doctor can recommend an antinausea medication. Dehydration brought on by motion sickness necessitates hospital care, during which the child is given fluids intravenously.

RELATED TOPICS: Dehydration; Vomiting

Mumps

Mumps is a moderately contagious infection caused by a specific virus that especially affects the salivary glands. It is contracted by contact with the saliva of an infected person. The incubation period (the time it takes for symptoms to develop once the child has been exposed to the virus) for mumps is 14 to 21 days. The disease can be passed on any time from two or more days before symptoms appear until all symptoms have gone.

One attack almost always provides lifelong immunity. If a child has had mumps, and similar symptoms subsequently develop, the problem is most likely not mumps but some other disease of the salivary glands.

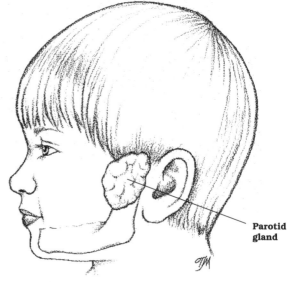

Mumps is caused by a virus that infects the salivary glands, particularly the parotid glands, which results in swelling.

Complications of mumps include meningitis, encephalitis, permanent deafness, and orchitis (inflammation of the testes, or male sex glands). The disease may also involve the ovaries (female sex glands) or cause an infection of the pancreas.

A vaccine is available to prevent mumps. It is usually given in combination with the vaccines against measles and rubella (German measles) at around 12 to 15 months of age. This vaccine is 95 percent effective in preventing mumps.

SIGNS AND SYMPTOMS

Typical symptoms include fever (101°F to 104°F), loss of appetite, and headache. One or two days after the onset of these symptoms, one or more of the salivary glands become painfully swollen; the swelling lasts about a week.

The diagnosis of a typical case of mumps is obvious from the swelling of one or both of the parotid salivary glands, which lie behind, below, and in front of the earlobe. If the earlobe is at the center of the swelling, then it is the parotid gland that is swollen. Other salivary glands, such as those that lie under the edge of the jaw, may be swollen with or without swelling of the parotid glands. Swelling may occur on one or both sides of the face.

Accurately diagnosing mumps may be difficult if complications of mumps develop before, or sometimes even without, swelling of the salivary glands. If the pancreas or ovaries are involved, the child will have abdominal pain. If the testes are involved, they will be swollen and tender. The symptoms of encephalitis include stiff neck, headache, and fever. In the absence of swelling of the salivary glands, these other symptoms may be difficult to link with mumps.

HOME CARE

Rest and isolation are recommended until all symptoms have gone. Acetaminophen may be given to reduce pain and fever. Avoid feeding the child spicy foods.

PRECAUTIONS

■ Routine immunization against mumps is strongly advised.
■ If a child who has not been vaccinated against mumps is exposed to the disease, he or she can receive the vaccine shortly after exposure to prevent becoming ill with mumps.
■ If a mother is immune to mumps (because she has had it or has been vaccinated against

it), her baby acquires some temporary immunity before birth. This immunity lasts only until the infant is four to six months old.
■ In an adult man, inflammation of the testes caused by mumps can result in sterility (the inability to father a child). That is why it is important for males to be vaccinated against mumps in childhood.
■ Consult your doctor if a child who has already had mumps seems to have it again. The problem is most likely not mumps, but rather inflammation of a parotid salivary gland, a stone in the salivary duct, or a bacterial infection of the gland.

MEDICAL TREATMENT

If complications are suspected, your doctor may order a spinal tap to test for meningitis or encephalitis or may order blood tests to measure the number of mumps antibodies in the blood. (Antibodies are protective substances that the body produces to fight against disease.) Doctors do not follow any specific treatment for mumps but may hospitalize a child to arrive at a diagnosis or to provide supportive treatment.

RELATED TOPICS: Encephalitis; Immunizations; Meningitis

Nephritis

There are many forms of nephritis (inflammation of the kidneys), but the form that is most common in children usually follows a streptococcal infection, such as strep throat, scarlet fever, or streptococcal impetigo. The first symptoms of nephritis develop one to three weeks after the onset of a strep infection, and these symptoms are usually mild. In fact, most cases of nephritis probably go unnoticed (or undiagnosed) and pass without treatment. Occasionally, however, nephritis starts abruptly and the illness is severe. Most children recover completely from nephritis, but chronic kidney disease may develop.

SIGNS AND SYMPTOMS

In most cases, the first sign of nephritis is urine that is a smoky color or brownish-red and tinged with blood. The child may have puffy eyes and run a fever of 101°F to 102°F for several days. In severe cases, the illness produces high fever, headache, vomiting, high blood pressure, and convulsions; urination ceases almost completely, and the urine the child does produce contains a lot of blood. An analysis of the urine will confirm the diagnosis. Positive cultures of nose and throat secretions for strep bacteria support the diagnosis.

HOME CARE

If the symptoms are severe enough to be recognized, do not attempt home treatment. The child should be examined by a doctor.

PRECAUTION

■ Nephritis may follow streptococcal impetigo or a strep throat, whether or not the strep infection has been treated with antibiotics.

MEDICAL TREATMENT

In a case of suspected nephritis, the doctor will examine the child thoroughly and measure the blood pressure. The doctor may take a throat culture to identify a strep infection and order urine and blood tests. If the child does have nephritis, the doctor will usually prescribe penicillin or erythromycin for ten days. The doctor will monitor the child's blood and urine until they are normal again. The child should stay in bed only during the acute phase of the disease.

In a severe case, the child may have to be hospitalized for observation and treatment of high blood pressure or convulsions. Medication may be continued for several months, throughout the recovery period and even afterward.

RELATED TOPICS: High blood pressure; Impetigo; Strep infections; Urinary tract infections

Nightmares

Some experts distinguish bad dreams from nightmares and night terrors. For all practical purposes, however, all three have the same cause and treatment; they differ only in degree. In a nightmare, the mind relives the fears and anxieties that were experienced during the waking hours. Occasionally, a nightmare may be the result of the usual stresses a child encounters in daily life. Frequent nightmares, however, are abnormal and indicate that there are unreasonable pressures on the child.

High fever and illness (for example, measles) have been known to induce nightmares. When this happens, the condition resembles delirium; it should not recur once the child is well again. If no illness is involved, a nightmare is easily identified.

SIGNS AND SYMPTOMS

A child experiencing a terrifying dream may wake up screaming, frightened, and wild-eyed. The child may be confused or frantically active for several minutes and may not immediately recall the details of the dream. Often the incident will be forgotten by the next morning. Nightmares may also cause the child to sleepwalk.

HOME CARE

Immediate treatment involves holding and hugging the distraught child and speaking calmly and soothingly. Do not try to rouse the child to full consciousness too quickly. Sleepwalkers must be protected from falls and other injuries.

The basic home treatment is to identify and relieve the stress that is causing the child to have nightmares. Some situations that commonly underlie such stress include the following: school problems (fear of failure, teacher-student conflicts); problems in relating with peers (playing with older children, being bullied, sexual experimentation); and family pressures (marital friction, alcoholism, physical or emotional abuse, divorce, hospitalization, death). Watching too much television—or the wrong type of program—can also cause enough anxiety to give a child nightmares.

PRECAUTIONS

■ Be aware of school, social, and family pressures that can cause a child to have nightmares.
■ Be sure you know how much television your child is watching and what kinds of programs.
■ Protect a sleepwalking child from injury.

MEDICAL TREATMENT

Your doctor will try to uncover the cause of your child's anxieties by getting the child to talk about his or her daily relationships and experiences. The doctor may ask for assistance from school personnel in identifying the reason for the child's nightmares.

Nosebleeds

Nosebleeds are as inevitable a part of childhood as scraped knees and bruised shins. Ninety-nine percent of nosebleeds are caused by the rupture of tiny blood vessels in the septum, the midline partition of the nose, which is located about one-quarter inch in from the nostrils. These small blood vessels are easily broken by a minor blow to the nose, and the scab that forms during healing is easily disturbed by rubbing or picking, which starts the bleeding again. This sequence of events may be further aggravated by having an allergic reaction or a head cold that causes the blood vessels in the nose to dilate; by breathing heated air, which dries out the nasal membranes; by sneezing, coughing, and blowing the nose; or by rubbing and scratching the nose, especially during sleep (most nosebleeds start at night).

SIGNS AND SYMPTOMS

Since the two sides of the nose are joined in back and also join with the throat and the esophagus (which lead to the stomach), blood may flow from both nostrils and from the mouth, and the child may also vomit blood.

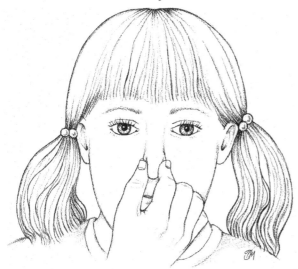

Teach your child to control a nosebleed by pinching the entire soft portion of the nose between thumb and forefinger for ten minutes.

HOME CARE

Teach your child at an early age how to stop a nosebleed. Tell the child to remain calm and to sit upright with the head held high; this will decrease the pressure in the blood vessels.

Show the child how to grasp the whole lower half of the nose between the thumb and fingers and in this way compress both sides of the nose firmly against the septum. The child should hold the nose this way for ten minutes to allow time for the blood to clot. If bleeding recurs when the pressure is released, it probably means that a large clot in the nose is preventing the broken blood vessel from sealing. The child should blow the nose vigorously to dislodge the clot and then, after the clot has been removed, compress the nose again for 10 to 12 minutes.

To prevent recurring nosebleeds, put petroleum jelly or an antibiotic cream in the child's nose morning and evening for 7 to 14 days. Use a vaporizer or humidifier to add moisture to the air at night. (Be sure to keep it meticulously clean, however. Otherwise, it can become a source of infection if microorganisms are allowed to grow in it.)

PRECAUTIONS

■ To stop a nosebleed, do not merely pinch nostrils together, but compress the entire soft portion of the nose. Otherwise, the blood will dam up and run down the throat.
■ Do not lay your child down. Remaining upright will decrease the pressure in the blood vessels.
■ Stay calm, and reassure your child.
■ It is not necessary to use cold compresses, pressure on the upper lip, nose drops, and other household remedies.
■ Do not pack the nose with cotton or gauze.

MEDICAL TREATMENT

Generally, you need to consult your doctor only when home treatment is not effective. If the nosebleed is due to an allergy or a cold, your doctor will treat that condition. Your doctor will rarely need to pack the nasal passages or cauterize (seal off) the blood vessels in order to control recurring nosebleeds.

RELATED TOPICS: Common cold; Hay fever and other nasal allergies

Pigeon toes

Toeing in (turning inward of the front part of the foot), particularly when standing and walking, is known as pigeon toes. After birth, the position and shape of the feet and legs reflect the position they were in during the baby's last weeks in the mother's womb. Usually by one year of age, the baby's toes are in normal position.

Throughout infancy and early childhood, however, the position of the feet and legs can be influenced by the manner in which they are held while the child is sitting and lying down. Habitually sleeping facedown with the toes directed inward encourages the development of pigeon toes.

Pigeon toes also may result from a malformation of the foot (adductovarus deformity), of the lower leg (tibial torsion), or of the thighbone (femoral torsion, or femoral anteversion). Depending on the severity of the malformation, the child's toes will point inward to a greater or lesser degree. A child who has a marked malformation will tend to trip over the feet until he or she learns to compensate for the condition.

SIGNS AND SYMPTOMS

The turning in of the front part of the foot is easy to see. If the condition persists beyond the age of one year, it should be brought to the doctor's attention.

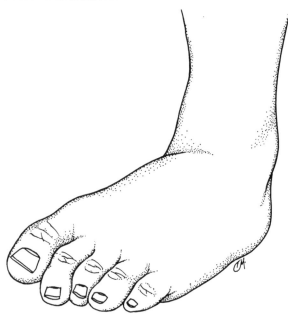

Pigeon toes may result from a malformation of the foot called an adductovarus deformity.

You can do a preliminary test for an adductovarus deformity of the foot by laying a straightedge along the outer border of the child's foot. If the outer border of the foot is not absolutely straight from the heel to the little toe, the child has adductovarus deformity.

As a preliminary home test to discern tibial torsion, place the infant or child on his or her back with the legs straight out, kneecaps pointed upward, and feet at right angles to the lower legs. If the toes point toward the midline instead of straight up, the child may have tibial torsion.

Your doctor will be able to detect whether your child has femoral torsion by manipulating the hips and thighs.

HOME CARE

By three months of age, your infant will prefer to sleep with the toes directed outward; this is normal and should be encouraged by placing the child's feet in this position as the child sleeps. When the child is old enough to sit upright, the feet should be straight or turned outward. Until 18 to 24 months of age, your toddler usually will walk with one or both feet turned outward; this is normal and gives the child a wider base and better balance. Toeing in after the age of one year should be called to your doctor's attention.

PRECAUTIONS

■ An uncorrected adductovarus deformity makes it very difficult to fit a child's shoes properly and may cause the development of a skewed foot and bunions in adolescence or adulthood.
■ A child who sits on the floor a lot should be taught to sit cross-legged, not on the haunches.
■ Corrective orthopedic shoes should be prescribed only by a medical professional, never by a shoe salesperson.
■ Most minor cases of pigeon toes correct themselves. Nevertheless, let a doctor judge if the condition is minor.

MEDICAL TREATMENT

Your doctor will observe the child while he or she stands and walks, both with and without shoes. The feet, the upper and lower parts of the legs, and the rotation of the hips will be examined. In the case of femoral torsion, the doctor may not start treatment until your child is a teenager; if the condition has not corrected itself by that time, surgery on the thighbones may be necessary.

Pinworms

The pinworm, a distant cousin of the earthworm, lives only in humans and apes. The adult pinworm is one-quarter to one-half inch in length, white in color, and about as thick as sewing thread. It lives in the large intestine and, moving with a caterpillarlike motion, comes out at night to lay microscopic eggs on the skin around the anus (the opening from the intestines to the outside of the body). The eggs are transmitted from the anus to the mouth on the child's hands, on toys, or in food that the child has touched. The child then swallows the eggs. The eggs hatch into larvae (the immature form of the pinworm). Two to six weeks later, the larvae have developed into mature, egg-laying adult pinworms, and the cycle continues. Pinworms can be transmitted to other children and to adults in the same manner.

SIGNS AND SYMPTOMS

A child with pinworms has few symptoms. The child may complain at night of itching or burning around the anal or genital area. Pinworms can also be a cause of a sudden onset of bedwetting. If the infestation is heavy, the child may have abdominal cramps. Pinworms can cause appendicitis (although this is rare), and they can work their way into a girl's vagina and urethra (the passageway from the bladder to the outside), causing inflammation.

The diagnosis of pinworms is usually made easily by examining the skin around the anus at night while the child sleeps or just after the child awakens. Pinworms head back into the anus if disturbed by light, so the search must be done quickly. A pinworm can be mistaken for lint on the skin; if the "lint" moves, it is a pinworm. Pinworms may occasionally be found in a bowel movement, but this is not a reliable way of making a diagnosis.

Another way to diagnose pinworms is the "Scotch Tape test." Place a loop of tape over the child's anus just before he or she goes to bed. If the child has pinworms, they will stick to the tape during their nocturnal travels.

HOME CARE

Vermifuges (worm medicines) are available both over the counter and by prescription. When one member of a family has pinworms, some doctors believe all members should be treated at the same time (the only exceptions are infants and pregnant women, for whom the physician must make special arrangements). Other doctors don't treat unaffected family members unless many family members are affected.

PRECAUTIONS

■ If there are symptoms of recurrent inflammation of the vagina or bladder (such as burning on urination or lower abdominal pain), suspect that pinworms may be the cause.
■ If one member of a family has pinworms, launder that person's underclothes, bed linens, and towels to destroy the worms' eggs. Also, cut and scrub his or her fingernails to remove any eggs.
■ Do not mistake lint or thread for pinworms; look for movement.
■ Do not blame household cats and dogs if your child has pinworms. These worms live only in humans and apes.

MEDICAL TREATMENT

Your doctor will investigate for pinworms using clear tape that will pick up any eggs that are on the skin. The tape is then examined under the microscope. If pinworms are found, the doctor will prescribe or recommend worm medication.

RELATED TOPICS: Appendicitis; Bedwetting; Stomachache, chronic; Urinary tract infections; Vaginal discharge

Pityriasis rosea

Pityriasis rosea is a common, harmless, long-lasting disease that goes unrecognized by most parents. It affects children and young adults most often, but it may occur at any age. The disease is probably caused by a virus, but the specific organism has not been identified. Pityriasis rosea is mildly contagious, but isolation is not considered necessary. One attack gives lifelong immunity.

SIGNS AND SYMPTOMS

In most cases of pityriasis rosea, the first sign is a single patch, called the herald patch, on the skin of the trunk or extremities. The patch is round or oval, the size of a nickel or a quarter, salmon-colored (pink or reddish), and slightly crinkled in the center; the edges are slightly scaly. The patch is not tender, but it may itch. It is occasionally accompanied by headache, lethargy, pain in the joints, and a sore throat. Five to 14 days after the appearance of the herald patch, spots break out on the body; each is similar in appearance to the original patch, but smaller. The rash generally does not affect the face, forearms, and lower legs of an older child, but in a younger child these areas may also be involved. The rash lasts for three to eight weeks, during which time the child feels fine.

The diagnosis is based on the characteristic appearance of the rash, which includes both round and oval spots.

HOME CARE

No treatment is necessary. Itching, if present, can be relieved by giving the child a nonprescription antihistamine by mouth. Bathing with a mild soap and exposure to sunlight apparently shorten the duration of the rash.

PRECAUTIONS

■ The appearance of the herald patch may suggest ringworm, eczema, or impetigo. If the patch does not respond to treatment for any of these conditions, it may be the first sign of pityriasis.
■ The condition may last for up to eight weeks but is harmless.

MEDICAL TREATMENT

No medical treatment is required.

RELATED TOPICS: Eczema; Impetigo; Rashes; Ringworm

Pneumonia

Pneumonia is an infection of one or more areas of the lungs. It is usually caused by bacteria or viruses, although there are other causes, such as fungi and parasites. The most common bacterial cause is the pneumococcus bacterium; less common causes are streptococcus and staphylococcus bacteria. Pneumonia may also be caused by mycoplasma organisms. Viral causes include the influenza and parainfluenza viruses, the respiratory syncytial virus, and adenoviruses.

To contract bacterial pneumonia, the child must be exposed to it at a time when he or she is particularly susceptible. Pneumococcus,

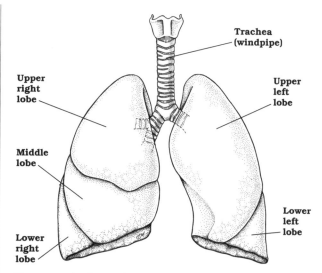

Pneumonia is an infection of one or more areas of the lungs.

streptococcus, and staphylococcus bacteria frequently are present in the nose and throat of a healthy child. Before these organisms can invade the lungs, however, the child's resistance must have been lowered by a cold or some other upper respiratory tract infection. Therefore, bacterial pneumonia is not considered contagious in the usual sense.

The types of pneumonia that are caused by viruses are known as "walking pneumonias" and are contagious. The incubation period (the time it takes for the symptoms to develop after the child has been exposed to the disease) for most types of viral pneumonia is two to five days.

SIGNS AND SYMPTOMS

The symptoms of bacterial pneumonia include a mild upper respiratory tract infection; the sudden onset of high fever, chills, cough, and rapid breathing; and sometimes pain on one or both sides of the chest. In infants, the respiratory distress may cause flaring of the nostrils, retractions (pulling in) of the soft spaces of the chest, and grunting sounds when the child breathes out.

The onset of viral pneumonia is gradual, accompanied by headache, fatigue, fever of variable degree (100°F–105°F), a sore throat, and a severe, dry cough.

HOME CARE

Many cases of viral pneumonia are mild and are not recognized as pneumonia at all. You may assume that the child has a cold and give cold remedies. The pneumonia then clears up on its own after 10 to 14 days.

If signs of respiratory distress are present, the child should be seen by a doctor.

PRECAUTIONS

■ Sudden worsening of a cold accompanied by high fever, cough, chills, chest pain, or rapid breathing suggests pneumonia.

■ In infants, flaring of the nostrils, pulling in of the chest, and grunting sounds when breathing out are serious symptoms and require **immediate medical care**.

■ In children, sputum (coughed-up discharge) tinged with blood may or may not be a sign of serious illness, but it indicates the need for a doctor's attention.

MEDICAL TREATMENT

Diagnosis depends on careful examination of the chest, X-ray studies, blood tests, and sometimes cultures of the blood and the sputum.

In the past, a child with pneumonia was always hospitalized; nowadays, only the youngest and the most severely ill are hospitalized. Most cases of bacterial pneumonia respond to antibiotics. A patient with pneumococcal pneumonia will generally recover rapidly once antibiotic therapy is begun. However, a patient with a streptococcal or staphylococcal infection may require in-hospital administration of antibiotics. Mycoplasma pneumonia responds to some antibiotics, but viral pneumonia does not. For viral pneumonia, your doctor will recommend rest, plenty of fluids, and patience while the condition runs its course.

RELATED TOPICS: Chest pain; Common cold; Coughs; Fever; G6PD deficiency; Sore throat

Poisoning

Young children, because of their curiosity and their inexperience, are constantly at risk for poisoning. Knowing what to do (and what not to do) in an emergency can save your child's life.

In a large enough quantity, any substance (even water) can be poisonous, but some substances are more apt to be swallowed in harmful amounts than others. In the United States, common causes of poisoning of children include soaps, detergents, cleaning products,

bleaches, vitamins, iron tonics, insecticides, plants, polishes and waxes, tranquilizers, hormones, and other prescription and over-the-counter medications (including aspirin and aspirin substitutes). Other common poisons include boric acid, oil of wintergreen, volatile hydrocarbons (gasoline, kerosene, turpentine, naphtha, cleaning fluids), strong acids, and alkalis (such as drain and oven cleaners). See page 331 for a list of poisonous substances commonly found in the home.

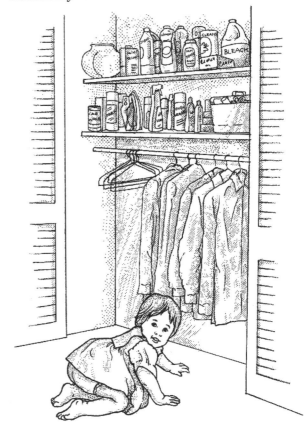

Prevent poisoning by keeping all poisonous substances out of the reach of children.

The first step in preventing poisoning is to keep all medications, cleaning substances, paints, and other hazardous substances in places where your child cannot get to them. Many poison control centers provide information on childproofing your house; some will send packets of "Mr. Yuk" stickers for labeling poisonous materials, so that your child can learn to identify and avoid these dangerous substances.

Another important way to be prepared for poisoning emergencies is to stock your medicine chest with syrup of ipecac. Syrup of ipecac is an emetic (a substance that makes one vomit). Periodically check the expiration date on the bottle to be certain of effectiveness. Some physicians also recommend that you keep activated charcoal (a special liquid form of charcoal) on hand. Activated charcoal works by being extremely absorbent—when swallowed, it will absorb a wide variety of substances from the stomach and prevent them from entering the bloodstream. Both syrup of ipecac and activated charcoal can be obtained without a prescription from any drugstore.

It is a good idea to contact your local poison control center **before** an emergency arises. Confirm the phone number and find out if the center is staffed with poison control specialists 24 hours a day. If not, try to find a facility that is, and keep the phone number handy.

SIGNS AND SYMPTOMS

It is often apparent when a child has taken a poison. The child may tell you, or you may see an empty bottle lying around. If your child is behaving strangely, suspect poisoning. The telltale signs of aspirin overdose are rapid breathing, ringing in the ears, nausea, overexcitement, and eventually unconsciousness. If your child consumes an acid or alkaline substance, there will usually be burns on the mouth and tongue. Many liquids have a distinctive odor that may be a tip-off. An overdose of an iron tonic produces abdominal pain and severe vomiting, often with blood in the vomited material, followed by collapse.

Not all poisons leave telltale signs, however. If you have any suspicion at all that your child has been poisoned, call the poison control center immediately. Do not wait for the appearance of definite symptoms.

HOME CARE

The first step in treating poisoning is to get the remaining poison away from your child. If there is any poison left in the child's mouth, try to get him or her to spit it out. Try to ascertain exactly what and how much the child consumed and when the poisoning occurred.

Immediately call your local poison control center—before you call your doctor, the hospital, or anyone else. Be prepared to tell them what your child ate or drank, how much, and when; your child's age and weight; whether the child has vomited or lost consciousness; and whether you have syrup of ipecac available. They can then tell you what to do next.

Treatment differs for different types of poisons. What is right for one poison may be wrong for another. Follow their instructions exactly.

Make every attempt to contact a poison control center, hospital, or doctor. If professional help is unavailable, however, follow these general guidelines before taking your child to the nearest emergency room:

Do not attempt any treatment if your child is unconscious or very woozy or is having a convulsion. Concentrate your efforts on getting the child to a medical facility.

Most poisons should be expelled from a child's stomach (by vomiting) as soon as possible; however, others are better left in the stomach temporarily because they will do additional damage as they come back up through the esophagus and the throat. As a general rule, if your child has taken a normally edible substance (such as a medication), induce vomiting with syrup of ipecac, but if the child has taken an acid or alkaline substance or any substance that is not normally edible (for example, gasoline, drain cleaner, or furniture polish), do not induce vomiting—just get the child to a hospital immediately. Read the label on the bottle or container of the substance that your child ingested; many product labels tell you if you should try to induce vomiting. Check the table on page 331 for a list of substances for which you should not induce vomiting.

Syrup of ipecac is the best medicine for inducing vomiting. For children under one year of age, give one to two teaspoonfuls of syrup of ipecac; for children over one year of age, give three teaspoonfuls. Follow the dose immediately with one or two glasses of water, and then leave for the nearest medical facility. Do not expect immediate results; it takes five to ten minutes for ipecac to work. If you get no results, give your child more water. Do not give your child milk; it may lessen the effectiveness of the ipecac and make it more difficult to see what is in the vomitus (the material thrown up). Do not use syrup of ipecac and activated charcoal together; the charcoal will absorb the ipecac before it can work. If there are no results in 20 to 30 minutes, repeat the ipecac dose (only if the child is over a year old). Once begun, vomiting may continue for 20 to 30 minutes.

Even if you think that the danger has passed—your child seems to have vomited all of the poison and to be feeling all right—take the child to a medical facility as soon as you can. (Bring a sample of the poison and the vomitus, if available.) Effects of poisons are not always immediately apparent, and delayed reactions are possible.

If your child inhales a poison (for example, carbon monoxide from car exhaust fumes or from a blocked chimney), immediately remove the child from the vicinity of the fumes to fresh air, and then contact the fire department or the emergency room of your local hospital.

PRECAUTIONS

■ Keep the telephone numbers of police and fire departments, your doctor, and the local poison control center near the telephone.
■ Always have syrup of ipecac in the house. Check the expiration date periodically to be certain of effectiveness.
■ Never induce vomiting in a child who is not fully conscious.
■ Be aware that treatment for poisoning depends on the substance taken, and that in the case of some poisons vomiting can worsen the child's condition.
■ The most important precaution is prevention. See that all poisonous substances are stored out of the reach of children, under lock and key if necessary.
■ Put safety locks on all cupboards that contain poisonous substances.
■ Never store a dangerous substance in anything but its original container.
■ Do not keep drugs in unlabeled bottles.
■ Insist on child-resistant caps on all bottles that contain poisonous substances. (However, don't be casual about storage of substances in containers with such caps. Remember that "child resistant" means only that *most* children cannot manage to open it.)
■ Many drugs and vitamin and mineral supplements look and taste like candy. Teach your child that medicine isn't candy, and don't present medicine or vitamins as a treat.
■ Be aware that more children are fatally poisoned by adult aspirin than by children's flavored aspirin.
■ Be careful with iron tablets. They taste sweet, look like candy, and can be deadly.
■ When visiting other people's homes, do not let your children explore until you are sure that there are no poisons within reach.
■ When guests visit you, be certain that their medications are out of reach of children.

COMMON HOUSE-HOLD POISONS			DO NOT INDUCE VOMITING IF YOUR CHILD HAS SWALLOWED:
Adhesives (such as glue and paste)	Fertilizers	Oven cleaner	Acids
Aftershave	Floor wax	Paint	Ammonia
Alcoholic beverages	Fungicides	Paint thinner	Benzene
Ammonia	Furniture polish	Perfume	Bleach
Antifreeze	Gasoline	Pet medications	Carbon tetrachloride
Art materials	Grease remover	Petroleum distillates	Cleaning fluid
Aspirin and acetaminophen	Hair-care products	Plant sprays	Correction fluid
Auto wax	Herbicides	Rodenticides (mouse and rat poisons)	Dishwasher detergent
Baby powder	Houseplants (some)	Room deodorizers	Drain cleaner
Batteries (including "button" batteries)	Ink	Rubbing alcohol	Furniture polish
Benzene	Insecticides and pest strips	Rust remover	Gasoline
Bleach	Insect repellent	Scabicides	Glue
Boric acid	Iodine	Shampoo	Insect spray
Carbon tetrachloride	Kerosene	Shoe polish	Kerosene
Charcoal lighting fluid	Laundry products	Soaps	Lye
Cleaning products	Laxatives	Solvents	Oven cleaner
Correction fluid	Lighter fluid	Swimming pool and aquarium chemicals	Paint thinner
Cosmetics	Lye	Tobacco	Petroleum distillates
Deodorants	Medications of any kind	Toilet bowl cleaner	Polishes
Dishwasher detergent	Moth repellents	Turpentine	Solvents
Disinfectants	Motor oil	Vitamin and mineral supplements	Tobacco products
Drain cleaners	Mouthwash	Weed killer	Turpentine
	Nail polish	Windshield washer solution	
	Nail polish remover		
	Naphtha		
	Oil of wintergreen		

MEDICAL TREATMENT

If the syrup of ipecac doesn't work, your child may need to have his or her stomach pumped. A flexible plastic tube will be inserted up into the nose and down into the stomach. Although the insertion is uncomfortable, it is necessary to allow the doctor to clean out the child's stomach. Further treatment varies with the substance taken and your child's condition.

Poison ivy

Rashes among children in the 2- to 12-year-old age group are generally due to contact with irritants, one of the most common of which is poison ivy. Contact with certain other plants, such as poison oak and poison sumac, can also cause a rash.

Poison ivy rash develops in sensitive children after direct contact with any part of the vine. It can also occur after the child has been exposed to smoke from the burning plant or to pets that have rolled in the plant. Poison ivy rash can be spread to any part of the body by the hands, the fingernails, and contaminated clothing and shoes; it is not spread by the fluid on the blisters. Poison ivy is often carried to a boy's penis by his hands.

SIGNS AND SYMPTOMS

Itching develops within 2 to 24 hours after contact with poison ivy. It is followed by swelling and reddening of the skin. Pin-sized, clear blisters develop and may merge to create blisters as large as one-half inch across. The rash often appears in straight lines where the plant has brushed against the skin or where the child has scratched. The rash may also be distributed generally over the skin and look like rashes caused by other agents.

HOME CARE

Bathe the child promptly with soap and water, and cut and scrub the child's fingernails; this will remove much of the irritating substance from the skin and hands. To relieve itching, apply calamine lotion to the rash or give the child nonprescription antihistamines. Launder contaminated clothing to remove the irritant.

PRECAUTIONS

■ Scratching can make the skin susceptible to impetigo. Watch for signs of infection.

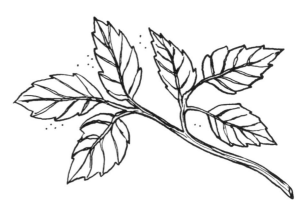

Poison ivy has three leaflets on each stem.

■ If poison ivy continues to spread after four to seven days, your child is still coming in contact with the plant, directly or indirectly. Try to find the source.
■ Teach your child to recognize and avoid poison ivy.
■ Make sure your child is dressed appropriately (in long pants and socks) when in the woods or around campsites.

MEDICAL TREATMENT

Your doctor will confirm the diagnosis, treat any secondary infection, and perhaps prescribe a steroid medication if the rash is severe. Desensitization shots are not very effective; preparations taken by mouth are even less helpful.

RELATED TOPICS: Impetigo; Rashes

Polio

Polio (also known as poliomyelitis and infantile paralysis) is an infection of the spinal cord by one of three related types of viruses. Recovery from attack by one type confers lifelong immunity against that type only. Therefore, it is possible to have three separate attacks of the disease.

The polio virus is found in the saliva and the stool of an infected person. It is transmitted by direct contact or through contact with something that has been contaminated by the virus carried in an infected stool (for example, food, toys, or the water in a swimming pool). The incubation period (the time it takes for the symptoms to appear after exposure to the virus) for polio is 3 to 14 days.

SIGNS AND SYMPTOMS

Of those children who are infected by one of the three types of polio viruses, 90 to 95 percent will have no symptoms but will develop immunity to that type. Four to five percent of those infected will experience a minor illness, with fever, general bodily discomfort, sore throat, and nausea for three to four days. One to two percent will have clinically recognizable polio, with symptoms of a minor illness plus sore, stiff muscles and a stiff neck and spine. Within this one to two percent are the children who may become paralyzed or die.

Minor cases may never be recognized as polio unless they occur as part of an epidemic. Diagnosis is based on examination of viral cultures and studies of antibodies (substances that the body produces to fight disease) in the blood. If the central nervous system (the spinal cord and the brain) is involved, the child will have a stiff neck and back and may not be able to sit up without supporting the trunk with both hands braced behind in a tripod fashion. The diagnosis is confirmed by the results of a spinal tap (in which spinal fluid is withdrawn from the spinal column), cultures, or antibody studies.

HOME CARE

Prevention through immunization is of the utmost importance. The live-virus (Sabin) vaccine, which is given by mouth, is effective against all three types of polio, and it confers long-lasting immunity. The risk of paralysis from present-day vaccines is less than one in ten million—a far cry from the one in a thousand risk of exposure to naturally occurring viruses. There is an injectable polio vaccine, the Salk vaccine. It is not used often, although it may be appropriate in certain situations.

PRECAUTIONS

■ An infant is temporarily immune to each of the three types of polio for four to six months after birth only if the mother is immune (because she has had the disease or been vaccinated against it). The child needs a full series of vaccinations by mouth to achieve long-lasting immunity.
■ Anyone who has received injections of the original, inactivated (Salk) vaccine must have boosters or a full series of the Sabin vaccine to guarantee immunity.

■ Polio virus still exists in this country, and polio is epidemic in many other countries of the world. Since it is not possible to avoid exposure to the disease, immunization is essential.

MEDICAL TREATMENT

Your doctor's diagnosis will be made on the basis of a physical examination and the results of a spinal tap. A child with a suspected or known case of polio will be isolated. A child who has not been immunized and has been exposed to the disease will be given gamma globulin to prevent or lessen the severity of the disease. A child who has contracted polio will be given aspirin, acetaminophen, or another painkiller and hot packs to reduce the pain. If polio causes paralysis, the child may need artificial respiration, a tracheotomy (the surgical creation of an opening into the windpipe through the neck), prolonged physical therapy, braces, or orthopedic surgery.

RELATED TOPICS: Immunizations; Viral infections

Puncture wounds

Wounds that pierce the skin are classified as abrasions (scrapes), lacerations (cuts), or punctures. A puncture is a wound that is deeper than it is long or wide. Most puncture wounds in children are made by nails, needles, pins, knives, or splinters.

Because of their small opening and their depth, puncture wounds are hard to clean and therefore are especially susceptible to infection. A puncture wound is an ideal site for tetanus to develop because the bacterium that causes tetanus thrives in the absence of air. Puncture wounds may also harbor foreign bodies that are difficult to detect.

SIGNS AND SYMPTOMS

The presence of a puncture wound usually is obvious. The important aspects of the diagnosis involve determining whether the puncture has penetrated into a deeper structure (such as a joint, the abdominal cavity, the chest cavity, the skull, or a tendon), whether it contains a foreign body (for example, a broken needle, a wood or glass splinter, or a shred of clothing), and whether it is infected.

HOME CARE

Wash the skin surrounding the puncture with soap and water and apply a nonirritating, non-stinging antiseptic, such as solution (not tincture) of Merthiolate antiseptic. Be sure your child has been immunized against tetanus within the last five years. Make sure that the object that made the wound is intact and has not broken off at the tip. Inspect and feel the wound to determine if a foreign body can be detected under the skin. If no foreign body is present, cover the wound with a sterile bandage and inspect it twice a day for signs of infection (redness, discharge, swelling, increasing pain, and tenderness). Soak the wound frequently in warm water to help keep it clean. If there is a foreign body in the wound, take the child to a doctor.

PRECAUTIONS

■ Puncture wounds in the head, neck, abdomen, or chest can be very serious. Take your child to a doctor **immediately**.
■ Punctures of a joint may cause infectious arthritis within hours. The knee joint is particularly susceptible. A puncture near a joint, especially the knee, should be seen by a doctor. Any signs of infectious arthritis (redness, swelling, increasing pain, inability to move the joint through its full range of normal motion) should be considered a **medical emergency**.
■ Do not remove an object from a puncture wound—not even if it is a knife blade, a nail, a splinter of wood or glass, or a needle. Let your doctor remove it. You might cause further damage if you try to remove the object yourself.
■ If a puncture wound remains tender for more than one or two days, it should be seen by your doctor.

MEDICAL TREATMENT

A puncture wound cannot be cleaned completely, even by a doctor. Your doctor will try to determine if any foreign bodies are present by feeling the wound or by X-ray examination. If there is anything in the wound, your doctor may want it to be removed surgically or may wait and observe the wound for a while, perhaps instructing you to soak it in Epsom-salts solution for five to ten minutes four times a day. Antibiotics will be prescribed if the wound is infected, and a tetanus toxoid injection will be given if the child's immunization status is not current. If a wound has penetrated a joint,

the abdomen, the chest, the skull, or a tendon, your doctor will hospitalize the child and explore the wound surgically.

RELATED TOPICS: Arthritis; Cuts; Immunizations; Scrapes; Tetanus

Rashes

A rash is a skin eruption that appears as red patches, blisters, or spots. It is often accompanied by itching. A rash can affect a limited area or be widespread over extensive areas of the body.

A rash can be caused by exposure to the sun, heat, cold, chemicals in household products, or certain fabrics, such as wool. Certain foods (for example, strawberries) also produce rashes in people who are allergic to them.

A rash can also appear as a characteristic symptom of a disease. For example, distinctive rashes appear as symptoms of many infectious diseases, such as measles, rubella (German measles), chicken pox, and shingles. Certain sexually transmitted diseases, such as herpes and syphilis, also display distinctive rashes.

A rash generally disappears when its underlying cause disappears or is successfully treated.

SIGNS AND SYMPTOMS

The rash itself is obvious, but the cause may not be so easily identified. A rash caused by a disease will be accompanied by other symptoms (such as fever or swollen lymph glands).

HOME CARE

You need not be too concerned about a rash that appears and then disappears within a couple of days and does not recur. If the rash causes itching, you can apply a soothing lotion like calamine or have the child take a warm bath.

A rash that recurs may indicate an allergy. If you cannot immediately identify the allergy-causing substance (a certain food, for instance), have the child examined by a doctor. You can avoid the allergy-causing substance in the future only if you know what it is. If the child has a rash accompanied by other symptoms, consult the doctor.

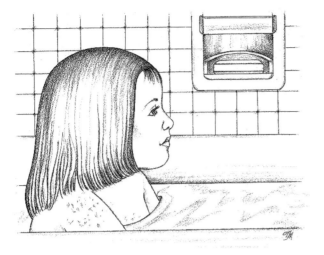

If a rash causes itching, it may help to have the child sit in a warm bath.

PRECAUTIONS

■ A rash that lasts for more than a few days and has no identifiable cause should be seen by a doctor.
■ Certain types of rashes are warning signs of specific infectious or sexually transmitted diseases.

MEDICAL TREATMENT

The doctor may prescribe a soothing lotion for minor itching caused by a rash. If an allergy is suspected, the doctor will try to identify the causative substance. If a disease is most likely the cause, the doctor will diagnose and treat it.

RELATED TOPICS: Chicken pox; Diaper rash; Eczema; Fifth disease; Food allergies; Hand, foot, and mouth disease; Heat rash; Herpes simplex; Hives; Impetigo; Measles; Molluscum contagiosum; Pityriasis rosea; Poison ivy; Ringworm; Rocky Mountain spotted fever; Roseola; Rubella; Shingles

Reye's syndrome

Reye's syndrome is a relatively rare but very serious noncontagious disease. Although it affects all organs and muscles of the body, it does the most damage to the brain and the liver, causing the brain to swell and fatty deposits to collect in the liver.

Reye's syndrome usually strikes children and teenagers who are recovering from a viral infection, most commonly influenza or chicken pox.

Children between the ages of 5 and 11 are at highest risk. Most of the reported cases occur from December through March.

It is not known precisely what causes Reye's syndrome. Some researchers think that, since it almost always follows a viral infection, Reye's syndrome may be caused by a virus, and that the virus, in conjunction with some other unknown substance, produces a toxin (poison) that damages the body. Recent research suggests that the swelling of the brain that accompanies Reye's syndrome may be caused by a defect in the body's metabolism that prevents substances harmful to the brain from being flushed out.

There is also evidence of a link between Reye's syndrome and the use of aspirin in treating the viral infections that generally precede its onset. Although it has not been proved that aspirin causes or promotes Reye's syndrome, doctors now caution against giving aspirin to children with viral infections, especially influenza and chicken pox.

If Reye's syndrome isn't diagnosed and treated early, it can cause permanent brain damage, coma, or death. About 25 percent of cases of Reye's syndrome are fatal.

SIGNS AND SYMPTOMS

Suspect Reye's syndrome if a child who has been recovering from a viral infection suddenly starts vomiting severely and becomes unusually drowsy, overactive, or confused. As the disease progresses, it can cause convulsions and unconsciousness.

HOME CARE

If you suspect that your child has Reye's syndrome, **consult a doctor immediately**. Do not attempt home treatment.

PRECAUTIONS

■ **Do not** give aspirin to a child with a viral infection, particularly chicken pox or influenza. Instead, sponge baths and aspirin substitutes such as acetaminophen can be used to treat fever and other symptoms. Aspirin substitutes have not been linked to Reye's syndrome.
■ Reye's syndrome is fatal in 25 percent of all cases. Early diagnosis and treatment are essential to the child's recovery.

MEDICAL TREATMENT

If the doctor suspects that your child may have Reye's syndrome, tests will be ordered to confirm the diagnosis. Blood tests may reveal abnormalities that suggest liver damage. Younger children may have a very low blood sugar level. A spinal tap may be done to rule out other diseases.

There is no known cure for Reye's syndrome, and treatment consists of supportive therapy to help the child withstand the disease until it runs its course. The child is usually hospitalized. As a rule, a child who survives for three or four days will recover completely.

RELATED TOPICS: Chicken pox; Convulsions without fever; Encephalitis; Fever; Influenza; Viral infections

Ringworm

Ringworm is a skin infection caused by a fungus, not a worm. Ringworm spreads by direct contact with an infected person or pet animal or by contact with contaminated objects, such as combs, pillows, towels, clothing, and even the floor.

SIGNS AND SYMPTOMS

Different fungi prefer different areas of the body. Ringworm of the scalp (*tinea capitis*) appears as scaly patches with stubs of broken-off hairs. Ringworm of the body (*tinea corporis*) shows up as round or oval, scaly, red patches that enlarge as healing proceeds from the center. Ringworm of the groin (*tinea cruris*), also known as jock itch, is characterized by a scaly, red or brown rash on the crotch and the genital area, with a sharply defined margin of spread. Ringworm of the feet (athlete's foot, or *tinea pedis*) sometimes affects the ankles and legs as well.

HOME CARE

Antifungal ointments (such as haloprogin, clotrimazole, tolnaftate, undecylenic acid, and Whitfield's ointments) can be applied to the infected area until the skin clears.

PRECAUTIONS

■ Several other common rashes resemble ringworm. If a rash does not improve after several days of home treatment, see your doctor.
■ The preparations used to treat ringworm may cause another rash on sensitive skin. If the rash worsens or changes in any way, stop home treatment and see your doctor.

MEDICAL TREATMENT

Your doctor can confirm a home diagnosis of ringworm by examining the rash under ultraviolet light and by culturing a skin scraping and examining the results under a microscope. The doctor may prescribe either an antifungal ointment to be applied to the skin or a medication, such as griseofulvin fungicide, for the child to take by mouth.

RELATED TOPICS: Athlete's foot; Pityriasis rosea; Rashes

Rocky Mountain spotted fever

Rocky Mountain spotted fever is a noncontagious disease transmitted by the bite of a wood tick, rabbit tick, or dog tick. The name of the disease is misleading; it occurs in all states and is just as common in eastern and midwestern states as in the Rocky Mountain states.

The disease is caused by a microorganism called a rickettsia, which is midway between a virus and a bacterium. The incubation period (the time it takes for the symptoms to develop once the child is exposed to the rickettsia) is two to eight days. Rocky Mountain spotted fever was fatal in as many as 40 percent of cases before the availability of antibiotics, but the mortality rate has decreased considerably since then.

SIGNS AND SYMPTOMS

Rocky Mountain spotted fever starts with vague symptoms of headache, fever, and loss of appetite. One to five days later, a rash appears on the ankles and wrists and spreads rapidly to involve the entire body. The pale, rose-colored, flat or slightly raised spots often become reddish-purple. As the disease progresses, the fever worsens and severe muscle pain develops.

The disease can be suspected if a rash and other symptoms follow a tick bite. The diagnosis cannot be confirmed, however, until the second week of the illness; a blood test at that time should show an increase in the number of antibodies (substances produced by the body in response to invasion) against the causative rickettsia. Usually, the illness lasts about two to three weeks.

HOME CARE

There is no home treatment. All you can do is watch carefully for symptoms of Rocky Mountain spotted fever in a child who has been bitten by ticks. If symptoms appear, take the child to the doctor at once.

PRECAUTIONS

■ If your dog has ticks, remove the ticks cautiously with tweezers, not with your fingers. A crushed tick can contaminate a scratch in the skin and transmit the microorganism that causes Rocky Mountain spotted fever.
■ Use tick repellents on pets.
■ Do not allow your child to handle wild rabbits.
■ If your child has been bitten by a tick, observe the child carefully for a week afterward.

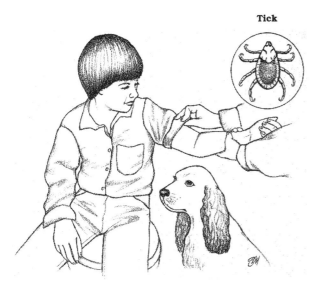

Tick

Children who are exposed to ticks should be checked carefully for signs of tick bites and symptoms of Rocky Mountain spotted fever.

MEDICAL TREATMENT

If there is a strong reason to suspect that your child has Rocky Mountain spotted fever, the doctor may start antibiotic therapy even before the diagnosis is confirmed. Tetracycline and chloramphenicol are the medicines used for initial treatment. The doctor may recommend that a child with Rocky Mountain spotted fever be hospitalized for up to ten days.

RELATED TOPICS: Insect bites and stings; Rashes

Roseola

Roseola is an infectious disease of sudden onset, which is characterized by a high fever followed by a rash. It is thought to be caused by a virus, although the causative organism has not yet been identified. Roseola occurs almost exclusively in children between the ages of six months and three years. The incubation period (the time it takes for symptoms to develop once a child has been exposed to the virus) is 7 to 17 days. One attack of roseola provides lifelong immunity.

SIGNS AND SYMPTOMS

Roseola begins suddenly with a fever of 104°F to 106°F. It is one of the more common causes of convulsions with fever, which occur at the onset of the disease. It rarely produces any other symptoms, although sometimes roseola can cause a runny nose, mild redness of the throat, and minimal enlargement of the lymph nodes in the neck. Generally, the fever persists for three or four days and cannot be kept down consistently. Meanwhile, the child appears to be less ill than the degree of fever suggests. The fever disappears abruptly; at the same time, a splotchy, red rash appears on the trunk and spreads to the arms and neck. Roseola is difficult to identify until the fever drops and the rash appears.

The rash disappears in one or two days, and the child is well again. Complications are rare.

HOME CARE

Give acetaminophen and lukewarm baths to help control the fever.

PRECAUTIONS

■ Another common illness that produces a high fever but few other symptoms is infection of the urinary tract, especially in girls.
■ Coughing, vomiting, diarrhea, discharge from the eyes or ears, and extreme fatigue or collapse are not associated with roseola. If these symptoms occur, consult a doctor.

MEDICAL TREATMENT

The doctor will conduct a careful physical examination and may order blood or urine tests to rule out other illnesses that cause a high fever. Usually, however, a few days' observation will confirm the diagnosis of roseola.

RELATED TOPICS: Convulsions with fever; Fever; Rashes; Urinary tract infections

Rubella

Rubella, or German measles, is one of the mildest contagious diseases of childhood. However, it can damage the fetus of a pregnant woman who contracts the disease. Women who contract rubella during the first three months of pregnancy have a 50-50 chance of bearing an infant who has cataracts, a cleft palate, or heart problems or who is permanently deaf or mentally retarded.

Rubella is caused by a specific virus and can be transmitted by direct contact with an infected person or by contact with articles contaminated by urine, stool, or nasal or throat secretions from an infected person. The incubation period (the time it takes for symptoms to develop once a person has been exposed to a disease) is 14 to 21 days.

One attack of rubella usually confers lifelong immunity, but reinfection is possible. For that reason, pregnant women and women who are planning to become pregnant should not assume that they are immune to rubella simply because they have had it in the past.

SIGNS AND SYMPTOMS

The characteristic first sign of rubella is swollen, tender lymph nodes in front of and behind the ears, at the base of the skull, and on the sides of the neck. In a day or two, a fine or splotchy dark-pink rash appears on the face. The rash then spreads over the rest of the body within 24 hours. The rash usually lasts about three days and may be accompanied by a low-grade fever (100°F to 101°F), slight reddening of the throat and the whites of the eyes, and slight loss of appetite.

The patient is contagious during the period from seven days before the onset of the illness until four or five days after the appearance of the rash. Infants born with rubella may be contagious for as long as 18 months after birth.

No other disease causes both a rash and tenderness and enlargement of the particular lymph nodes involved in rubella. Your doctor can confirm the diagnosis by identifying the virus on cultures of throat secretions, blood, or urine or by finding an increased level of anti-

bodies (protective substances that the body produces to fight infection) against rubella in the blood.

HOME CARE

Give acetaminophen to reduce fever or discomfort. Do not let your child come in contact with pregnant women.

PRECAUTIONS

■ Before becoming pregnant, a woman either should be immunized against rubella or should receive a blood test to find out if she is immune to the disease. If she is not immune, she should be immunized at least three months before trying to become pregnant.
■ All children should be immunized against rubella.
■ A pregnant woman who has been exposed to rubella should consult her doctor immediately.

MEDICAL TREATMENT

Because rubella is so mild, doctors generally do not need to treat it in children. Relief of symptoms is all that is necessary. However, the doctor will establish the diagnosis by means of a physical examination and laboratory tests.

RELATED TOPICS: Glands, swollen; Immunizations; Rashes

Scabies

Scabies is a skin infection caused by the mite *Sarcoptes scabiei*, a crawling insect barely visible to the eye. The mite burrows under the skin to lay eggs. The eggs hatch quickly, and the immature mites tunnel for two weeks until they mature. Mature mites congregate around hair follicles, mate, and begin the cycle all over again. Scabies is easily transmitted to others and can be spread by direct human contact. It is rarely spread by animals.

Infestation by mites typically occurs between the fingers and toes, on the palms of the hands and undersides of the wrists, in the armpits, at the waistline, and on the penis. Because mites may also attack the skin around a woman's nipples, scabies sometimes occurs on the face of a breast-fed infant.

In recent years, scabies has appeared in a new pattern. The rash is scattered over the entire body and not limited to specific areas.

SIGNS AND SYMPTOMS

The burrowing of the insects and the allergic reaction to their presence under the skin cause relentless itching. When the child scratches the skin to relieve the itching, secondary infection can set in.

The diagnosis is based on the appearance and location on the skin of the small, red dots that mark the openings to the mites' burrows and the gray or black lines that mark their tunnels. However, these signs on the skin can be obscured by scratching.

HOME CARE

Mites can be destroyed by applying an ointment or lotion containing lindane, gamma benzene hexachloride, or crotamiton. Before you use these medications, discuss them with your doctor. The medication is applied to all skin surfaces except the head and the face. If your infant appears to have scabies on the face, consult your doctor before applying any medication. Because scabies is so easily transmitted from person to person, all family members should receive treatment at the same time. Treatment can be repeated once or twice. Nonprescription antihistamines may be used for temporary relief of itching.

PRECAUTIONS

■ If marks on the skin and itching continue after treatment, reinfestation may have occurred, or there may be a persistent allergic reaction or secondary infection. Do not keep treating the condition in the hope that it will clear up; see your doctor.

■ Destroy mites on undergarments, bedding, and towels by thorough laundering.

■ In both ointment and lotion form, **lindane is poisonous**. Be sure to keep it out of the reach of children.

MEDICAL TREATMENT

Your doctor will prescribe oral antibiotics to treat a secondary infection and antihistamines to relieve an allergic reaction.

RELATED TOPICS: Head lice; Impetigo

Scoliosis

Scoliosis is also known as curvature of the spine, or the vertebral column. In profile (side view), a normal spine has the shape of an S curve from top to bottom; viewed from the front or the back, the spine is straight from top to bottom. In scoliosis, the spine can be seen to curve toward one side or the other when viewed from the rear. That curve toward one side produces a second, compensating curve in the spine to keep the head straight.

The idiopathic type of scoliosis, which more frequently affects girls than boys, has no known cause. It develops during adolescence and stops getting worse when the child stops growing. The other types of scoliosis can develop at any age and can be caused by damage to the vertebrae (bones of the spine) from an infection, a tumor, an injury, or radiation therapy; abnormal development of the vertebrae or ribs; or weakness in the muscles of the trunk. Scoliosis can also result from a difference in the length of the legs. Unlike other forms of the disease, this type of scoliosis does not result in a fixed curvature of the spine; the vertebral column straightens when the child lies down.

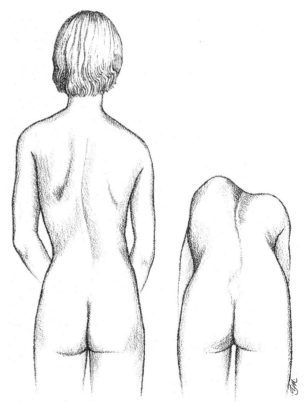

Severe scoliosis can be seen from the back when the child stands up, and even mild scoliosis is evident when the child bends forward at the waist. Bending forward causes the chest to rotate, making one side of the back prominent.

SIGNS AND SYMPTOMS

In severe cases of scoliosis, the curvature of the spine can easily be seen when the child stands up. Even a slight curvature may be easy to recognize because the child stands with one hip thrust forward. Scoliosis in almost any degree can be observed when the child bends forward at the waist with the knees straight; in this position, scoliosis causes the chest to rotate, making one side of the back prominent.

HOME CARE

Watch for the onset of the condition by observing your child's posture periodically, particularly during periods of rapid growth.

PRECAUTION

■ Any curvature of the spine toward one side or the other is abnormal. Since scoliosis can become severe in a matter of months, your child should be checked as soon as you notice any abnormality and then reexamined regularly.

MEDICAL TREATMENT

After confirming the presence of the condition, your doctor will often refer you to an orthopedist (bone specialist) who is skilled in treating scoliosis. X-ray films of the spine will be used to make the diagnosis.

Idiopathic scoliosis occasionally corrects itself during growth. However, it must be checked several times a year. Correction of idiopathic scoliosis may require the use of a back brace or surgery of the spine. Differences in leg length will be treated by placing lifts in the child's shoes or by surgery.

Exercise and physical therapy are not known to be helpful in treating any type of scoliosis.

Scrapes

A scrape, or abrasion, is a shallow break in the skin caused by an injury. Scrapes are distinguished from cuts and lacerations in that they are not as deep as they are long or wide. Scrapes are generally the most common and least dangerous injuries sustained by children. Most scrapes do not involve the loss of a full thickness of skin and heal with little or no scarring. However, any embedded dirt may be permanently sealed under the skin if it is not removed before the abrasion heals.

SIGNS AND SYMPTOMS

Scrapes are easy to identify. As long as the full thickness of the skin has not been injured, the surface of the scrape will bleed unevenly, and some areas will not bleed at all. When the surface of a scrape does not bleed uniformly, it is classified as a first- or second-degree abrasion and can be treated at home. A third-degree abrasion bleeds uniformly over its entire surface and must be seen by a doctor because it could leave a scar.

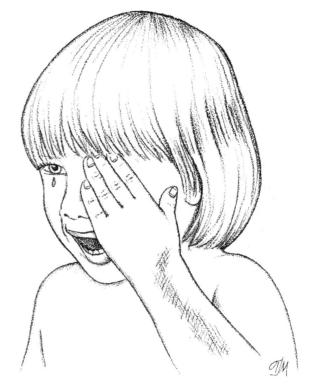

Scrapes are the most common childhood injuries.

HOME CARE

Wash the wound with soap and water, and then examine it for any embedded dirt or other foreign matter. Inspect the wound carefully under a good light—with a magnifying glass, if necessary. To stop the bleeding, place a square of sterile gauze over the scrape, and apply gentle pressure directly to the wound.

If there is no dirt in the wound, apply a nonstinging antiseptic, cover the scrape with a sterile bandage, and keep it covered until it heals completely and the scab falls off by itself.

If the abrasion is in an area that is moved constantly (at a joint, for example), periodically apply an antibiotic ointment to keep the scab flexible and to avoid cracking.

If dirt is embedded in the wound, scrub gently. Apply liberal amounts of antibiotic ointment twice a day during healing. Keep the area covered with a sterile bandage.

PRECAUTIONS

■ Do not treat a wound that involves the full thickness of the skin or is deeply soiled. Have the doctor look at it.

■ A scrape that bleeds evenly over its entire surface requires medical attention.

■ Remove dirt from an abrasion, both to guard against infection and to prevent the dirt from being permanently sealed under the skin.

■ It is unlikely, but not impossible, that tetanus will follow a scrape. Because minor abrasions are seldom treated by a doctor, take the precaution of keeping your child's tetanus immunization status up to date.

■ Impetigo may begin at the site of an abrasion.

MEDICAL TREATMENT

If an abrasion is deep and badly soiled, your doctor may apply a local anesthetic to the region and scrub out the dirt with a brush or a substance that will dissolve the dirt.

RELATED TOPICS: Cuts; Immunizations; Impetigo; Puncture wounds; Tetanus

Shingles

Shingles is an acute infection that produces crops of blisters on the skin. It is caused by the same virus that causes chicken pox. Shingles almost always develops in people who have had chicken pox at some time in the past; presumably, the virus lies inactive in the body until, for some reason, it is reactivated to cause shingles. Shingles is unusual in children under ten years of age, but it becomes increasingly common with age. One attack of shingles usually provides lifelong immunity.

SIGNS AND SYMPTOMS

The initial symptoms of shingles are listlessness, fever, and pain and tenderness along the path of a nerve. Shingles usually erupts on the chest, back, or abdomen, but it can occur along a nerve in the head or face, and it can involve an eye. In a few days, red pimples appear on the skin, and nearby lymph nodes enlarge. The

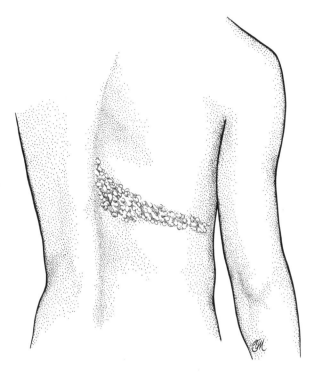

Shingles is a viral infection characterized by a blistering skin rash that follows the path of the affected underlying nerve or nerves.

pimples turn into blisters that dry out and form scabs in five to six days. New outbreaks may continue to appear for up to a week; both the rash and the pain disappear within one to five weeks.

The diagnosis is based on the typical appearance of the rash, which is confined to the length of one or two nerves, and the pain. Before the rash appears, the pain, which is sometimes intense, may be similar to that caused by pleurisy (inflammation of the lining of the chest cavity), an acute abdominal condition, or heart pain. In doubtful cases, the diagnosis of shingles is made on the basis of the results of blood tests.

HOME CARE

The only effective treatment consists of giving acetaminophen—not aspirin—to reduce the pain.

PRECAUTIONS

■ If shingles involves the eye, consult an ophthalmologist (eye specialist).

■ People who have shingles may transmit chicken pox. If a child has been exposed to shingles and would be placed at special risk by the possible complications of chicken pox (for example, if the child is taking steroids, which suppress the body's immunity to disease), consult your doctor.

■ Giving aspirin to a child with shingles *may* increase the risk of Reye's syndrome, which is a life-threatening illness.

MEDICAL TREATMENT

If chicken pox would present a special risk to a child who has been exposed to shingles, your doctor may administer zoster immune globulin or immune serum globulin.

RELATED TOPICS: Chest pains; Chicken pox; Glands, swollen; Rashes; Stomachache, acute

Shock

Shock is the term used to describe a sudden drop in blood pressure or a collapse of the circulatory system, which seriously reduces the blood supply to all parts of the body. Shock is an extremely dangerous condition; if it is not treated quickly, it is usually fatal.

Generally, shock occurs when a great deal of blood or other body fluids has been lost. It can also occur when blood vessels dilate (expand) and cause blood to pool or collect in one part of the body instead of circulating normally. The danger of shock exists in virtually every case of serious accident, injury, burn, or poisoning. Shock may also be associated with severe infections, wounds or broken bones, hemorrhage (severe, uncontrolled bleeding), insect stings (in people who are allergic to the insect's venom), excessive vomiting or diarrhea, heart attacks, and reactions to certain drugs.

SIGNS AND SYMPTOMS

Signs of shock include weakness; faintness; rapid, weak pulse; paleness; cold, clammy skin; cold sweat; chills; dry mouth; nausea; rapid, shallow breathing; restlessness; and confusion. Without treatment, the victim may lose consciousness.

HOME CARE

Shock is a **medical emergency** that requires immediate professional attention. After giving immediate life-saving first aid—for example, taking steps to stop bleeding and making sure that the child's airway is open—you must call for professional help. If there is a head injury,

have the child lie flat without elevating the feet; otherwise, keep the child lying flat with the legs raised. Keep the child warm. Do not give food or water.

PRECAUTION

■ Shock is a very dangerous condition, which is usually fatal if not treated immediately by professionals. If you suspect that your child is in shock, call at once for emergency help.

MEDICAL TREATMENT

Emergency medical treatment for shock will probably include administration of blood or other fluids into a vein and hospitalization.

RELATED TOPICS: Burns; Diarrhea in young children; Diarrhea in older children; Fractures; Insect bites and stings; Poisoning; Vomiting

Shortness of breath

Breathing is the process by which the body is supplied with oxygen and relieved of the waste product carbon dioxide. When the body's demand for oxygen is not met or it retains too much carbon dioxide, shortness of breath results. Shortness of breath usually follows prolonged physical exertion, but it also may accompany fever because the elevated temperature speeds up the body's chemical reactions, which in turn increases the amount of carbon dioxide in the body and the demand for oxygen.

Shortness of breath also may be a sign of disease. It indicates that something is interfering with the intake and transport of oxygen. It may be due to croup, inflammation of the bronchial tubes or the epiglottis in the throat, asthma, pneumonia, inhalation of a foreign body, or pneumothorax (spontaneous collapse of a lung). Shortness of breath may signal the presence of heart disease, severe anemia, or carbon monoxide poisoning from automobile exhaust fumes or a defective heater.

A rapid rate of respiration may be a consequence of aspirin poisoning, which stimulates the respiratory center in the brain, or of uncontrolled diabetes and dehydration (loss of body fluids). Anxiety sometimes causes hyperventilation, creating a false sensation of shortness of breath.

Shortness of breath and wheezing that occur only with exertion may be the only sign of asthma. Children with exercise-induced asthma don't wheeze or have any other symptoms of asthma until they exert themselves; then they develop wheezing. Many professional athletes have exercise-induced asthma.

SIGNS AND SYMPTOMS

The diagnosis of shortness of breath depends on the rate of breathing. To determine if your child is actually short of breath, count the number of breaths per minute when the child is at rest. The average normal rate of breathing for newborns is 40 breaths per minute; for one-year-olds, it is 30; and for children over eight years old, it is 20. If the rate of breathing for your child at rest is double the normal rate, he or she is short of breath.

Your child's fever may hinder your ability to judge whether the rate of breathing is normal. If your child seems to be short of breath and has a fever, allow two or three extra breaths per minute for each temperature degree above normal, or time the breathing after the temperature has returned to normal.

HOME CARE

Unless "air hunger" is caused by anxiety, no home treatment for shortness of breath should be attempted. Ask your doctor's advice.

PRECAUTIONS

■ A fever increases a person's rate of breathing. If a fever is treated with too much aspirin, the rate of breathing will increase even more. If your child is taking aspirin and becomes short of breath, double-check the dose to see if it is too high.
■ Rapid breathing while your child is resting often signals a serious problem. Contact your doctor promptly if it occurs.

MEDICAL TREATMENT

Your doctor will perform a complete examination, paying particular attention to the lungs, heart, throat, and blood pressure. Chest and neck X-ray studies will be performed. Blood and urine tests will be used to determine if the underlying cause of the shortness of breath is diabetes. You may be asked whether your child has been exposed to poisonous gases, such as carbon monoxide, and whether the child is being treated with aspirin for some other health

condition. The specific treatment of shortness of breath depends on its cause.

Most children with exercise-induced asthma are treated with inhaled medications, which eliminate the wheezing.

RELATED TOPICS: Anemia; Asthma; Croup; Dehydration; Diabetes mellitus; Fever; Hyperventilation; Pneumonia; Poisoning

Sickle cell anemia

Sickle cell anemia, also called sickle cell disease, is an inherited blood disease. It is caused by an abnormality in the hemoglobin, a special protein that helps the red blood cells carry oxygen through the bloodstream. The abnormal hemoglobin makes the red blood cells become rigid and sickle-shaped (hence the name hemoglobin S). The deformed blood cells have difficulty passing through the blood vessels. Blood cells are constantly being destroyed and replaced by the body, but these abnormal, deformed cells are destroyed more quickly than normal ones. The replacement process cannot keep up with the destruction of the sickled cells, causing recurrent anemia. Sickle cell trait and sickle cell disease are most common among persons of African descent but are also found in persons from certain areas of India, Greece, Italy, and the Middle East.

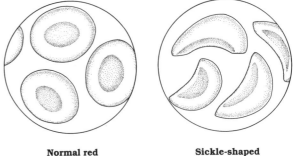

Normal red blood cells **Sickle-shaped red blood cells**

Sickle cell anemia is a blood disorder in which normally round red blood cells become deformed, sickle-shaped cells that tangle and interfere with blood circulation.

A child may be born with sickle cell trait, rather than sickle cell disease itself. The red blood cells of a child with sickle cell trait have about 40 percent hemoglobin S and 60 percent normal hemoglobin. The child will function normally and will show no signs of sickle cell disease. However, the child carries the trait in his or her genes, and either the trait or the disease may appear in the next generation. If the child eventually marries someone who also has the trait, the chances of their child having the disease are greatly increased.

SIGNS AND SYMPTOMS

In a child who has sickle cell disease, almost all the hemoglobin is hemoglobin S. The child may often show symptoms of anemia, which include weakness and constant tiredness. In certain circumstances, such as when the child has an infection, a sickle cell crisis may occur. Crises may also occur for no apparent reason, or as a result of flying in an unpressurized airplane or traveling to altitudes over 6,000 feet. Other stresses on the body, such as injuries or surgery, can also cause a sickle cell crisis.

In a sickle cell crisis, the abnormal red blood cells are destroyed rapidly, causing severe anemia. At the same time, sickled cells may lodge in the blood vessels, causing swelling of the joints and severe pain. Sickle cell crises can damage body organs, and such damage can eventually cause death.

To find out if a child has this disease, a blood test called a "sickle prep" is first performed to look for sickled cells in the blood. If abnormal cells are found, a more complicated test is done to identify the types of hemoglobin in the blood. The amount of hemoglobin S relative to the amount of normal hemoglobin indicates whether the child has the trait or the disease.

HOME CARE

Sickle cell anemia requires medical treatment.

PRECAUTIONS

■ All black parents, as well as other parents who know that there have been cases of sickle cell disease in their families, should have their children tested for the disease before they are a year old.
■ All infections should be treated immediately, and high fevers should also be reported to the doctor right away.
■ A child with this disease should have frequent checkups and may need special treatment before having dental work or surgery.
■ A child who has sickle cell trait needs no special treatment.

MEDICAL TREATMENT

Periodically, the doctor will carefully examine the child's liver, kidneys, heart, lungs, nervous system, and eyes. The doctor will probably prescribe antibiotics immediately if the child gets any infection. Blood transfusions may be needed to prevent anemia, and a vaccination against pneumococcal infection may be given.

In a sickle cell crisis, the child should be hospitalized. Intravenous fluids and pain medications will be given until the crisis passes.

RELATED TOPIC: Anemia

Sinusitis

Sinusitis is inflammation or infection of the sinuses, the air-filled cavities in the face that connect with the nasal passages. Around the nose are four pairs of sinuses—the maxillary, frontal, sphenoidal, and ethmoid sinuses. The maxillary sinuses (which lie below the eyes) and the ethmoid sinuses (which lie between the eyes) are present in infancy. The sphenoidal sinuses (located behind the roof of the nose) become fully developed between the ages of three and five years; the frontal sinuses, situated above the eyes, between six and ten years.

Because the sinuses are continuations of the nasal cavity, they are affected by any viral infection of the nose or any allergic reaction

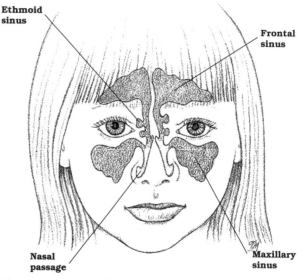

Sinuses are air-filled cavities in the face that connect the nasal passages. (The sphenoidal sinuses are located behind the ethmoid sinuses.)

that occurs in the nose. Either condition can lead to a bacterial infection within the sinuses, as can a bacterial infection of the nose.

SIGNS AND SYMPTOMS

The symptoms of sinusitis include fever (sometimes as high as 105°F), pain, stuffy nose, and cough. Depending on the location of the infection, headache may occur in the back of the head (infection of a sphenoidal sinus), at the temples and over the eyes (infection of the ethmoid and frontal sinuses), or above and below the eyes (infection of the maxillary sinuses). Small children who have an infection in the ethmoid sinuses develop red and swollen eyelids.

The key to diagnosing sinusitis is the discharge from the nose. With sinusitis, discharge from the nose is yellow, milky, or opaque. Pus in the sinuses can be revealed on an X-ray examination, but it is easily confused with a thickening of the lining of the sinuses because of a common cold or an allergy.

HOME CARE

You can promote sinus drainage and protect against sinus infection by treating a cold with decongestants (taken by mouth) and nose drops, or by treating an allergy with antihistamines taken by mouth. These measures also encourage drainage after sinusitis has developed. Consult your doctor about the type and duration of such treatment. To relieve pain and fever, heat may be applied over the affected sinuses, and acetaminophen may be given to the child.

PRECAUTIONS

■ A high fever (103°F to 105°F) accompanied by signs of sinusitis indicates a potentially serious infection. See your doctor.
■ A puslike discharge or signs of sinusitis on one side of the nose suggest that a foreign object may be lodged in the nose or that the inside of the nose may be deformed. See your doctor.

MEDICAL TREATMENT

If a bacterial infection is identified, the doctor may prescribe antibiotics for the child to take by mouth. Suction may be used to drain the sinuses of older children with sinusitis. Surgical drainage is rarely indicated in children.

RELATED TOPICS: Common cold; Coughs; Fever; Headaches

Sore heels

Painful heels are a common complaint before and during adolescence. Almost 90 percent of the time, the pain is due to injury of the bony growth plate near the back of the calcaneus (heel bone). This condition is called Sever's disease and may be due to a direct blow, such as might be caused by the heels pounding the ground, or to the pull of the calf muscles on the Achilles tendon and the back of the heel bone.

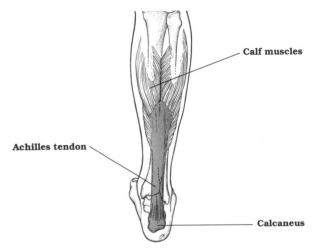

Heel pain may be due to injury to the bony growth plate near the back of the calcaneus, which may be caused by the pull of the calf muscles on the Achilles tendon and calcaneus.

SIGNS AND SYMPTOMS

In Sever's disease, one or both heels hurt when the child walks and are tender to the touch on both sides and on the bottom of the heel bone (about one-half inch to one inch away from the back of the heel). The heels are not swollen or red; the skin over the heels shows no abnormality. The diagnosis is based on the presence of pain and tenderness at the heel and the absence of other symptoms.

Other problems that cause pain at the heel are associated with other symptoms. For example, infection of the heel bone produces severe pain that intensifies over time, redness and swelling of the infected heel, and a low-grade fever. Blisters, plantar warts, and wounds in the heel area can also cause sore heels.

HOME CARE

To relieve pain from Sever's disease, pad the heels of all of your child's shoes with a quarter-inch heel pad and temporarily restrict activities that involve running and jumping. Even if a child has pain in only one heel, be sure to pad the heels of both shoes.

PRECAUTIONS

■ If your child cannot move the affected foot up and down (by rising on tiptoe), he or she may have a torn Achilles tendon. Do not attempt home care. The child should be seen by a doctor.

■ With the proper home treatment, Sever's disease should subside in four to six weeks, and the pain should cease as soon as the heels of the shoes are padded. If the pain isn't promptly eased, you should take your child to the doctor.

MEDICAL TREATMENT

Your doctor will perform a careful examination to rule out possible causes of pain. If Sever's disease is severe, the doctor will temporarily immobilize the ankles. X-ray studies are seldom required.

RELATED TOPICS: Blisters; Puncture wounds; Warts

Sore throat

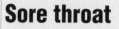

In theory, a sore throat should be one of the simplest childhood medical problems to diagnose and to treat. Medical textbooks state that a sore throat is usually caused by a virus and, therefore, does not require treatment with antibiotics because viral infections do not respond to medication. A sore throat that is not caused by a virus is generally due to streptococcus bacteria. These organisms can be identified by culturing throat secretions, and a strep throat can be treated with penicillin or, if the child is allergic to penicillin, with erythromycin.

In practice, however, the diagnosis and treatment of a sore throat are not so straightforward. Viral infections sometimes are complicated by streptococcal infections. A throat culture may isolate streptococcus organisms, even though they are not the cause of the illness. Furthermore, about five percent of throat cultures will not show streptococcus organisms even when they are present and are, in fact, the cause of the sore throat. Some bacterial illnesses that cause a sore throat will respond to

antibiotics, but the infecting bacteria cannot be identified with the use of an ordinary throat culture.

SIGNS AND SYMPTOMS

It is difficult to be certain that an infant or toddler has a sore throat because the child cannot communicate, but swollen glands in the neck and difficulty in swallowing are clues. Determining the cause of a sore throat depends on the results of blood tests and a throat or other type of culture, as well as on the doctor's skill in performing the physical examination, knowledge of the illnesses in the community, and professional judgment.

HOME CARE

All children should drink extra fluids and eat their usual diet if they can. Older children may gargle with warm salt water to relieve a sore throat. Give acetaminophen to reduce pain or fever, and isolate the child from other children, particularly infants, until the cause of the problem has been found.

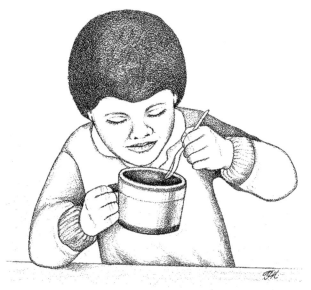

All children should consume extra fluids when they have a sore throat.

PRECAUTIONS

■ Take the child to a doctor if a sore throat is accompanied by any of the following symptoms: moderately or severely swollen and tender lymph nodes in the neck, difficulty in swallowing that cannot be relieved by acetaminophen, puslike discharge from the eyes or nose, moderate or severe earache, tenderness over the sinuses, breathing difficulty, chest pain, reddish-purple rash or a rash resembling scarlet fever

(fine, slightly raised red spots resembling coarse red sandpaper), stiff neck, weakness or exhaustion, confusion, or repeated vomiting.
■ If a sore throat and a fever continue to worsen after 24 to 36 hours, consult a doctor.

MEDICAL TREATMENT

Your doctor will conduct a complete physical examination and a rapid strep screen. Some doctors order a throat culture if the rapid strep screen is negative, other doctors do not. Depending on the results of these tests, your doctor may treat a sore throat with antibiotics. Regardless of the treatment prescribed, you should report any new symptoms to your doctor. Also consult the doctor if there is no improvement in the child's condition after 48 hours.

RELATED TOPICS: Chest pain; Common cold; Coughs; Croup; Diphtheria; Earaches; Fever; Glands, swollen; Gonorrhea; Infectious mononucleosis; Meningitis; Pneumonia; Rashes; Sinusitis; Strep infections; Tonsillitis

Speech problems and stuttering

Children learn to speak by imitation, but they learn at different rates depending on their intelligence, their hearing, and their control of the muscles involved in speaking. Speech may be delayed or impaired if the speech centers in the brain are not normal or if there is any abnormality of the larynx (voice box), throat, nose, tongue, or lips. Speech development also depends on how often a child hears speech and how much he or she is encouraged to speak. Because of the wide range of individual differences in learning to speak, parents should not be unduly alarmed if their child does not reach a certain stage exactly "on schedule."

A general timetable for speech development includes the following milestones: By the age of four to six months, most babies have begun to babble and to make letterlike sounds. By eight months, most children have achieved a typical baby vocabulary, using such "words" as "goo," "ba-ba," and "da-da." By 12 months, most babies will be using two-syllable "words" meaningfully ("ma-ma" for mother, "ba-ba" for bottle), and by two years old will be connecting words purposefully ("go bye-bye," "want cookie"). A child of five years can generally speak five-word sentences, and by the age of six can make all the sounds of the alphabet, except perhaps the sounds for s and z.

Children between two and five years of age often lack fluency and may stutter or stammer at times. If the lack of fluency or the stuttering or stammering continues, the child may have a speech problem. Speech that does not develop normally may also be due to partial or complete deafness, mental retardation, inadequate exposure to language, brain damage, physical abnormalities, or malfunction of the speech centers.

SIGNS AND SYMPTOMS

Any impairment of speech or marked delay in a child's achieving speech should raise the suspicion of a speech or hearing problem.

HOME CARE

If your baby is to learn to speak adequately, he or she must be spoken to and listened to. Incorrect speech should be corrected, but a child should not be scolded, deliberately ignored, or forced to practice speaking. Stuttering in children aged two to five years can be disregarded unless it is still a problem several months after its onset. It should not provoke anger or anxiety, suggestions that the child speak more slowly or more clearly, or laughter and taunts from brothers and sisters. Stuttering warrants professional attention if it is severe, constant, or prolonged.

PRECAUTIONS

■ If your child's speech does not develop more or less in accordance with the general timetable, consult your doctor.
■ Do not refuse to understand your child or try to force him or her to speak more clearly.
■ Do not call the child's attention to stuttering.
■ Read, sing, and speak to your child whenever possible.
■ If your child speaks only in a monotone or with a marked nasal quality or if the vocabulary and ability to pronounce words are diminishing instead of improving, consult your physician.

MEDICAL TREATMENT

Your doctor will perform a complete physical examination, checking the child's throat, palate, and tongue, and testing the child's hearing. If your child is under the age of five years, you may be referred to a speech pathologist for evaluation and treatment if stuttering is severe, constant, or unduly prolonged; if the child seems to be severely frustrated in his or her efforts to speak clearly; or if you need assistance in handling your child's development of speech. If your child substitutes sounds or stutters after the age of five or six, your doctor may suggest that he or she be seen by a speech specialist.

RELATED TOPIC: Deafness

Sprains and dislocations

All joints of the body are surrounded by ligaments (the tough connective tissues that link bones together). These ligaments can be partially or completely torn when the joint is forcibly twisted beyond its normal range of movement. A partial or complete tear of a ligament is called a sprain. If the ligaments are badly torn, the bones of the joint may become dislocated (slip out of position). In addition to the usual symptoms of a sprain, a dislocation causes a visible malformation of the area, as well as marked or total loss of function of the dislocated parts. Even after the dislocation has been corrected, the joint may remain unstable for weeks.

Sprains are common during childhood, but dislocations (other than those of the elbow) are rare. Sprains most often occur in the fingers ("jammed" or "baseball" fingers), toes, ankles, neck, and back. Dislocations can occur in the fingers, toes, kneecaps, shoulders, elbows, and hips.

SIGNS AND SYMPTOMS

A sprain causes swelling, tenderness, decreased movement of the joint, internal bleeding, and pain, which is sometimes severe. A mild or moderate sprain generally can be suspected if a joint is tender after it has been twisted or overextended.

Because dislocations produce a visible malformation, they are seldom missed. Furthermore, the inability to use the joint is an obvious sign of a dislocation. Fractures of the bones of the joint cannot be ruled out without an X-ray examination.

HOME CARE

A dislocation should not be treated at home. Minor sprains, particularly those of the fingers, toes, and ankles, may be treated safely at home by immobilizing the hand or foot involved and then resting it. The sprained part should be kept elevated. Cold compresses applied for one to four hours after injury help minimize swelling. Aspirin or acetaminophen should temporarily relieve the pain. If a sprain does not improve rapidly, a bone may be fractured. In such a case, the child should be seen by a doctor.

PRECAUTIONS

■ Do not attempt to correct a dislocation, even of the fingers. Dislocations are often accompanied by a fracture.
■ What appears to be a sprained wrist in a child may actually be a fracture of the forearm bones near the joint, and what appears to be a sprained thumb may actually be a fractured navicular bone in the hand.
■ A severe sprain may take as long as a fracture to heal and, if not treated properly, can result in a permanently weak joint.
■ A sprain is not healed if it is still swollen or if it is painful to move.
■ Elastic bandages do not adequately support or protect a sprained ankle.

MEDICAL TREATMENT

Your doctor will carefully examine the injured joint and will order an X-ray examination if a dislocation or a fracture is suspected. If a sprain appears to be minor, the doctor may choose to simply immobilize the joint and observe its rate of healing; if the rate of healing is not rapid enough, an X-ray will then be ordered.

RELATED TOPICS: Dislocated elbow; Dislocated hips; Fractures; Knee pains

Stomachache, acute

The abdomen contains the stomach, small and large intestines, liver, spleen, pancreas, kidneys, urinary bladder, gallbladder, and organs of reproduction. Disease or injury involving any of these organs can cause abdominal pain. Consequently, a "stomachache" can test the diagnostic ability of parent and doctor alike.

Fortunately, almost all stomachaches in children are caused by one of four problems: constipation, acute digestive tract upset (caused by viruses, bacteria, or improper diet), emotional stress, or urinary tract infection.

Other less frequent causes of a stomachache are appendicitis, pneumonia, infectious mononucleosis, and hepatitis.

SIGNS AND SYMPTOMS

The first step in diagnosis involves ruling out appendicitis. If appendicitis can be ruled out, consider other possibilities.

Your child probably is constipated if he or she has not had a bowel movement recently or has had only a hard bowel movement, if the pain is intermittent and crampy on the left side of the body and follows eating, and if the abdomen is not tender to the touch.

Your child probably has digestive tract upset if he or she has eaten too much or has been exposed to someone who has acute gastroenteritis, if the pain is intermittent and occurs around the upper abdomen or navel, or if diarrhea follows vomiting.

Your child's stomachache is probably due to emotional stress if he or she is or has been upset and if the pain does not worsen.

Your child's stomachache may be due to urinary tract infection if the child has a fever and frequent, painful urination. The child should be seen by a doctor.

If your child's pain cannot be explained by any of these causes, take the child to the doctor.

HOME CARE

Treat constipation with a change in diet. Foods that prevent constipation are fruit juices and fruits (particularly those eaten with the skin on) except bananas; vegetables (especially if eaten raw) except peeled potatoes; and unrefined grains (whole-grain cereals and breads). A glycerin suppository may also be used to treat constipation.

Unless it is severe (acute pain lasting for more than 24 hours), digestive tract upset will usually go away on its own. An antinausea medication (ask your doctor for suggestions) can relieve the vomiting, and mild heat applied to the abdomen can relieve the pain.

A stomachache due to emotional stress will ease with relief from the stress, but one that arises from a urinary tract infection requires the attention of a physician. If any stomach pain persists or worsens, see the doctor.

PRECAUTIONS

■ Never give a child a laxative or place ice on the abdomen to treat abdominal pain.
■ Steady, worsening pain usually is more serious than intermittent, crampy pain. However, severe and regular crampy pain may indicate a serious problem, particularly if there is also blood or mucus in the child's stools.
■ Abdominal pain that forces a child to bend forward as he or she walks is a cause for concern.
■ Abdominal pain combined with fever and a cough suggests pneumonia.
■ Severe, worsening abdominal pain that follows an injury to the abdomen or lower chest suggests internal injury and requires a doctor's attention.

MEDICAL TREATMENT

Your doctor's first task is to determine the cause of the pain by taking a detailed medical history, performing a complete physical examination, and, in many cases, ordering a series of laboratory tests and X-ray studies. If the diagnosis remains uncertain, your doctor may observe your child for a few hours or ask for a consultation with another physician.

RELATED TOPICS: Appendicitis; Constipation; Diarrhea in older children; Diarrhea in young children; Dysentery; Food poisoning; Gastroenteritis, acute; Hepatitis; Infectious mononucleosis; Pneumonia; Shingles; Stomachache, chronic; Strep infections; Urinary tract infections; Vomiting

Stomachache, chronic

Intermittent, crampy abdominal pain is quite common in children and may continue for weeks, months, or years. In some cases, the pain occurs as often as two or three times a day; in others, much less frequently. To further complicate diagnosis, one of a series of recurrent stomachaches may seem to be a bout of acute abdominal pain, and some conditions that cause abdominal pain can recur again and again.

Chronic stomach pain usually is due to constipation, intolerance to cow's milk due to lactase deficiency, or emotional stress. Less common causes are urinary tract problems (such as obstruction and chronic infection), peptic ulcer, sickle cell anemia, lead poisoning, ulcerative colitis, regional enteritis (Crohn's disease), tumors, ovarian problems, worm infestations, intolerance to foods other than milk, and internal hernias. Recurrent abdominal pain is not due to appendicitis.

SIGNS AND SYMPTOMS

To pinpoint its cause, recurrent abdominal pain must be associated with other symptoms, such as vomiting, diarrhea, constipation, blood or mucus in the stools, fever, failure to gain weight, painful urination, pica (ingestion of inedible substances), and anemia. Also important is the pattern of the pain—where it is, when it occurs, and how long it lasts.

In general, recurrent abdominal pain that is accompanied by no other symptoms or has no set pattern is probably not serious.

HOME CARE

If constipation is the cause of the pain, correct it by changing your child's diet. Foods that prevent constipation are fruit juices and fruits (particularly those eaten with the skin on), with the exception of bananas; vegetables (especially if eaten raw), with the exception of peeled potatoes; and unrefined grains (whole-grain cereals and breads). A glycerin suppository may also be used to treat constipation.

If you have any reason to believe that milk intolerance may be causing the stomachaches, ask your doctor if you should remove milk and milk products from your child's diet for one or two weeks. At the end of that period, you may then add milk and milk products to the diet again and observe the effects.

Try to eliminate emotional stress if that may be responsible for the stomachaches.

Most important, note and record the pattern of recurrent abdominal pain and any other symptoms before consulting your doctor.

PRECAUTIONS

■ Recurrent abdominal pain due to emotional stress is real and requires treatment just as much as pain due to an identifiable physical condition.
■ Do not try to relieve stomach pain by giving laxatives or placing ice on the stomach.

MEDICAL TREATMENT

Your doctor will take a careful history of your child's recent health and perform a complete

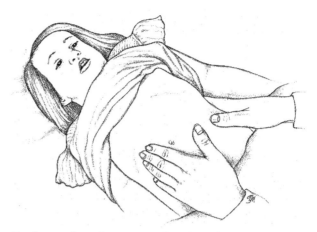

To determine the cause of a chronic stomachache, your doctor will carefully examine your child's abdomen as part of a complete physical evaluation.

physical examination. Frequently the doctor will order urine, stool, and blood tests. If the cause of the pain still has not been identified, X-ray studies of the stomach, large and small intestines, and urinary tract may be required. If these studies provide no clues to the problem, your child may be hospitalized for extensive blood tests and an internal abdominal examination.

RELATED TOPICS: Anemia; Constipation; Diarrhea in older children; Diarrhea in young children; Food allergies; Hernia; Lead poisoning; Pinworms; Sickle cell anemia; Stomachache, acute; Ulcers; Urinary tract infections; Vomiting

Strep infections

There are at least 60 different types of streptococcus ("strep") organisms. After a strep infection, one is immune to further attacks by the type of streptococcus organism that caused the illness, but not against other types.

Strep throat is a highly contagious infection of the throat, usually caused by the group A strain of beta-hemolytic streptococcus bacteria. Although some strep germs do not cause rashes, most types can produce a toxin (poison) like the one that causes the rash that is characteristic of scarlet fever (also commonly called scarlatina), which is another type of strep infection. A streptococcal infection can be serious. Among its complications are rheumatic fever, nephritis (inflammation of the kidneys), middle ear infection, sinusitis, pneumonia, and transient (temporary) arthritis.

The incubation period (the time it takes for symptoms to develop once the child has been exposed to the bacteria) of strep throat is two to five days. The disease is passed from child to child by means of throat or nasal secretions from an infected person. It may also be spread by a carrier who has no symptoms of the illness. At times, as many as half the children in any one area may be carriers of strep infection.

SIGNS AND SYMPTOMS

The onset of strep throat is sudden. It begins with a headache, fever (up to 104°F), sore and red throat, vomiting, abdominal pain, and swollen lymph nodes in the neck.

If a strep infection is caused by a rash-producing type of organism, a rash will develop within 24 to 72 hours. The rash of scarlet fever typically has fine, slightly raised red spots resembling coarse red sandpaper. It appears on the base of the neck, in the armpits and groin, and then on the trunk and extremities. The child's face is flushed, but the lips are pale. When the rash subsides in 3 to 20 days, the skin flakes and peels.

The diagnosis of strep throat cannot be confirmed without a throat culture that isolates streptococcus organisms. However, cultures are only 90 to 95 percent reliable. The diagnosis of scarlet fever is based on the appearance of the rash.

HOME CARE

The only home treatment recommended is to give aspirin or acetaminophen to relieve fever and pain. A streptococcal infection should be treated by your doctor.

PRECAUTIONS

■ Infants are immune to the scarlet fever toxin for four to six months after birth only if their mothers are immune. Infants are not immune to other streptococcal infections, which may be very serious but may not produce typical symptoms. Consequently, keep infants away from groups of children, some of whom may be carriers of streptococcus bacteria.

■ Give the full course of antibiotic treatment prescribed by your doctor, even if the child seems to be well before all the medicine is finished.

■ If your child is being treated with antibiotics for a strep infection but the condition does not improve within 24 to 48 hours of starting the

medication, inform your doctor. The child may have infectious mononucleosis as well.

MEDICAL TREATMENT

Strep throat is diagnosed on the basis of physical examination findings and the results of a throat culture. Penicillin (or another antibiotic for those who are allergic to penicillin) is usually prescribed for ten days to treat a streptococcal infection. Antibiotics prevent rheumatic fever and may prevent inflammation of the kidneys. Hospitalization may be necessary if complications develop.

RELATED TOPICS: Arthritis; Earaches; Fever; Glands, swollen; Headaches; Infectious mononucleosis; Nephritis; Pneumonia; Rashes; Sinusitis; Sore throat; Stomachache, acute; Vomiting

Styes

Styes are boils that occur in the oil or sweat glands in the upper or lower eyelids. Styes are usually caused by staphylococcus bacteria and can spread from person to person through direct contact. Styes tend to occur in crops, because the bacteria in the pus that forms in the stye spreads easily to infect other glands in the eyelids.

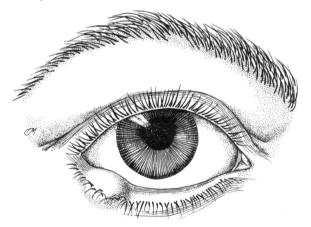

A stye is a boil that occurs in the oil or sweat glands in the upper or lower eyelid.

SIGNS AND SYMPTOMS

Styes develop like boils. The area at the edge of the eyelid becomes increasingly red, painful, tender, and swollen. After two to three days, pus forms, and the stye "points" (that is, a yellow head appears at the edge of the lid near the base of the eyelashes). Styes usually break spontaneously, drain, and heal. Occasionally, a stye will heal without pointing or draining.

Styes differ from insect bites and cysts in that styes are painful and tender. They occur near the margins of the eyelids, and they usually come to a head. Insect bites itch, are usually not painful, and do not come to a head. Cysts are lumps or swellings that show through the undersurface of the eyelids as pink or pale yellow spots. They usually are not tender. Sometimes, however, they become infected and, like styes, are red, tender, and painful. Unlike styes, cysts persist for some time and do not come to a head.

HOME CARE

Place cotton balls or a washcloth soaked in warm water on the eyelids for 10 to 20 minutes several times a day. Give aspirin or acetaminophen to reduce pain. Do not treat cysts unless they are infected; then, treat them in the same way you would a stye.

PRECAUTIONS

■ The whites of the eyes do not become red as a result of a stye. Consult your doctor if redness appears.
■ Your child should be seen by a doctor if he or she has one large or several small recurring styes or if the child has a stye that is accompanied by fever, headache, loss of appetite, or lethargy.
■ Styes can be contagious. Keep the infected child's towels and washcloths separate from those used by other family members.

MEDICAL TREATMENT

Your doctor may prescribe an antibiotic to treat one large or several small recurring styes. It is rarely necessary to open and drain a stye. The doctor may take a culture of the nose and throat secretions to find out where the bacteria are located.

Your doctor may surgically remove an infected cyst. However, cysts often disappear spontaneously in months or years. An infected cyst is treated in the same way as a stye.

RELATED TOPICS: Boils; Conjunctivitis; Insect bites and stings

Sudden infant death syndrome

All babies sometimes have periods when they stop breathing for a second or two. Occasionally, the nonbreathing periods will last for a longer time; this is called "periodic breathing." But if the infant's automatic breathing mechanism does not start again, and if no one is there to revive the baby, the child will die. This condition is called sudden infant death syndrome (SIDS) because the cause is not understood well enough to give it a more specific name.

Deaths due to SIDS usually occur at night, when the infant is asleep, and are most common between the ages of one and four months. SIDS is most common in the winter months and affects boys more often than girls. Although the cause of death is not known, some experts believe SIDS is related to abnormality or underdevelopment of the respiratory control center in the brain.

There are several factors that make some babies more susceptible to SIDS than others. If a child's parents are under 20 years of age when the child is born or if they are poor, the risk of SIDS is increased. If the mother did not receive medical care during the pregnancy, was ill during the pregnancy, or smoked or abused drugs during the pregnancy, the risk is also increased. Infants of multiple births and infants who are born prematurely or whose birth weight is below normal are especially susceptible. Although SIDS is not actually inherited, the risk is greater for infants whose parents have lost a child to SIDS before and for infants from families in which SIDS has occurred before.

SIGNS AND SYMPTOMS

There are no warning signs. A diagnosis of SIDS can be made only after death, when an autopsy does not reveal any other cause of death.

If an infant has ever stopped breathing and then been revived or is considered at risk for other reasons, the doctor may recommend that the child undergo pneumography. In this test, a machine is attached to the infant for 48 hours to record breathing patterns. The periods of nonbreathing are evaluated based on their number, their length, and how often they occur. The doctor can then determine if special treatment is necessary.

HOME CARE

There is no specific treatment for SIDS, unless a diagnosis of a high-risk condition has been made.

PRECAUTION

■ Every parent should know how to revive an infant who has stopped breathing. The best way to learn the proper technique is to take one of the courses in cardiopulmonary resuscitation (CPR) that are offered by local hospitals and community organizations. If, for some reason, taking such a course is not possible, ask your doctor to demonstrate the technique.

MEDICAL TREATMENT

If your baby is in a high-risk category (for example, if he or she has ever stopped breathing or turned pale or blue, or if a pneumogram has shown abnormal breathing patterns), there are two ways to protect the baby from SIDS.

The first is to attach monitors to the infant whenever he or she is put down to sleep. Each time the infant stops breathing for an amount of time set on the monitor, an alarm goes off. These devices are not completely reliable, and they can be disruptive to the whole family if they are used at home.

The second possibility is for the doctor to prescribe regular doses of a drug called theophylline, which stimulates the respiratory center of the brain and is usually used to treat asthma. In some infants, use of theophylline protects against nonbreathing periods. The long-term results of giving theophylline to infants are not yet known, so the drug must be prescribed with caution. An infant who is being given theophylline as protection against SIDS must be watched closely and have blood tests and pneumograms regularly.

Sunburn

Sunburn is a heat burn, usually of the first degree. Babies and children who have fair complexions are particularly susceptible to sunburn, even on cloudy days or in the shade. Occasionally, sunburn causes a skin rash that resembles hives or the rash caused by poison ivy. This condition is called sun poisoning.

SIGNS AND SYMPTOMS

Sunburn causes the skin to become inflamed, blistered, and painful, and the diagnosis is usually immediately obvious. The rash caused by sun poisoning, however, may not appear for several days after exposure to the sun.

HOME CARE

Apply cold water compresses to the burned area, followed by cocoa butter, commercial burn ointments, or a paste made of baking soda and water. Do not break the blisters. Give the child aspirin or acetaminophen to relieve pain and nonprescription antihistamines to reduce itching.

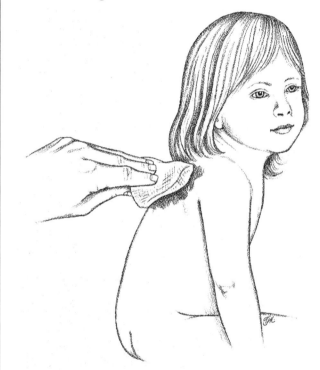

Apply cold-water compresses to the sunburned area, followed by cocoa butter, commercial burn ointments, or a paste made of baking soda and water.

PRECAUTIONS

■ The most important aspect of home treatment is prevention. A child should be protected from the sun as much as possible, and exposure to the sun should begin slowly and be gradually increased.

■ Apply sunscreens to filter out damaging rays of the sun, but remember that sunscreens offer only limited protection; the child who is out in the sun for too long can still get sunburned. For a child, select a sunscreen that contains

UNDERSTANDING YOUR CHILD'S CONDITION   353

para-aminobenzoic acid (PABA), titanium dioxide, or sulisobenzone.

■ Remember that most sunscreens wash off when the child goes swimming or even perspires. Follow the instructions on the product's package for reapplying the sunscreen.

■ Sunscreens may cause a mild rash on some people. If a rash appears, switch products.

■ Infants and children may receive a severe burn from sunlight coming through open windows, especially in the car. Be sure that children are protected by sunscreens.

■ Sunburn medication applied to large areas can be absorbed into the body and produce side effects. Use such medications sparingly.

■ Injury to the skin from overexposure to ultraviolet light from sunlamps is common among teenagers.

■ Some medications (for example, tetracycline, chlorpromazine, griseofulvin, and coal-tar ointments) increase the sensitivity of the skin to sunburn. Ask your doctor if a medication your child is taking has this effect. If your child is taking one of these medications, be extra careful about protecting the child from the sun by using a sunscreen and limiting the child's exposure to the sun.

■ Take the child to a doctor if he or she has a sunburn plus a fever or extreme fatigue and weakness.

MEDICAL TREATMENT

Your doctor will treat your child's sunburn the same as any other type of burn. A child who has a severe burn will be hospitalized for treatment.

RELATED TOPICS: Blisters; Burns

Swallowed objects

Over 95 percent of the penny-, nickel-, and dime-sized foreign objects that are swallowed by children cause no trouble and pass from the body in the child's stool. However, objects that are the size of a quarter or larger may become lodged in the esophagus. Sharp objects (pins, needles, bones, matchsticks, nails, glass splinters) may lodge in the tonsils, throat, or esophagus. Objects longer than a toothpick may not be able to pass out of the stomach and may have to be removed surgically.

SIGNS AND SYMPTOMS

Depending on where the object is lodged, it may cause choking or inability to breathe or cry (see the section on *Choking* on pages 71-72 immediately), gagging, pain, discomfort in the throat or chest, or difficulty in swallowing. Once a foreign object has passed into the stomach, it does not produce any symptoms unless it obstructs or penetrates the digestive tract, in which case abdominal pain, vomiting, and fever may develop. If the child has swallowed a metal object, it will be visible on an X-ray examination, but wooden, plastic, or glass objects may not. Usually, however, the diagnosis is suggested by the circumstances and the symptoms that do appear.

HOME CARE

Ask your doctor whether immediate medical attention is necessary. If the swallowed object is small and smooth, it should pass out of the body without treatment; if the object is long, sharp, or large, it may not. Examine the child's stools carefully for several days to be sure that the object has passed from the body. Each bowel movement should be passed through a sieve until the object has been passed. If the child has been toilet trained, place a basin fashioned of window screening in the toilet bowl. Then, after the child has passed a stool, wash it through the screening with hot water.

PRECAUTIONS

■ An object lodged in the esophagus must be removed **within hours** by a doctor.

■ No food, drink, or medication will speed up the passage of a foreign object through the body.

■ If an object has not passed from the child's body within one week, see your doctor. Try to bring a duplicate of the swallowed object to show your doctor.

■ Do not give your child a laxative in an effort to speed passage of a swallowed object.

■ As with choking, prevention is most important. Examine all toys for loose eyes and other small parts that might be swallowed. Keep other small objects out of the reach of babies and toddlers.

MEDICAL TREATMENT

Your doctor will carefully inspect the throat and observe the way your child swallows. X-ray examinations of the throat, neck, chest, or abdomen may be ordered. If an object is

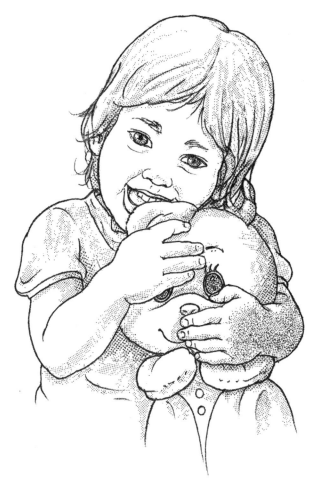

Examine all toys for loose eyes and other small parts that might be swallowed.

wedged in the throat or esophagus, your doctor will remove it with a surgical instrument. If the object is in the stomach, the doctor may watch the child's condition for three or more weeks before trying to remove it surgically. If the object is in the intestines and does not pass within a week, the doctor may remove it surgically.

RELATED TOPIC: Choking

Swimmer's ear

Irritation or infection of the ear canal is known as swimmer's ear. Swimmer's ear may arise from a middle ear infection that has caused the eardrum to rupture and allowed pus (infected material) to drain into the outer canal. The condition can also occur if an injury to the ear canal becomes infected. Usually, however, swimmer's ear is caused by swimming in fresh water or pools. The frequent and sustained presence of moisture in the ear softens, swells, and cracks the ear canal, allowing germs to penetrate the canal and cause infection.

SIGNS AND SYMPTOMS

An itching, clogged ear canal, with or without discharge, may indicate a mild case of swimmer's ear; hearing may be diminished. A severe case may cause intense pain, fever, and swollen, tender lymph nodes in front of, behind, and below the ear.

HOME CARE

Your doctor may direct you to treat a mild case of swimmer's ear by administering eardrops containing antibiotics and steroids. Give aspirin or acetaminophen or apply warm compresses to the outside of the ear to reduce pain. If your child has had several bouts of swimmer's ear, dry the ear canals at the end of each swimming session by dropping in a few drops of rubbing alcohol or glycerin. This may prevent the condition from recurring.

PRECAUTIONS

■ If a child has severe pain, fever, or swollen lymph nodes or does not respond to home treatment in a few days, take the child to your doctor.
■ Rubber earplugs will not keep water out of the ear canals.
■ Do not attempt to clean ear canals by using any object (including a cotton swab).
■ If eardrops do not penetrate deeply into the ear canal, they will not be effective. After administering the drops, be sure to keep the child's head tilted for a little while to give the drops time to penetrate properly.

MEDICAL TREATMENT

The doctor will carefully examine your child to rule out other possible causes of the symptoms. In the absence of discharge from the ear canal, the diagnosis is based on internal examination of the ear. In addition to eardrops, your doctor may prescribe antibiotics for the child to take by mouth. If the ear is not too tender, the doctor will clean the ear canal.

RELATED TOPICS: Draining ear; Earaches; Glands, swollen

Teething

A baby usually cuts 20 teeth during the first three years of life. All 20 are temporary (primary) and are partly formed within the gums at birth. The age and sequence of the eruption of the teeth vary from child to child. Usually, however, the lower central incisors (front teeth) are the first to break through the gums. This can occur before birth or as late as one year of age. The four upper central incisors and the lower lateral incisors usually follow. The four one-year molars appear next (toward the rear of the mouth), followed by the four canines (the cone-shaped pointed teeth on either side of the upper and lower incisors), and finally the four two-year molars.

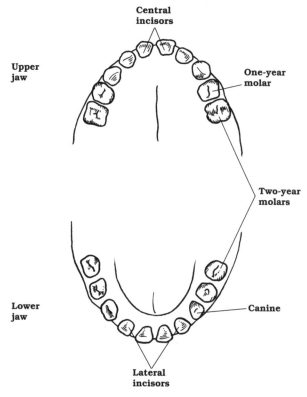

A baby usually cuts 20 teeth during the first three years of life.

SIGNS AND SYMPTOMS

Teething commonly is accompanied by drooling, fretfulness, wakefulness at night, unwillingness to eat, discomfort, or chewing on the fingers or objects. The drooling and chewing are quite normal; fretfulness, wakefulness, and unwillingness to eat can have many causes.

A few days before teeth erupt, they push at the gum ahead of them and can be seen or felt. Before molars erupt, they frequently cause a blue blood blister at the site of the tooth.

HOME CARE

Teething pain can be eased by rubbing the baby's gums with a cold object. Biting on zwieback toast, teething biscuits, and teething rings helps the teeth erupt, and biting on cold objects (such as frozen teething rings) numbs the gums and eases the pain of teething. Aspirin or acetaminophen also may help relieve pain. In the daytime, keeping the child amused and occupied may help the child forget the pain.

PRECAUTIONS

■ Young children cut teeth on and off for three years. During this period, do not assume that every symptom the child has is due to teething; look for other possible causes.
■ Fever, cough, and nasal discharge are not symptoms of teething.
■ Diarrhea and constipation are related to teething only if there is an extreme change in the child's diet.
■ If the child's eating and drinking habits change during teething, do not try to force-feed.
■ Drooling because of teething may produce chapping on the face, but rashes are not related to teething.
■ Overuse of commercial teething ointments and solutions that contain local anesthetics can cause anemia (deficiency of red blood cells).
■ **Never** apply aspirin directly to the gums. (This practice can cause a chemical burn.)

MEDICAL TREATMENT

Before assuming that symptoms are caused by teething, your doctor will check for other causes.

RELATED TOPICS: Anemia; Toothache

Testis, torsion of

For unknown reasons, a testis (one of the male sex glands) may become twisted, shutting off its blood supply. Although the condition is more apt to affect boys who have an undescended testis, it also occurs in boys whose testes are in the normal position in the scrotum (the pouch of skin behind the penis). The condition may also follow a minor injury.

SIGNS AND SYMPTOMS

A testis that is twisted first becomes slightly swollen and tender. Within a few hours it is intensely painful and very tender and swollen. The testis and the surrounding skin become discolored (red or blue), and the boy may be nauseated or vomit and have lower abdominal pain and a fever.

Torsion (twisting) of a testis that has descended into the scrotum may be confused with orchitis (inflammation of one or both testes), a strangulated hernia, or a bruise of the scrotum. Torsion of a testis that has not descended and lies in the groin may be confused with a strangulated hernia, an injury, or infected lymph nodes in the groin. Torsion of an undescended testis that lies within the abdominal cavity is difficult to diagnose but may be suspected whenever abdominal pain occurs. This is an **emergency** situation and requires immediate medical treatment. Torsion of a part of a testis called the appendix of the testis causes similar, although less intense, symptoms. Nevertheless, this too is considered an emergency.

HOME CARE

Do not attempt home treatment. Torsion of the testis is an emergency that requires immediate surgical correction.

PRECAUTIONS

■ Take your child to a doctor immediately if pain near a testis increases and the testis is tender, swollen, or discolored. **Do not delay;** hours count.

■ Suspect torsion of the testis in a boy with an uncorrected, undescended testis if he has lower abdominal pain or groin pain.

■ An injury or a bruise of the scrotum and testis is not uncommon and will cause instant pain that gradually subsides. If pain increases following an injury or a bruise, it may be caused by torsion of the testis.

MEDICAL TREATMENT

Your doctor will arrange immediate surgery to untwist the testis and to anchor it in the scrotum in order to prevent further episodes. If surgery is not performed within 24 hours of the onset of symptoms, the testis may be damaged permanently.

RELATED TOPICS: Bruises; Glands, swollen; Hernia; Testis, undescended

Testis, undescended

In the male fetus, the two testes (sex glands) develop just beneath the kidneys. Before birth, the testes usually travel down into the groin and come to rest in each side of the scrotum. In one to two percent of full-term male infants and 20 to 30 percent of premature male infants, one or both testes have not completed their descent by the time the baby is born. The testis or testes are then referred to as "undescended."

An undescended testis may lie within the abdomen or the groin. In a boy's first months or years of life, an undescended testis may successfully complete its migration to the scrotum.

A testis that remains undescended is at risk of becoming twisted, injured, or cancerous. If the condition is not corrected by the time a boy reaches the age of four years, an undescended testis may be damaged by the heat of the body; it may atrophy (shrivel) and lose its ability to produce sperm.

SIGNS AND SYMPTOMS

The condition exists if one or both testes do not rest in the scrotum at birth. However, an undescended testis must be distinguished from a migratory, or retractile, testis. A migratory testis has completed its descent into the scrotum but has risen temporarily into the groin. A migratory testis returns to its normal position as a boy matures, and it needs no correction. If the size of the scrotum is normal, the testis is most likely migratory; if it is small, the testis is probably undescended. An undescended testis sometimes can be felt in the groin, but it may be mistaken for a hernia or a swollen lymph node.

HOME CARE

If a testis appears to be missing from the scrotum after birth, check periodically to see if it has descended. To check for an undescended testis, place the child in a tub of warm water and pull his knees up toward his chest. If the testis is migratory, it will often descend into the scrotum; if the testis is undescended, it will not descend.

PRECAUTIONS

■ Don't worry the child by discussing the condition. An undescended testis can usually be corrected.

■ Do not postpone correction of an undescended testis. It should be corrected before the boy is four years old.

■ A boy with an undescended testis has an increased chance of an inguinal (groin) hernia.

MEDICAL TREATMENT

Your doctor will examine the child's scrotum and groin carefully and check for the presence of a hernia, which often accompanies an undescended testis. Some doctors give hormone injections to encourage the testis to descend, but most prefer to perform surgery.

RELATED TOPICS: Glands, swollen; Hernia; Testis, torsion of

Tetanus

Tetanus (lockjaw) is a disease of the nervous system and is caused by the *Clostridium tetani* bacterium. This germ grows in the absence of oxygen and normally lives in soil, dust, and the intestines and wastes of animals and humans. It easily enters the body through puncture wounds or cuts but can also enter through a scratch, scrape, burn, or insect bite. The time between exposure to the bacteria and the development of symptoms is 3 to 21 days. Tetanus is frequently fatal.

SIGNS AND SYMPTOMS

Once the infection is full-blown, it causes muscle stiffness, especially of the jaw and neck (giving rise to the name lockjaw); difficulty in swallowing; pain in the extremities; muscle spasms throughout the body; and convulsions. When a child has muscle spasms and convulsions days or weeks after sustaining a wound, the child probably has tetanus. However, in newborn infants, tetanus may be confused with a disorder called neonatal tetany (a generally harmless condition), and in older children, it may be confused with a drug reaction, poisoning, meningitis, encephalitis, or rabies. The diagnosis can be confirmed by laboratory tests to isolate the *Clostridium tetani* bacterium.

HOME CARE

Prevention is the key to home care. Keep your child's tetanus immunization status up to date, and be sure to take proper care of wounds, even minor ones, until they heal.

PRECAUTIONS

■ If a mother has not been immunized against tetanus, her newborn baby is susceptible. If a mother is immune, her baby may be temporarily immune.

■ In newborns, the tetanus germ can enter the body through the stump of the umbilical cord. If a baby is delivered at home, be certain that strict antiseptic techniques are employed during and immediately after the birth.

■ Be certain that all members of the family have received the initial series of tetanus immunizations and the necessary boosters.

■ In general, someone who receives a relatively "clean" wound (such as one from a kitchen utensil) should have had a tetanus booster within the previous ten years, and someone who receives a relatively "dirty" wound (such as one from a nail or barbed wire or any other wound that occurs out-of-doors) should have had a booster within the previous five years. For example, if your child has a puncture wound from stepping on a nail in the backyard, be certain that the child has received a booster within the previous five years.

MEDICAL TREATMENT

Your doctor will take prompt care of a wound that may be infected with tetanus. The doctor will also administer a tetanus booster to a child who has not been fully immunized or tetanus immune globulin (a substance that contains antibodies to fight tetanus) to a child who has not been immunized at all. If tetanus has developed, your doctor will hospitalize the child and order intensive treatment, including tetanus toxoid, tetanus immune globulin or antitoxin, antibiotics, sedation, and intravenous fluids. Recovery from tetanus does not confer immunity; the patient should receive the full course of immunizations and boosters.

RELATED TOPICS: Animal bites; Burns; Cuts; Encephalitis; Immunizations; Insect bites and stings; Meningitis; Poisoning; Puncture wounds; Scrapes

Thrush

Thrush is a mouth infection caused by the *Candida albicans* fungus. It is common in babies immediately after birth and in infants and toddlers. Thrush frequently follows antibiotic treatment and accompanies nutritional deficiencies and chronic illnesses.

SIGNS AND SYMPTOMS

Thrush causes white, flaky plaques that resemble milk curds to appear on the tongue, the roof of the mouth, the gums, and the insides of the cheeks and lips. These plaques do not easily wipe away. Generally, thrush produces no other symptoms. The diagnosis is confirmed by laboratory tests to identify the *Candida albicans* fungus.

HOME CARE

To treat thrush, the doctor will prescribe nystatin solution and show you how to place the recommended dose into each of the child's cheeks four times a day after the child has nursed or eaten. To prevent reinfection, sterilize objects that are placed in the baby's mouth. A nursing mother may have to use nystatin cream on her breasts to avoid reinfecting the baby.

PRECAUTIONS

■ White plaques confined to the tongue are probably not due to thrush. They are normally the result of nursing.
■ If thrush occurs with a fever or cough, see your doctor.
■ If thrush recurs frequently, it may be because objects that are placed in the baby's mouth are not being adequately sterilized. Consult your doctor.
■ Treat thrush only with products recommended by your doctor. Overuse of nonprescription products can burn the membranes of the mouth.

MEDICAL TREATMENT

Your doctor will try to determine if the child has some condition that increases his or her susceptibility to thrush. The nursing mother may be examined and treated for diseases of the nipples or vagina that may reinfect the infant. (The *Candida albicans* fungus causes what is commonly known as a vaginal yeast infection, and a mother can pass the infection to the baby.)

Thyroid disorders

The thyroid gland is located in the neck just below the Adam's apple. It produces hormones that control the body's temperature, energy production, growth, and fertility. The thyroid gland may become underactive (resulting in hypothyroidism) or overactive (resulting in hyperthyroidism). Either condition can occur in infancy or at any age thereafter.

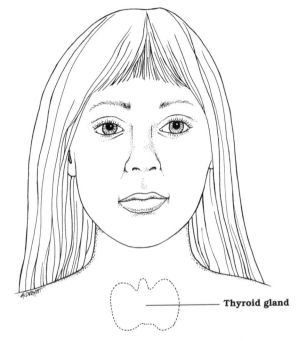

Thyroid gland

The thyroid gland is located in the neck, just below the Adam's apple.

SIGNS AND SYMPTOMS

Hypothyroidism. When the thyroid is underactive at birth, it is not usually apparent for a few weeks; then it causes excessive sleepiness, choking while nursing, severe constipation, and noisy breathing. After three to six months, it is obvious that the child's growth rate is retarded. In addition, the child has a protruding tongue; thick, dry skin; and a hoarse cry. When the thyroid becomes underactive later in childhood, it slows growth and causes constipation, sleepiness, and thick, dry skin. An underactive thyroid may or may not be associated with goiter (enlargement of the thyroid gland).

Hyperthyroidism. Overactive thyroid usually develops between the ages of 10 and 15 years. Sometimes, however, it may occur in children as young as one or two years. An overactive thyroid causes irritability, restlessness, behavior problems, tremors of the hands, increased appetite without weight gain, excessive sweating, and protruding eyeballs. Overactive thyroid is sometimes accompanied by goiter.

Because all symptoms of overactive and underactive thyroid can result from other conditions not related to the thyroid, laboratory tests are essential to the diagnosis. Newborn infants are routinely tested for congenital hypothyroidism (a disorder of the thyroid gland that causes abnormalities of mental and physical development) before leaving the hospital.

HOME CARE

Home care involves taking your child to the doctor for routine checkups and watching for the symptoms of thyroid malfunction.

PRECAUTIONS

■ Symptoms of underactive thyroid may occur in older children, especially adolescents, who have normal thyroid function. Only your doctor can determine if the thyroid is malfunctioning.
■ A cyst on the neck should be seen by a doctor. It could be an abnormally positioned thyroid gland.

MEDICAL TREATMENT

Your doctor will establish the diagnosis on the basis of a physical examination, including measurement of the child's blood pressure, and laboratory tests that measure the levels of thyroid and pituitary hormones in the blood. The doctor may also order a test to determine how well the thyroid absorbs radioactive iodine; this test is used to evaluate function and to look for tumors of the thyroid.

Treatment of an underactive thyroid usually involves prescribing synthetic thyroxine (a thyroid hormone) for the child to take by mouth. Treatment of an overactive thyroid involves either medication or surgical removal of part of the thyroid gland.

RELATED TOPIC: Goiter

Tics

Repeated, jerky, spasmodic movements of isolated groups of muscles are called tics. Tics often occur in preschool and school-age children as a result of undue pressure and emotional stress. They increase when a child is upset or excited and stop temporarily when he or she is distracted or asleep.

SIGNS AND SYMPTOMS

Usually, tics involve twitching the mouth, wrinkling the forehead, blinking the eyes, sighing, coughing, or sniffing. Tics must be distinguished from allergic responses, which often lead to twitching the nose, blinking the eyes, and coughing as well. Tics can also cause the head, shoulders, hands, or arms to jerk uncontrollably. Tics can happen several times a minute or only once or twice a day, and they may persist for weeks or months.

A serious but rare condition called Gilles de la Tourette's disease is characterized by tics at the outset, but it progresses to violent twitching of the face and arms and sometimes other parts of the body. The spasmodic movements are accompanied by explosive sounds, such as barking and shouting obscene words. Because Gilles de la Tourette's disease is so unusual and because it is fairly mild at the beginning, early diagnosis is not possible.

HOME CARE

Do not pay undue attention to tics. You may aggravate or prolong the condition if you react by calling your child's attention to the tics, demanding that the child stop, nagging, or punishing the child. Your best plan is to identify and then relieve any obviously stressful situations at home, at school, or among your child's friends.

PRECAUTIONS

■ Ignoring tics requires the cooperation of brothers and sisters, parents, relatives, neighbors, and teachers.
■ If tics are the only sign of emotional tension in a child, they may be due to the customary stresses of childhood. However, if tics persist for more than a few weeks or occur with other symptoms or patterns of disturbed emotional behavior, they may signal a potentially serious problem. Seek professional advice.

MEDICAL TREATMENT

Your doctor will examine the child carefully to make sure that the tics are not due to a physical illness. The doctor will evaluate stressful situations in your child's life and advise you on how to handle them. Your doctor may recommend consultation with a neurologist (a specialist in nervous-system disorders).

RELATED TOPIC: Hay fever and other nasal allergies

Tonsillitis

The tonsils (located in the throat) and the adenoids (located in the back of the nose) are part of the lymphatic system. Their function—to destroy disease-causing organisms—places them at risk for becoming infected themselves with germs from a common cold, strep throat, infectious mononucleosis, diphtheria, or tuberculosis.

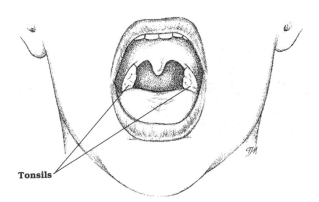

Tonsils

The tonsils are small masses of tissue in the throat. Their job is to destroy disease-causing germs.

SIGNS AND SYMPTOMS

The child will complain of a sore throat and will have a fever. The throat will appear red, and sometimes there will be white or yellow spots on the tonsils. Acute infection of the tonsils is diagnosed from the appearance of the throat and the results of a throat culture or blood cell count. This enlargement of the tonsils rarely produces symptoms by itself but, in extreme cases, can make it hard for the child to swallow. Enlargement of the adenoids can result in mouth breathing, hearing loss, middle ear infection, snoring, nasal speech, and bad breath. Adenoids can be examined with special instruments and can be seen on an X ray.

One form of infection of the tonsils is quinsy sore throat (known medically as peritonsillar abscess). In quinsy, a large abscess (a cavity containing pus and surrounded by inflamed tissue) forms behind a tonsil, producing intense pain and a high fever (103°F or 104°F). The abscess eventually pushes the tonsil across the midline of the throat. The child will have difficulty speaking ("hot-potato speech") and swallowing and will drool. A peritonsillar abscess requires treatment by a doctor.

HOME CARE

In general, treat tonsillitis as you would treat a common cold or a sore throat. The child should drink a lot of liquids but should eat only if he or she wants to eat. Give acetaminophen for fever or pain. Bed rest is not necessary, but most children will prefer it. Older children may gargle with warm salt water to relieve the sore throat. Inhaling steam may also ease the discomfort of the sore throat.

PRECAUTIONS

■ If drooling occurs with a sore throat, the child should be seen by a doctor **immediately**.
■ Enlarged adenoids and tonsils are common in healthy children three to nine years of age.
■ A white, cheesy material on the tonsils is normal and does not indicate infection.
■ Tonsils and adenoids may be infected without becoming enlarged.
■ Enlarged tonsils do not cause poor eating habits.

MEDICAL TREATMENT

The decision to perform a tonsillectomy (surgical removal of the tonsils) or an adenoidectomy (surgical removal of the adenoids) requires careful evaluation. Some doctors insist that they should never be removed; others recommend routine removal. Both groups are mistaken.

The tonsils can be removed as part of the treatment of a quinsy sore throat. Other indications for tonsillectomy include frequent infections (for more than a year) of the tonsils, a tonsillar tumor, or infection of the tonsils by the organisms that cause diphtheria.

Upper airway obstruction resulting in sleep apnea (a temporary halt in breathing) is an indication for adenoidectomy. The adenoids can also be removed to stop snoring or to correct a nasal voice or a nasal obstruction that has led to facial peculiarities, such as a pinched face, narrow nostrils, or a constantly open mouth. In some cases, it may be wise to have the adenoids removed if their enlargement is causing hearing loss or frequent middle ear infections. Alternatives to adenoidectomy include prolonged use of decongestants and antibiotics.

Your doctor will treat a peritonsillar abscess with antibiotics; surgical drainage is occasionally necessary.

RELATED TOPICS: Common cold; Diphtheria; Earaches; Fever; Frequent illness;

Glands, swollen; Hay fever and other nasal allergies; Infectious mononucleosis; Sore throat; Strep infections

Toothache

Like earaches and the onset of labor, children's toothaches seem always to happen at the least convenient time—after pharmacists have closed their doors and doctors and dentists have closed their offices.

A toothache can be caused by an injury to a tooth, an infection between the gum and the tooth, or an abscess (a cavity containing pus and surrounded by inflamed tissue) of the root of the tooth due to extension of a cavity (even a filled one) into the tooth's pulp (central portion).

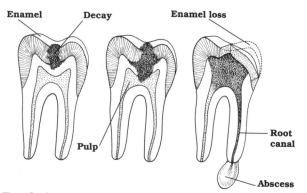

Tooth decay can progress from the enamel covering the tooth through the pulp to the root canal, forming an abscess (puss-filled cavity).

SIGNS AND SYMPTOMS

The cause of a toothache is obvious if the gum near the tooth is red, swollen, and tender or if a cavity is visible. If the source of the pain is in doubt, tapping gently with the handle of a spoon will cause sharp pain in the affected tooth.

HOME CARE

Temporary treatment is to ease the pain of the toothache with aspirin or acetaminophen. An ice pack on the jaw may help. Heat may make the toothache worse. Call your dentist.

An important part of home treatment is prevention. Your child should see a dentist regularly, beginning at age two or three years. The child should brush his or her teeth at least once daily and use floss. Through adolescence, fluoride must be provided each day. If you live in an area where the water is not fluoridated,

supplementary fluoride is needed. Talk to your doctor or dentist about this.

PRECAUTIONS

■ Do not apply heat to the site of a toothache.
■ Take your child to a dentist regularly to help avoid emergency situations involving toothache.
■ **Never** apply aspirin directly to the site of a toothache. (This practice can cause a chemical burn.)

MEDICAL TREATMENT

Your doctor may prescribe a painkiller or, if infection is present, an antibiotic. Treatment of the tooth is left to the dentist.

RELATED TOPICS: Gumboils; Teething

Toxic shock syndrome

Toxic shock syndrome (TSS) is a rare and sometimes fatal disease that occurs when a toxin (poison) produced by the *Staphylococcus aureus* bacterium enters the bloodstream. The toxin causes leaks in cell membranes that allow blood to seep into the tissues of the body. This seepage can lead to a dangerous drop in blood pressure, shock, and possibly death.

TSS develops very suddenly and progresses rapidly. Although most of the victims recover, a severe case of TSS can lead to liver and heart damage. This damage occurs because low blood pressure and weakening of the cell membranes allow foreign substances to invade the heart and liver.

TSS was first officially defined in 1975 and is considered by many to be a new disease. Since the *Staphylococcus aureus* bacterium can be present in the body without producing the toxin, it is still not known what triggers the disease.

TSS has been linked to the use of tampons during menstruation, but scientists are still trying to determine what the link is. It is known that the tampons themselves do not cause TSS. However, they may promote the growth of the causative bacteria if they are left in too long or if they swell so much that they block blood flow, creating a breeding ground for bacteria. It is also possible that the tampon applicators scratch the vagina, allowing bacteria to enter the bloodstream.

This disease, however, is not limited to menstruating girls and women. It also has been seen in nonmenstruating women, in men, and in children. Women who have just had a baby are at greater risk because the vagina is more susceptible to bacteria at that time. TSS also affects those recovering from surgery or burns and persons suffering from boils or abscesses. Thus, the bacteria can enter the body via routes other than the vagina.

SIGNS AND SYMPTOMS

Symptoms of TSS include high fever, vomiting, diarrhea, a rash that resembles sunburn, peeling of the skin on the soles of the feet and the palms of the hands, blurred vision, and confusion. Because the disease frequently occurs during or just after menstruation, these symptoms in a girl who menstruates should be brought to the immediate attention of a doctor.

HOME CARE

If a child or adolescent has symptoms resembling those of TSS, consult a doctor at once.

PRECAUTIONS

■ This disease is not restricted to menstruating girls and women; it can also occur in men, children, and nonmenstruating women; it can also occur with certain medical conditions.
■ Tampon use is clearly a risk factor for the disease. A girl who is using tampons should change them every three to four hours and use tampons alternately with sanitary napkins whenever possible. She should not wear tampons through the night as she sleeps.

MEDICAL TREATMENT

Because there is no quick and definite test for TSS, diagnosis depends largely on the doctor's ability to recognize the symptoms. It is possible to test for the presence of the *Staphylococcus aureus* bacteria, but the presence of the bacteria does not necessarily mean that the person has the disease. If TSS is identified, it can usually be treated successfully. In most cases, the patient is hospitalized for supportive treatment similar to that used in cases of poisoning. The treatment may include intravenous (into a vein) administration of fluids and blood transfusions to raise the blood pressure. An ice blanket may be used to bring down the fever, and antibiotics may be prescribed.

RELATED TOPICS: Boils; Burns; Shock

Toxoplasmosis

Toxoplasmosis afflicts all mammals (including people), many birds, and some reptiles. It is caused by a one-celled parasite called *Toxoplasma gondii*, which is one-third the size of a red blood cell. Although blood tests show that as many as half the adults in this country have had the infection at one time or another, few persons outside the medical community are even aware of it. Like rubella (German measles), toxoplasmosis can severely damage the fetus during the first three months of pregnancy; however, it is rarely serious for any other age group.

Toxoplasmosis is contracted by eating raw or undercooked meat or by direct contact with the feces of chickens, cats, or dogs. The disease is not spread among humans, except from a pregnant woman to her unborn child.

A woman who contracts toxoplasmosis during the first three months of pregnancy can transmit the infection to the fetus. As a result, she may miscarry, the baby may be stillborn, or the infant may be born with hydrocephalus ("water on the brain") or microcephaly (an abnormally small head). The newborn may be mentally retarded or have convulsions, anemia, jaundice, or eye damage.

SIGNS AND SYMPTOMS

Most people with toxoplasmosis have no symptoms. Some have temporary swelling of the lymph nodes, and a few have symptoms resembling those of infectious mononucleosis. Rarely is the illness severe. When it is, it causes a high fever (103°F or 104°F) and can lead to pneumonia, encephalitis, and heart disease. One attack, however mild, seems to give lifelong immunity.

Toxoplasmosis is not usually diagnosed. It may be suspected from a blood cell count that shows numerous white blood cells of a certain type, but it can be confirmed only by complicated tests that evaluate the blood levels of the antibodies (protective substances) that the body produces to fight against the *Toxoplasma* organisms.

HOME CARE

Prevention is the best method of home care. However, congenital (present at birth) toxoplasmosis transmitted to the fetus during pregnancy is so rare that many experienced physicians have never seen a case. It hardly seems necessary, therefore, for a pregnant woman to avoid eating meat altogether or to get rid of household pets.

PRECAUTIONS

■ A pregnant woman should not expose herself to *Toxoplasma* organisms by eating raw or undercooked meat.
■ A pregnant woman should not change a cat's litter box or acquire a new pet during the first three months of her pregnancy.

MEDICAL TREATMENT

Drugs are available to treat severe cases of toxoplasmosis, but they are highly toxic (poisonous) and cannot be given to pregnant women.

RELATED TOPICS: Glands, swollen; Infectious mononucleosis

Ulcers (open sores on an internal surface of the body) are less common in children than in adults, but they are by no means rare and may even occur in newborns. Like adults, children get ulcers in the stomach or in the duodenum (the first part of the small intestine). Duodenal ulcers, in fact, are five times more common than stomach ulcers.

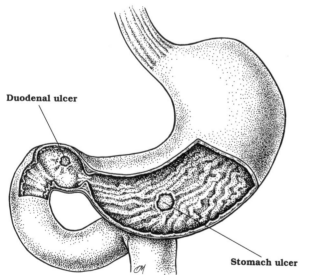

Duodenal ulcer

Stomach ulcer

The most common ulcers are those that affect the stomach or the duodenum (the beginning section of the small intestine).

Ulcers are more common in intense, highly motivated children, particularly those who have family conflicts. Ulcers also can be caused by prolonged treatment with steroid medications, extensive burns, diseases of the brain, blood poisoning, or severe infections, such as meningitis.

SIGNS AND SYMPTOMS

An older child with ulcers generally has upper abdominal pain before meals or at night; the pain is often relieved by eating. Preschoolers with ulcers usually have pain near the navel; the pain comes and goes and is aggravated by eating. Children of any age may vomit bright red or dark brown blood or have blood in the stools (as evidenced by black, tarry stools). Ulcers are seldom the cause of ordinary stomachaches in children.

The definitive diagnosis of an ulcer can be made only with an X-ray study called an upper gastrointestinal series ("upper GI") or with endoscopy, which is a procedure that allows direct viewing of the stomach by means of an instrument passed down the esophagus (the passageway from the mouth to the stomach).

HOME CARE

Temporary relief for pain can be provided by giving the child antacids by mouth. Other home treatment is not recommended. The child should be under a doctor's care.

PRECAUTIONS

■ Not all black, tarry stools contain blood. Taking iron supplements and eating some foods can cause black stools. The stools should be tested.
■ Abdominal pain in a child who is under emotional stress is more likely to be caused by the stress than by an ulcer.
■ Several members of a family may have ulcers because they share the family's lifestyle and tensions, not because ulcers are hereditary.

MEDICAL TREATMENT

Your doctor will take a careful health history of your child and perform a physical examination. An upper gastrointestinal series may be ordered. Your child's doctor may refer your child to a gastroenterologist (a doctor who specializes in the digestive system) for an evaluation and possible endoscopy. The child's stools will be tested for blood, and a blood cell count will be performed to seek evidence of secondary anemia. The doctor will probably prescribe antacids between meals and at bedtime. There are a number of different drugs that decrease acid secretion, help coat the stomach, or increase the secretion of the mucus that lines the stomach. The doctor will also advise you on changes in the diet and ways to relieve the child's emotional stress.

A new theory on the cause of ulcers is that they are really the result of an infection with *Helicobacter pylori*. The treatment includes two antibiotics and a bismuth preparation.

Changes in the diet usually involve avoiding caffeine (found in cola drinks, cocoa, tea, and coffee) and aspirin (including that found in some cold remedies). Treatment usually can be discontinued in a few weeks or months.

RELATED TOPICS: Anemia; Blood poisoning; Burns; Meningitis; Stomachache, chronic

Urinary tract infections

The urinary tract is a series of connecting structures, and an infection in one part easily spreads to another. For this reason, it is difficult to distinguish among pyelonephritis and pyelitis (infections of the collecting basins of the kidneys), cystitis (infection of the bladder), and urethritis (infection of the tube that leads from the urinary bladder to the outside of the body).

In many cases, except during infancy, there is no physical abnormality to account for the development of a urinary tract infection (UTI). However, in five percent of girls and more than 50 percent of boys with a UTI, it is due to an underlying anatomical abnormality somewhere along the urinary tract that results in a partial or total blockage of the flow of urine.

Most UTIs are caused by organisms that do not cause disease in other locations of the body. For example, *Escherichia coli* bacteria live harmlessly in the bowels of all children and adults but cause infection when they enter the urinary tract. Other causes of UTI are inflammation of the vagina, foreign bodies in the bladder or urethra, and possibly severe constipation.

Beyond infancy, UTIs occur ten times more frequently in girls than in boys. About five percent of all girls will have one or more UTIs before reaching maturity.

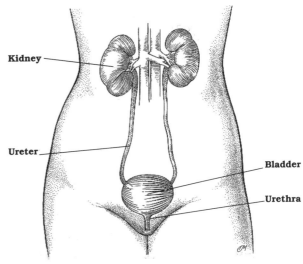

Female urinary tract

The urinary tract is a series of connecting structures, which makes it difficult to distinguish among infections of the kidneys, the bladder, and the urethra.

SIGNS AND SYMPTOMS

A UTI may produce either no symptoms at all (silent UTI) or any combination of the following symptoms: urgency or frequency of urination; painful urination; dribbling of urine; bed-wetting; daytime incontinence (inability to control urination); fever; abdominal or back pain; vomiting; chronic diarrhea; redness of the external genitals; or foul-smelling, cloudy, or bloody urine. If the infection is untreated, the symptoms often disappear in a few days or weeks but are likely to return later.

The diagnosis of UTI depends on the findings from a careful physical examination and urine tests. In boys, the diagnosis involves a search for an obstruction in the urinary tract. In girls, the search for an obstruction usually is undertaken only after two or three bouts of UTI or one bout with a UTI that is resistant to treatment. In an infant, whether a boy or a girl, investigation for the underlying cause should always be undertaken immediately.

HOME CARE

Any attempt at home treatment is potentially dangerous and may result in a low-grade, destructive infection with no outward symptoms. The child should be seen by a doctor.

PRECAUTIONS

■ A UTI, particularly one of a series of infections, commonly produces fever but few or no other symptoms. The doctor's physical examination may reveal nothing unusual.

■ To obtain an uncontaminated urine specimen for analysis or culture, cleanse the genitals and collect the sample at the midpoint of urination.

MEDICAL TREATMENT

Your doctor will perform a complete physical examination, including taking your child's blood pressure, and will order urine tests. If the urine specimen shows an infection, the doctor will prescribe antibiotics for 10 to 14 days. Urine samples will be retested during and after the course of antibiotics.

After your child has recovered from a UTI, the doctor may recommend an X-ray or ultrasound examination to determine if there is a physical abnormality. Sometimes, further X-ray studies and direct examination of the urethra and bladder are necessary. To treat recurrent UTIs that are not due to obstruction, your doctor may prescribe the use of antibiotics continuously or on and off for months or years. Surgery may be necessary to correct an obstruction.

RELATED TOPICS: Bed-wetting; Constipation; Diarrhea in older children; Diarrhea in young children; Fever; Nephritis; Stomachache, chronic; Vaginal discharge; Vomiting

Vaginal bleeding

The most common cause of vaginal bleeding is, of course, menstruation, which begins at puberty. Precocious (occurring before its usual time) puberty may begin before age nine, even as early as five or six years of age. With both normal menstruation and precocious puberty, the first menstrual flow is preceded by development of the breasts.

A baby girl may have a bloody discharge from the vagina during the first two weeks of life; this is usually due to the withdrawal of her mother's hormones after birth. Vaginal bleeding any time after the immediate postbirth period in a girl whose breasts have not yet developed or bleeding between menstrual periods is most often due to injury. Wounds in the vaginal area, even those of considerable size, usually heal rapidly with no infection or scarring.

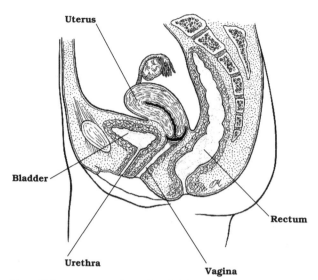

Possible causes of vaginal bleeding (other than menstruation) include inflammation of the vagina, a foreign body in the vagina, prolapse (slipping from the usual position) of the urethra, and tumors of the vagina or uterus.

Girls whose mothers received the drug diethylstilbestrol (DES) during pregnancy may have vaginal adenosis, an abnormality that causes bleeding. All girls with vaginal adenosis should be carefully monitored.

Whether or not they have vaginal bleeding, all girls whose mothers took DES should be examined by a gynecologist (a specialist in disorders of the female reproductive system) at the beginning of puberty. Although the medical profession originally overestimated the chances that a girl whose mother took DES would get cancer, the possibility does exist.

Less common causes of vaginal bleeding are inflammation of the vagina, a foreign body in the vagina, prolapse (slipping from the usual position) of the urethra (the tube leading from the urinary bladder to the outside of the body), and tumors of the vagina or the uterus.

SIGNS AND SYMPTOMS

The sign of bleeding is obvious. Diagnosis of the cause of abnormal vaginal bleeding often can be made by inspecting the vaginal area. The inspection should determine whether blood is coming from the vaginal opening, the urethra, a laceration of the surrounding tissues, or the rectum.

HOME CARE

Unless bruises and lacerations of the vagina and the surrounding area are extensive or due to sexual molestation, they usually can be treated at home. No antiseptic is necessary, and burning on urination can be minimized by having the child urinate while in a bathtub of water (to dilute the urine) and then bathe in fresh water.

All other causes of vaginal bleeding require your doctor's attention.

PRECAUTIONS

■ If a girl is less than nine or ten years old and has vaginal bleeding with or without breast development, she should be seen by a doctor.

■ If there is any suspicion of sexual molestation, contact your doctor immediately.

■ Any girl whose mother took DES during pregnancy should be seen by a gynecologist at the beginning of puberty whether or not vaginal bleeding is present.

■ A baby girl may have a bloody discharge from the vagina during the first two weeks of life. This is usually a normal response to the withdrawal of the mother's hormones, but mention it to your doctor.

MEDICAL TREATMENT

Treatment of vaginal bleeding depends on its cause. Your doctor will determine what is causing vaginal bleeding by performing a careful examination, sometimes including the rectum. A culture of any vaginal discharge and an X-ray examination of the pelvis may be performed. A girl whose mother received DES will be referred to a gynecologist. A prolapsed urethra may require surgical correction.

RELATED TOPICS: Bruises; Menstrual irregularities; Vaginal discharge

Vaginal discharge

Mucous discharge from the vagina is normal during the first two weeks of a baby girl's life and during the one to two years before a girl starts menstruating. Such vaginal discharge may be quite heavy, but it does not have an unpleasant odor and does not irritate the skin.

Vaginal discharge that irritates nearby membranes, smells foul, and causes itching, soreness, or pain may be caused by using chemicals in the bathwater (for example, bubble bath and water softeners) or vaginal hygiene sprays, wearing panties made from synthetic materials, or practicing poor toilet habits. It

can also result from pinworms, a urinary tract infection, masturbation, foreign bodies in the vagina, or poor hygiene. Discharge can also be caused by vaginitis (vaginal infection) due to viral or bacterial microorganisms or yeasts.

Girls whose mothers received the drug diethylstilbestrol (DES) during pregnancy may have vaginal adenosis, an abnormality that causes bleeding and discharge. All girls with vaginal adenosis should be carefully monitored. Whether or not they have vaginal bleeding, all girls whose mothers took DES should be examined by a gynecologist (a specialist in disorders of the female reproductive system) at the beginning of puberty. Although the medical profession originally overestimated the chances that a girl whose mother took DES would get cancer, the possibility does exist.

SIGNS AND SYMPTOMS

Vaginal discharge that occurs during puberty and is not irritating or foul smelling is normal. Vaginal discharge that is puslike, irritating, foul smelling, or bloody is not normal. The cause of the problem must be determined by your doctor.

HOME CARE

Some of the causes of abnormal vaginal discharge can be prevented. Have your daughter wear cotton rather than synthetic underpants, wipe herself from front to back after going to the bathroom, and avoid using chemicals in the bathwater. Look for signs of pinworms or urinary tract infections. Taking sitz baths in a tub of shallow water to which a cup of vinegar has been added may be helpful.

PRECAUTION

■ Any girl whose mother took DES during pregnancy should be seen by a gynecologist at the beginning of puberty.

MEDICAL TREATMENT

Your doctor will take a detailed health history and conduct a physical examination, including inspection of the vaginal area and the rectum. A culture of the discharge, an X-ray examination of the pelvis, and urine tests may be performed.

Treatment depends on the cause of the problem, but it may involve the use of antibiotics, worm medicine, fungicides, medicated suppositories, or hormone ointments.

RELATED TOPICS: Gonorrhea; Herpes simplex; Menstrual irregularities; Pinworms; Toxic shock syndrome; Urinary tract infections; Vaginal bleeding

Viral infections

A virus is an organism, smaller than a bacterium, that can live only within a living cell. Many common illnesses are caused by particular viruses, among them mumps, chicken pox, measles, rubella, infectious mononucleosis, cat scratch fever, hepatitis, warts, molluscum contagiosum, and roseola. Two large groups of other viruses—the respiratory viruses and the intestinal viruses—cause a variety of similar illnesses in children.

The respiratory viruses include the adenoviruses, parainfluenza viruses, rhinoviruses, influenza viruses, and the respiratory syncytial virus. The intestinal viruses (also called enteroviruses) are divided into Coxsackie viruses (of which 30 varieties are known so far), the so-called ECHO viruses (of which there are more than 30 known types), and the three polio viruses.

Coxsackie viruses are responsible for hand, foot, and mouth disease; herpangina; and pleurodynia. Hand, foot, and mouth disease is characterized by the presence of blisters and sores in the area of the mouth and throat and blisters on the hands and feet. Herpangina lasts three to six days and produces a fever, sore throat, swollen lymph nodes in the neck, and painful ulcers (open sores) on the soft palate, tonsils, and throat. Pleurodynia is an inflammation of the muscles between the ribs, which causes intense pain, aggravated by breathing, on one side of the chest.

Coxsackie and ECHO viruses may cause symptoms of a common cold, a fever with or without a rash, encephalitis (inflammation of the brain), or paralysis. ECHO viruses may cause diarrhea.

Infections by the Coxsackie and ECHO viruses have an incubation period (the time it takes for symptoms to develop after exposure to the organisms) of three to five days or more, and they can be spread via the mouth or in the stool. Immunity against any one of them is short-lived. Therefore, a child can have one viral infection right after another.

SIGNS AND SYMPTOMS

Because of the large number of viruses and the multiplicity of symptoms, diagnosis of the specific type of viral infection is very difficult and usually not necessary. Herpangina can be identified by the look and location of the ulcers. Pleurodynia resembles pleurisy and pneumonia, but it produces no cough. A rash due to a virus tends to be generalized, flat, and pink rather than red and splotchy; however, rashes vary considerably from child to child.

HOME CARE

Only the symptoms caused by intestinal viruses can be treated. Because of the association between Reye's syndrome and use of aspirin, it is generally recommended that acetaminophen, rather than aspirin, be given to reduce pain and fever accompanying a viral illness. In particular, **do not** give aspirin to a child with chicken pox or influenza.

PRECAUTIONS

■ **Do not** give aspirin to a child with chicken pox or influenza.
■ Call the doctor immediately if your child has any of the following symptoms: stiff neck or back, severe headache and vomiting, extreme weakness or collapse, or confusion.
■ Consult your doctor if any of the following symptoms appears: rash resembling red sandpaper or red goose bumps; puslike discharge from eyes, nose, or ears; reddish-purple spots; tender, red, enlarging lymph nodes; severe earache; blood in the stools; severe cough; or breathing difficulty.

MEDICAL TREATMENT

A diagnosis may be difficult to reach. It usually depends on a careful history and physical examination, aided by knowledge of what illnesses are currently going around in the community. Blood studies and throat cultures may be needed to exclude other illnesses. A chest X-ray examination or a spinal tap may also be necessary. Viral cultures and antibody studies confirm the presence of specific diseases, but the results of these tests take days or weeks.

RELATED TOPICS: Cat scratch fever; Chicken pox; Common cold; Diarrhea in older children; Diarrhea in young children; Encephalitis; Fever; Glands, swollen; Hand, foot, and mouth disease; Hepatitis; Infectious mononucleosis; Measles; Meningitis;

Molluscum contagiosum; Mumps; Polio; Rashes; Reye's syndrome; Roseola; Rubella; Warts

Vision problems

By the age of four or five years, five to ten percent of all children have a problem with vision. By the end of adolescence, that figure has climbed to 30 percent.

The vision problems that occur most often among children and adolescents are myopia (nearsightedness, or the inability to see distant objects clearly), hyperopia (farsightedness, or the inability to see near objects clearly), amblyopia ex anopsia ("lazy eye," or loss of vision from lack of use), and astigmatism (a defect in the ability to focus light rays, which causes blurred vision at all distances).

Nearsightedness is hereditary; it is rarely present at birth but develops as the child grows. Lazy eye develops during the first six or seven years of life. Farsightedness and astigmatism occur at an early age and usually do not grow worse with time.

SIGNS AND SYMPTOMS

At birth, a baby who has normal eyes can focus on an object and visually follow movement. If an infant's eyes seem to make random, searching movements, the infant may have defective vision.

Beyond infancy, there are several symptoms that may indicate poor vision. If your child habitually tilts his or her head or looks out of the corners of the eyes, if the eyes cross, or if the child squints or is excessively sensitive to bright lights, there could be a vision problem. Holding objects close to examine them, failing to recognize familiar people at a distance, suffering headaches after use of the eyes, having problems in school, and disliking reading may also signify poor vision.

Vision can be tested at different ages in a variety of ways. During the first week of life, an infant should be able to fix his or her eyes on a bright light. By two months of age, the child's eyes should follow that light as it moves through a 180-degree arc. By seven or eight months, the child should be able to recognize and respond to facial expressions. After age three, a child's eyes can be tested by having the child focus on charts that use pictures or the

letter E pointed in different directions. Finally, around the age of five or six years, the child's eyes can be tested using a standard Snellen eye chart (a chart of rows of letters in diminishing sizes).

HOME CARE

Be alert to the symptoms that can indicate impaired vision, and have the child's eyes examined periodically.

PRECAUTIONS

■ A child who cannot see the television screen from a distance or who holds books close to the eyes may be nearsighted.

■ A child's vision should be checked annually, beginning no later than the age of four years.

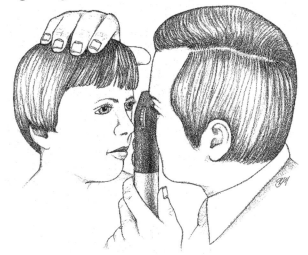

At each checkup, the doctor will examine the insides of your child's eyes using an instrument called an ophthalmoscope.

MEDICAL TREATMENT

At each annual eye checkup, your doctor will examine your child's eyes inside and out with an instrument called an ophthalmoscope and will test the child's vision with an eye chart. If an abnormality is suspected, your doctor will refer you to an ophthalmologist (an eye specialist) for more detailed examination and correction of the problem.

RELATED TOPICS: Crossed eyes; Lazy eye

Vomiting

Vomiting is a common occurrence during childhood. In most instances, it is merely a nuisance, but it can hinder the work of medications, cause the child to lose so much fluid that dehydration occurs, or indicate a problem that requires medical attention.

Most infants spit up and occasionally vomit. If this vomiting does not hinder weight gain, it is neither harmful nor abnormal. Excessive vomiting, however, may indicate intolerance to formula, milk, or some other food. Frequent, forceful vomiting during an infant's first two months suggests an obstruction at the end of the stomach.

In infants and children, coughing may be followed by vomiting; this is not abnormal. In children, gastroenteritis or intestinal flu (both viral infections of the digestive tract) or an infectious disease elsewhere in the body can cause vomiting. Other causes include abnormalities of the brain (for example, concussion, migraine, meningitis, encephalitis, and tumors), poisoning, appendicitis, severe emotional distress, jaundice, foreign bodies in the digestive tract, abdominal injuries, and motion sickness.

SIGNS AND SYMPTOMS

The vomiting itself is obvious. The doctor concentrates on identifying its cause. It is also important to evaluate the degree of dehydration caused by persistent vomiting.

HOME CARE

If your child is vomiting, avoid giving solid foods and aspirin tablets. Do not give cow's milk or cow's-milk-based formula. These substances aggravate vomiting. Allow the child sips of cold, clear liquids, such as ice water, carbonated beverages, tea with sugar, flavored gelatin water, apple juice, and commercial electrolyte solutions (available from your pharmacist). Commercial preparations of orthophosphoric acid, fructose, and glucose (also available from your pharmacist) may be used as well. If the child can keep down a teaspoonful of liquid every five minutes, he or she will retain two ounces of fluid in an hour. Gradually increase the amount of fluids given as the child's tolerance increases.

PRECAUTIONS

■ Prolonged or severe vomiting can cause dehydration. The younger the child, the more serious dehydration can be. Call your doctor if an infant has been vomiting for more than 12 to

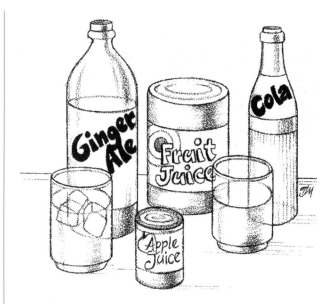

A child who has been vomiting should be encouraged to sip ice water, carbonated beverages, and juices.

24 hours or if an older child has been vomiting for more than two to three days.
■ Consult your doctor if vomiting is accompanied by abdominal pain, fever, or headache.
■ If vomiting and diarrhea occur at the same time, control the vomiting first.
■ Some phenothiazine drugs that are used to control vomiting in adults may cause serious side effects in the central nervous system in children; do not use them for children.
■ Remember that abdominal pain accompanied by vomiting could indicate appendicitis.

MEDICAL TREATMENT

Your doctor will determine the cause of the vomiting by obtaining a detailed health history and performing a thorough physical and neurologic examination. The presence and degree of dehydration will be assessed; if the child is seriously dehydrated, he or she will be hospitalized for administration of intravenous fluids.

RELATED TOPICS: Appendicitis; Concussion; Dehydration; Diarrhea in older children; Diarrhea in young children; Encephalitis; Food allergies; Gastroenteritis, acute; Headaches; Jaundice in children; Jaundice in newborns; Meningitis; Motion sickness; Poisoning; Stomachache, acute; Stomachache, chronic; Swallowed objects; Viral infections

Warts

A wart is a growth on the skin caused by a specific virus. Although warts may differ in appearance, they are caused by the same type of virus.

Warts can be spread by direct contact or by scratching. *Plantar warts*, which appear on the soles of the feet, can be contracted by walking barefoot where someone who has them recently walked.

In most cases, warts disappear spontaneously within two or three years; in almost all cases, they are gone within ten years. Still, some warts must be treated. Plantar warts usually require treatment because they cause pain. Warts that extend under the nails may produce permanent deformities if they are not treated. Warts on the face and eyelids are removed for cosmetic reasons. Most other warts are harmless and can be ignored unless they are annoying, bleed frequently, or become infected.

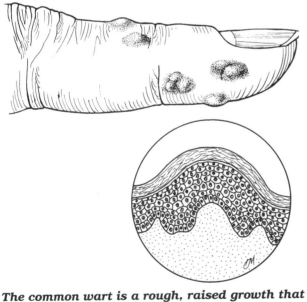

The common wart is a rough, raised growth that ranges in size from one-eighth inch to one inch in diameter and occurs anywhere on the skin.

SIGNS AND SYMPTOMS

The common wart is a rough, raised growth that ranges in size from one-eighth inch to one inch in diameter and occurs anywhere on the skin. A juvenile wart is a small (one-sixteenth to one-fourth inch in diameter), smooth, pinkish wart that is common on the hands. Plantar warts may be pressed into the foot (sometimes

to a depth of a quarter-inch or more) and are often surrounded by a callus. Groups of plantar warts are known as *mosaic warts*. Many warts are unmistakable, but some are not. When they are tiny, plantar warts may be mistaken for small, brown splinters on the sole of the foot. Also, you may not be able to see them if they are surrounded by a callus.

HOME CARE

As a rule, leave warts alone. If they have to be removed, it is safest to have a doctor do it or instruct you in the use of an appropriate medication. Usually, treatment must continue for many days or weeks.

PRECAUTIONS

■ If excessive pain or redness occurs on the surrounding skin, stop treatment.
■ Do not treat any warts on the face or eyelids at home.
■ Warts that involve the cuticles or that extend under the nails should not be treated at home.

MEDICAL TREATMENT

No treatment is successful in all cases. Treatment may even spread warts, or they may recur after treatment. In general, your doctor will remove warts by application of acids, podophyllin, liquid nitrogen, solid carbon dioxide, or phenol or by electric cauterization (burning away) or curetting (surgical removal).

RELATED TOPIC: Viral infections

Whooping cough

Whooping cough is a highly contagious infection of the respiratory tract, usually caused by the bacterium *Bordetella pertussis*, but sometimes by *Bordetella parapertussis* or *Bordetella bronchiseptica*. Whooping cough caused by one type of bacteria does *not* provide immunity against whooping cough caused by the other two types, and the vaccine that is available provides immunity only against infection from the most common organism, *Bordetella pertussis*.

The incubation period (the time it takes for symptoms to develop once the child has been exposed to the disease) is 7 to 14 days. Whooping cough can be extremely serious in infants under one year; as many as 50 percent of infants who contract whooping cough die. Newborns are not immune.

SIGNS AND SYMPTOMS

In a child who has not been immunized, the diagnosis is virtually unmistakable. Whooping cough begins with a runny nose, a low-grade fever (100°F to 101°F), and a cough that gradually worsens over the following two to three weeks. The cough then becomes characteristic: it is worse at night than during the day, and it is paroxysmal (the child coughs several times in succession without inhaling in between). At the end of a coughing spell, the child makes a "whoop," or strangling sound, as air is sucked into the lungs; vomiting of thick mucus follows. The severe, strangling cough persists for another two to three weeks and gradually subsides in three to six more weeks, but it may return with new respiratory infections.

The diagnosis may not be obvious, however, in infants in whom the characteristic "whoop" does not develop. And in an immunized child, the diagnosis may be impossible to make. (Remember that the child who has been immunized may have only partial immunity, and that without boosters the immunity declines over the years.) A child who is partially immune may have a mild case of whooping cough that produces none of the identifiable symptoms of whooping cough.

In the absence of the characteristic symptoms, laboratory tests do not help much. The organisms that cause whooping cough are difficult to grow on cultures. Because it may be difficult to diagnose and because many doctors and parents mistakenly believe that the disease is rare, over 90 percent of cases of whooping cough are never detected or even suspected.

HOME CARE

A child who has whooping cough should be isolated from others, especially young children. If the vomiting is severe, feed the child several small meals a day, rather than three large ones.

PRECAUTIONS

■ Make sure that your child is immunized against whooping cough. The risks from the disease far outweigh the risks from the immunization. Infants are not naturally immune to the disease, and the mortality (death) rate among infants who contract whooping cough is high.

■ A child who has a mild cough may have a mild form of whooping cough, in which case he or she can spread the disease. Avoid unnecessary exposure to others.
■ If your child has been exposed to whooping cough, have the child seen by your doctor.
■ Report to your doctor any cough that is getting progressively worse at the end of two weeks.

MEDICAL TREATMENT

Your doctor will try to establish a diagnosis with the help of blood studies and cultures of the secretions from the nose and throat. Most often, though, diagnosis is based on the child's medical history and the doctor's clinical judgment.

All infants with whooping cough are hospitalized. An older child may or may not be, depending on his or her condition.

Your doctor may prescribe the antibiotic erythromycin for 10 to 14 days to make the disease less contagious. If given early enough, the medication may shorten the course of the illness. If your child has been exposed to whooping cough, he or she can be given erythromycin by mouth, a booster shot of vaccine, or a large dose of human antipertussis serum.

RELATED TOPICS: Coughs; Immunizations; Vomiting

Index